Earth and Environmental Sciences Library

Series Editors
Abdelazim Negm, Faculty of Engineering, Zagazig University, Zagazig, Egypt
Tatiana Chaplina, Antalya, Türkiye

AF781129

Earth and Environmental Sciences Library (EESL) is a multidisciplinary book series focusing on innovative approaches and solid reviews to strengthen the role of the Earth and Environmental Sciences communities, while also providing sound guidance for stakeholders, decision-makers, policymakers, international organizations, and NGOs.

Topics of interest include oceanography, the marine environment, atmospheric sciences, hydrology and soil sciences, geophysics and geology, agriculture, environmental pollution, remote sensing, climate change, water resources, and natural resources management. In pursuit of these topics, the Earth Sciences and Environmental Sciences communities are invited to share their knowledge and expertise in the form of edited books, monographs, and conference proceedings.

Magdy T. Khalil · Wiame W. M. Emam ·
Abdelazim Negm
Editors

Climate Changes Impacts on Aquatic Environment

Assessment, Adaptation, Mitigation, and Road Map for Sustainable Development

Springer

Editors
Magdy T. Khalil
Department of Zoology
Faculty of Science
Ain Shams University
Cairo, Egypt

Wiame W. M. Emam
Department of Zoology
Faculty of Science
Ain Shams University
Cairo, Egypt

Abdelazim Negm
Department of Water and Water Structures Engineering
Zagazig University
Zagazig, Egypt

ISSN 2730-6674 ISSN 2730-6682 (electronic)
Earth and Environmental Sciences Library
ISBN 978-3-031-74899-8 ISBN 978-3-031-74897-4 (eBook)
https://doi.org/10.1007/978-3-031-74897-4

© The Editor(s) (if applicable) and The Author(s), under exclusive license to Springer Nature Switzerland AG 2025

This work is subject to copyright. All rights are solely and exclusively licensed by the Publisher, whether the whole or part of the material is concerned, specifically the rights of translation, reprinting, reuse of illustrations, recitation, broadcasting, reproduction on microfilms or in any other physical way, and transmission or information storage and retrieval, electronic adaptation, computer software, or by similar or dissimilar methodology now known or hereafter developed.
The use of general descriptive names, registered names, trademarks, service marks, etc. in this publication does not imply, even in the absence of a specific statement, that such names are exempt from the relevant protective laws and regulations and therefore free for general use.
The publisher, the authors and the editors are safe to assume that the advice and information in this book are believed to be true and accurate at the date of publication. Neither the publisher nor the authors or the editors give a warranty, expressed or implied, with respect to the material contained herein or for any errors or omissions that may have been made. The publisher remains neutral with regard to jurisdictional claims in published maps and institutional affiliations.

This Springer imprint is published by the registered company Springer Nature Switzerland AG
The registered company address is: Gewerbestrasse 11, 6330 Cham, Switzerland

If disposing of this product, please recycle the paper.

Preface

Welcome to *Climate Changes Impacts on Aquatic Environment: Assessment, Adaptation, Mitigation, and Road Map for Sustainable Development*, the latest addition to the Earth and Environmental Sciences Library Book Series. Climate change is no longer a distant threat; it is a present reality with profound consequences for our planet. From rising global temperatures to ecosystem disruptions, the impacts of climate change are far-reaching and multifaceted. This volume delves into the intricate relationship between human activity and the environment, exploring how our actions indelibly affect the Earth's climate and the resulting repercussions.

The chapters are meticulously crafted to offer a comprehensive examination of climate change's multifaceted impacts. We begin by exploring the Human Imprint and its Consequences on Climate Change, recognizing the pivotal role of human activities in driving environmental shifts. We then navigate through the consequences, from the Impact of Climate Change on Public Health to the effects on Aquatic Biodiversity and the phenomenon of Lessepsian Migration.

As we progress, we confront the challenges posed by climate change on critical sectors such as water resources, fisheries, aquaculture, and agriculture, exploring both vulnerabilities and opportunities for adaptation and resilience-building. Innovative approaches, including breeding climate-resilient plants and enhancing carbon sequestration in Egyptian wetlands, are examined for their potential to mitigate and adapt to climate change.

Additionally, we scrutinize the role of Marine Protected Areas (MPAs) in strengthening climate resilience and discuss the broader implications for sustainable development. Finally, we present a strategic roadmap for enhancing the resilience of Egypt's aquatic ecosystems, aligning with national and international sustainability targets.

This book is not just a collection of chapters; it is both a testament to the urgency of the climate crisis and a practical guide for action. It reminds us that the choices we make today will shape the world we inhabit tomorrow. As we embark on this journey through the complexities of climate change and its myriad impacts, may we be inspired to embrace innovation, collaboration, and stewardship of our planet for the betterment of current and future generations.

Together, let us explore these challenges and opportunities, armed with knowledge, determination, and a collective resolve to forge a path toward a more sustainable and resilient future.

Cairo, Egypt Magdy T. Khalil
Cairo, Egypt Wiame W. M. Emam
Zagazig, Egypt Abdelazim Negm

Acknowledgments

This book, *Climate Changes Impacts on Aquatic Environment: Assessment, Adaptation, Mitigation, and Road Map for Sustainable Development*, represents a significant achievement of the Center for Consultations and Scientific Studies of Nature Reserves (CCSSNR) at Ain Shams University. As one of the center's key output activities, this work reflects CCSSNR's unwavering commitment to advancing research and developing practical solutions to address the pressing challenges of climate change.

The leadership and vision of CCSSNR have been instrumental in bringing this book to fruition. The center's dedication to scientific excellence and sustainable development has guided this project from its inception to its completion, ensuring that it aligns with the mission to promote resilience and innovation in the face of global environmental challenges.

This book would not have been possible without the collective efforts of the researchers, contributors, and staff at CCSSNR. Their commitment to excellence and their tireless work have been essential in realizing this publication.

We also wish to express our gratitude to Ain Shams University for fostering a supportive academic environment that encourages impactful research. The university's support has been crucial in enabling the success of this project.

This volume is not just a scholarly contribution; it is a testament to CCSSNR's ongoing efforts to drive positive change and foster resilience in the face of global climate challenges.

Contents

Human Imprint, Climate Change, and Public Health Connectivity

Climate Change and Human Imprint Consequences

Safwat H. Shakir Hanna

Abstract Climate change is a long-term change in the average weather patterns that define Earth's local, regional, and global climates. These changes may occur naturally, such as changes in the solar cycle, or due to human activities. By mid-2024, the world population has reached 8.2 billion and is still growing. This rapid population growth raises concerns about whether the Earth's natural resources can meet everyone's needs. The growing population requires a greater supply of services and products, which in turn exerts strain on natural resources and contributes to the escalation in the use of energy derived from fossil fuels, leading to higher emissions of greenhouse gases. Accordingly, this chapter aims to assess climate change as a consequence of the increasing global human footprint and predict the impacts of climate change due to the growing human population. As changes in the global human imprint and growth, climate change causes the following points:1) Increase in global temperature; 2)Decrease in the availability of natural resources to suffices the global human population; 2) Loss of freshwater resources; 3) Intensive farming practice; and 4) Loss of economic growth, development and loss of sustainability.

Keywords Climate change · Human imprint · Scientific model exploring

1 Introduction

Climate change is a significant issue nowadays due to the appearance of global environmental problems such as the warming of the Earth through extreme temperatures, drought, excessive rains in some places, hurricanes, and other phenomena related to changes in the climate globally. The increasing human activities have induced global climate change and are also associated with the rising human population in an

S. H. Shakir Hanna (✉)
Emeritus Professor of Chemical and Environmental Engineering, Prairie View A&M University, Prairie View, TX 77446, USA
e-mail: shshakir@pvamu.edu; safwat_shakir@yahoo.com

© The Author(s), under exclusive license to Springer Nature Switzerland AG 2025

M. T. Khalil et al. (eds.), *Climate Changes Impacts on Aquatic Environment*, Earth and Environmental Sciences Library, https://doi.org/10.1007/978-3-031-74897-4_1

alarming situation; it reached 8 billion people globally in November 2022. Consequently, the increasing demands for natural resources are limited to cover the needs of all human populations and their global imprints.

Extreme temperatures leave many impoverished families with less food, less clean water, lower incomes, and worsening health. Additionally, droughts and flooding can destroy crops and cut access to clean Water (https://www.savethechildren.org/us/what-we-do/emergency-response/climate-change). Therefore, the climate crisis magnifies inequality, poverty, and displacement and may increase the likelihood of conflict.

- 90% of diseases resulting from the climate crisis are likely to affect children under five.
- By 2050, **a further 24 million children are projected to be undernourished** as a result of the climate crisis.
- By 2040, it is estimated that **one in four children will be living in areas with extreme water shortages**.
- Almost **160 million children are exposed to increasingly severe and prolonged droughts**,
- **The climate crisis disrupts the education of around 38 million children each year**.
- The climate crisis is forcing families to migrate. By 2050, **there could be 143 million more migrants** due to the climate crisis.

According to the United Nations Environmental Program, it is predicted that climate change can affect all global human people in one way or another. Climate change is expected to have unprecedented implications on where people can settle, grow food, build cities, and rely on functioning ecosystems for the services they provide. In many places, temperature changes and sea-level rise are already putting ecosystems under stress and affecting human well-being [24].

To this end, this chapter aims to assess climate change as the consequence of the increasing global human imprint and predict the impacts of climate change due to the increasing human population and imprint activities.

2 Materials and Methods

2.1 Data Collection and Analysis

Data on climate change, global human population, and ecological data were collected from various series published by many agencies worldwide, such as the United Nations Environment Program (UNEP), United Nations Food and Agriculture Organization [9, 8], United Nations Development Program (UNDP), World Development, World Bank, WRI [39], WRI [40, 41]. Additionally, data were collected from WWF reports from [29–36]. Furthermore, data on human population and other resources were gathered from published series from different agencies such as the World Bank, NOAA [12], United States Department of Agriculture [26, 28], and World Bank Data (1960–2023 series) [37, 38].

The data were analyzed using regression, correlation, and statistical methodologies with SigmaPlot Software (Version 8, Version 11.2, and Version 13), 2D software of SPSS SCIENCE 2002 [16], STELLA software [17], and SAS [15].

2.2 Construction of a Simulation Model with Stella Software

The simulated model was developed using several parameters such as human population, annual increase in population, biological capacity of ecosystems, water resources, CO_2, air temperature (in °C), sea level, and demands from nature. The data was converted to global hectares. The model was used to predict the ecological human imprint of the existing resources' demands and the ecosystems' biological and environmental capacities that will support sustainable development for the next one hundred years. In this respect, STELLA software was used to create the executable program using the second- or fourth-order Runge–Kutta integration method. The model predicts the changes in ecological footprint demands and footprint capacities according to human population change, fertility changes, factors impacting population growth, cropped lands, grazing lands, fisheries, built-up lands, carbon dioxide in the air, air surface temperature, vegetative lands, water resources, and more. The model provides annual predictions for the next century, fifty-year predictions, and decadal forecasts. The model considers both relaxed and accurate assumptions of changing data parameters. The model was developed using different thinking and hypothesis techniques. In the present paper, the calculated results for human population, CO_2, and the increase in air surface temperature are presented as derived from the developed model in the results section.

Why is Climate Change Important?

Climate change is interfering with all aspects of human survivability. By mid-2024, the human population has reached nearly 8.2 billion. Human activities are evident from the increasing greenhouse gas concentrations in the atmosphere, positive radiative forcing, and observed warming. Climate models reproduce observed continental-scale surface temperature patterns and trends over many decades, including the more rapid warming since the mid-twentieth century and the cooling immediately following significant volcanic eruptions.

Climate change is the most essential factor in the following issues:

1. Climate change is a problem that threatens human beings' survival
2. The climate crisis is a child rights crisis, particularly impacting those brunts of inequality and discrimination: the wealthiest 50% of states are responsible for 86% of emissions, while the poorest are responsible for just 14% (https://www.wpf.org.).

3. Climate change forces are responsible for food shortages and threaten food security.
4. Climate change is causing the displacement of many people due to increasing hurricanes and other events.
5. Climate change can impact the natural resources that supply the raw materials that can be factors for creating the production of goods and services that are dependent on them.

3 Results and Discussion

According to United Nations estimates, the global population is increasing by approximately 80 million people—the size of Germany—each year [23]. The current population increase is estimated at 67 million people per year (UNICEF, 2021). The annual growth rate peaked in the late 1960s at around 2% (Worldometer, 2023). By mid-2024, the world population reached 8.2 billion. On the other hand, the United Nations projects the world population to reach 9 billion in 2037 and 10 billion in 2058. Currently, the global population is increasing at a rate of approximately 0.98% per year. Although this rate is expected to decrease slightly, it remains an alarming trend (Worldometer, 2023).

Analysis of Human Population Impacts on Climate Changes

The human population, both globally and within individual countries, has been impacted by climate change, affecting various aspects of human life. Figures 1, 2, 3, and 4 highlight the significant impact of human activities, particularly population growth and CO_2 emissions, on global climate change.

Climate change can impact the ecosystem's natural resources to replenish and renew or regenerate ecosystems' capabilities to provide services and resources to humanity (Fig. 5). On the other hand, the growing human population's demand for goods and services is alarming [21]. It will increase demand more than the supplies from the ecosystem products and services humans depend on to survive. Consequently, reducing social help will be beyond the ecosystems' abilities to provide the required goods and services for humans to support their survivability despite improving technologies and other tools and mitigations to combat climate change. The growing human population beyond the balance [19] between the human population and the required needs which will not solve the climate change impacts, despite the excellent and perfect struggle to combat this issue. The critical point is to produce reasonable measures of the needs of ecosystems to support the globe with goods and services and the balance of human population needs. For example, a vital issue of water resources, such as rising water demands, outweighs global warming in defining the state of global water systems in the near future [27]. Also, climate change tends to increase potential irrigation water consumption on irrigated lands with other detrimental effects in regions with significant irrigation. The climate change signal on

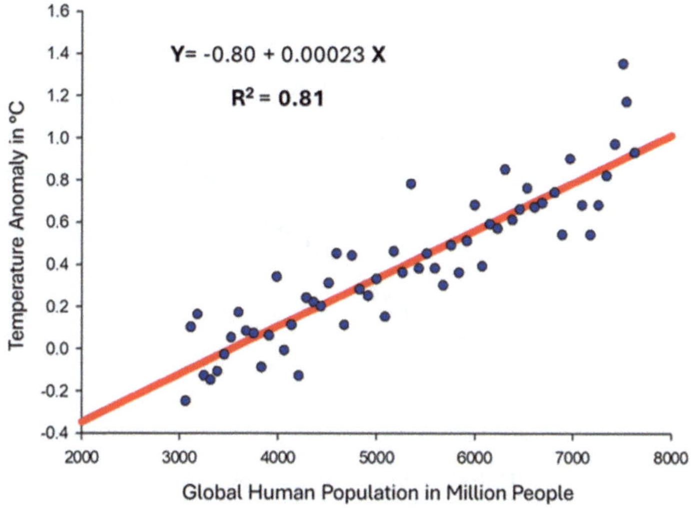

Fig. 1 Relationship between global human population and temperature anomaly

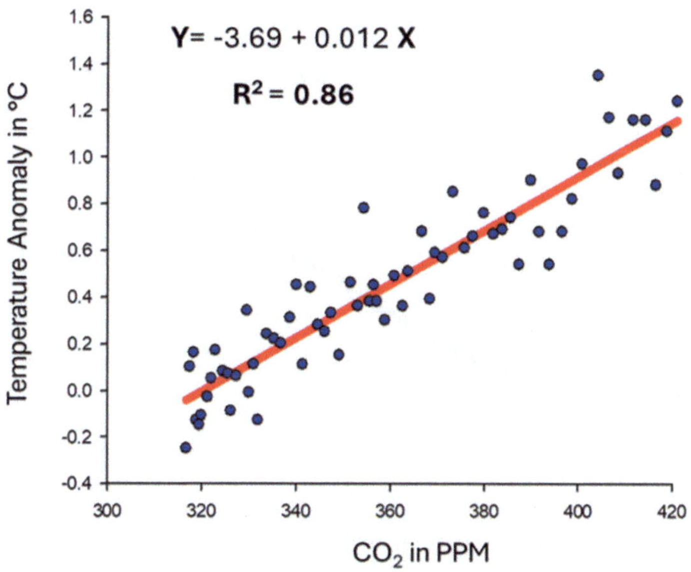

Fig. 2 Relationship between global CO_2 and temperature globally anomaly

runoff can be positive or negative and hence has the potential to alleviate or aggravate irrigation water scarcity. Globally, the relationship between actual and potential irrigation water consumption is expected to decrease, indicating increased water scarcity.

The impacts of human activities on the environment include:

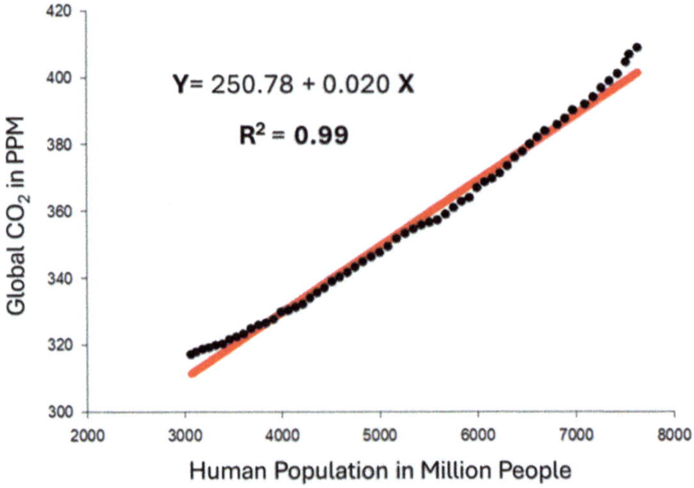

Fig. 3 Relationship between human population in million and global CO_2 in part per million

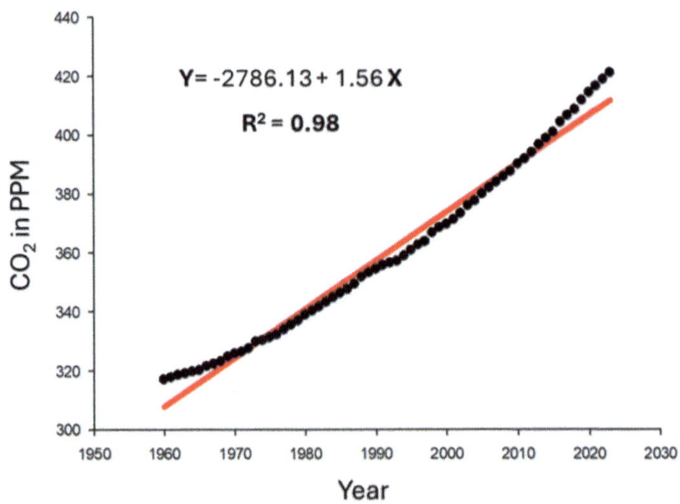

Fig. 4 Relationship between years and CO_2 in PPM

1. **Increasing Global Temperature**: Overpopulation means more people, vehicles, industries, and air travel, which increases greenhouse gas emissions. This results in the trapping of CO_2 in the atmosphere, leading to climate change and global warming [7] (Figs. 1 and 5).
2. **Resource Consumption**: The consumption of resources such as land, food, water, air, fossil fuels, and minerals increases with overpopulation.

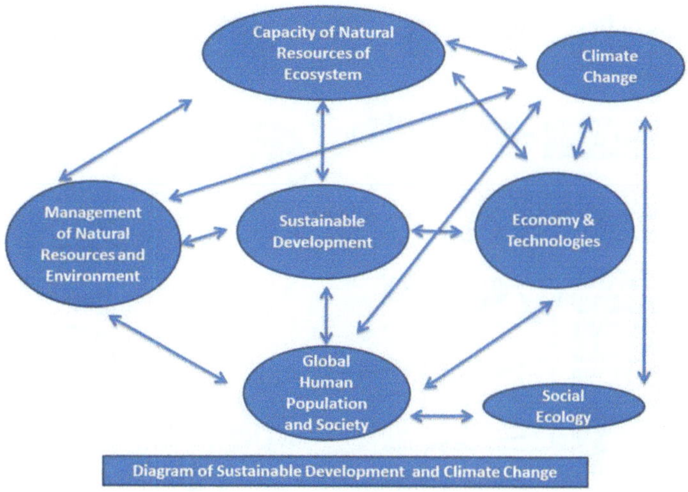

Fig. 5 Diagram explains the sustainable development and climate change

3. **Waste Products**: Increased consumption leads to waste products that include air and water pollutants, toxic materials, and greenhouse gases [1].
4. **Quality of Life**: Overpopulation can decrease the quality of life due to inadequate resources such as food, water, and shelter. This can lead to an increase in diseases and a decrease in life expectancy [7].
5. **Emergence of New Pandemics and Epidemics**: Overpopulation can lead to the emergence of new pandemics and epidemics due to overcrowding and poor sanitation [7].
6. **Intensive Farming Practices**: Overpopulation can lead to intensive farming practices that can cause soil degradation, deforestation, and water pollution [13].
7. **Rise in unemployment, crime rate, and violence**: overpopulation can lead to a rise in unemployment rates due to a lack of jobs. This can lead to an increase in crime rates and violence [7].

Figures 6, 7, and 8 provide the concept of climate change as a threat multiplier from an increase human population in an alarming status causing hungry, undernourished people, extreme weather events, health problems, displacement of people and loss their homes, including loss of communities, loss of biological diversity, migration impacts for other countries and regions, decreasing of clean water availability, security, poverty and undermining sustainable development without achieving U.N. the goals of U.N. for sustainability by 2030. Furthermore, since the early 1990s, the number of life-threatening weather-related disasters has doubled. Harvests have decreased, and food prices have risen as a result. The climate crisis is fueling the hunger crisis, and with our food systems more global than ever, humanity will lose this battle. Climate models predict higher average temperatures worldwide and hotter extremes, rising sea levels in coastal areas, and more frequent droughts in other areas. The Horn of Africa is currently experiencing its worst drought in 40 years. Millions

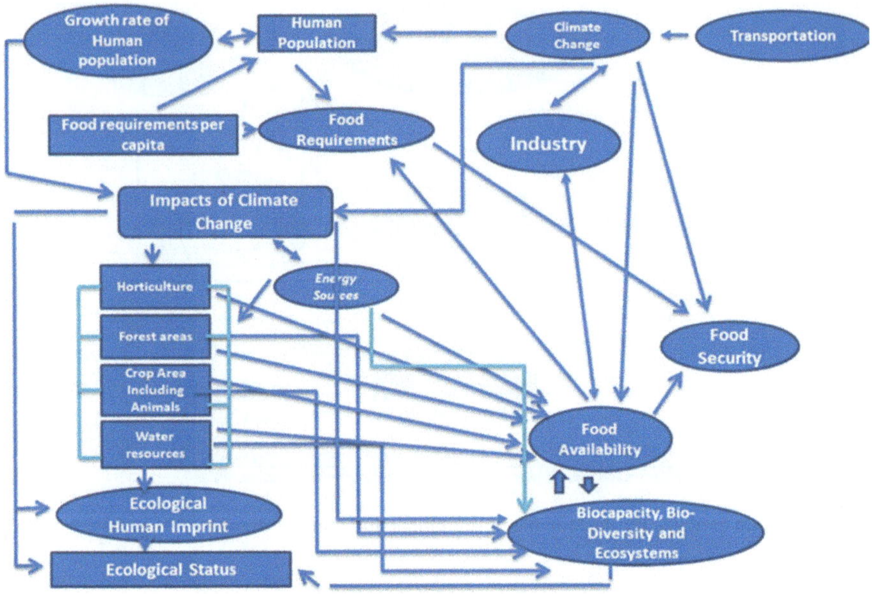

Fig. 6 Diagram explains the impacts of climate change globally and human imprint

of people go to bed hungry. As a result of global warming. Here are four ways that climate change and hunger go hand-in-hand, and as scientists, we are concerned for the future of humanity. In this respect, higher temperatures, water scarcity, droughts, floods, and greater CO_2 concentrations in the atmosphere affect staple crops worldwide. Corn and wheat production has recently declined due to extreme weather events, plant diseases, and a global water crisis (Accessed on 5/23/2023 https://www.concernusa.org).

Impacts of Climate Change on Global Water Loss

The global water crisis as related to climate change and growing human population showed the following concerns:

- According to UN-Water, 2.3 billion people live in water-stressed countries.
- According to UNICEF, 1.42 billion people—including 450 million children—live in areas of high or extremely high-water vulnerability.
- 785 million people lack access to basic water services.
- The WHO reports that 884 million people lack access to safe drinking water.
- Two-thirds of the world's population experience severe water scarcity during at least one month of the year [11].
- The Global Water Institute estimates that 700 million people could be displaced by intense water scarcity by 2030.
- 3.2 billion people live in agricultural areas with high water shortages or scarcity.
- Approximately 73% of people affected by water shortages live in Asia.

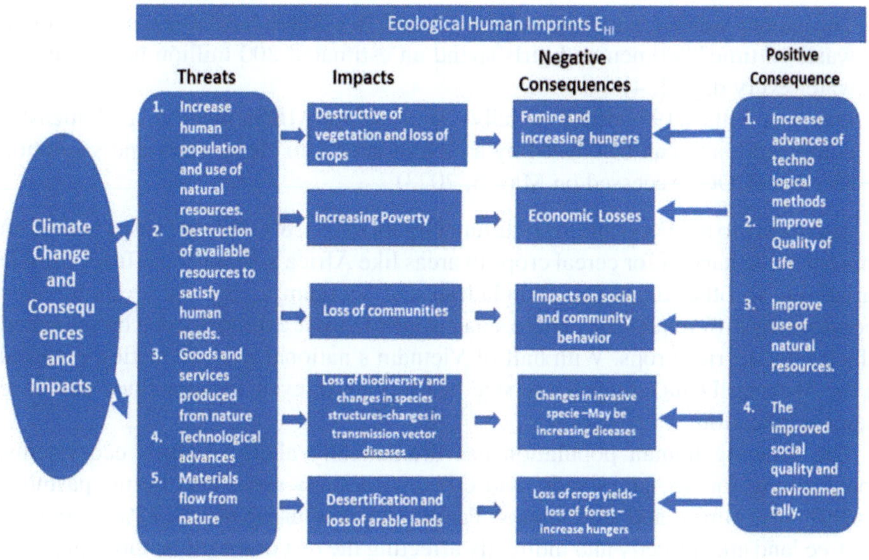

Fig. 7 Diagram explains the impacts of climate change and human imprint and analysis

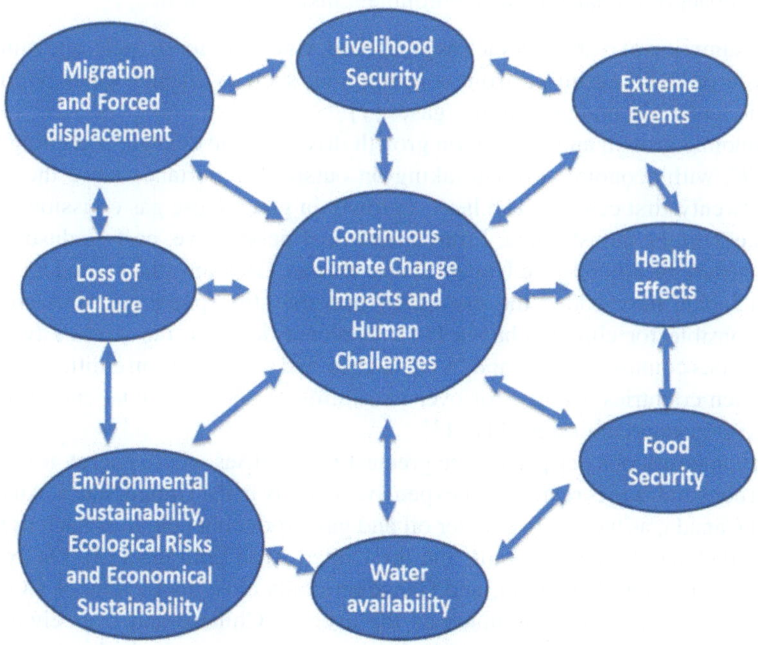

Fig. 8 Diagram explains climate changes impacts, human challenges and processes

- The global water crisis is a women's issue: In what UNICEF calls "a colossal waste of time," women and girls spend an estimated 200 million hours hauling water every day [3, 4]
- Diarrhea kills 2195 children daily—more than AIDS, malaria, and measles combined—and can be caused by a lack of access to clean water and sanitation services (CDC, Accessed on May, 5, 2023).

According to the Food and Agriculture Organization, 80% of the causes behind an unpredictable harvest for cereal crops in areas like Africa's Sahel come from climate variability. In other areas like Bangladesh and Vietnam, rising sea levels threaten food security differently [10]. There, coastal farmlands are often flooded by saltwater, which kills off rice crops. With half of Vietnam's national rice production centered in the Mekong Delta (roughly the size of Maryland), even a minor flood can have major implications.

The growing human population has dramatically altered Earth's ecosystems, transforming forests, grasslands, and other wilderness areas into farms, pastures, timberlands, mines, and settlements. People are now using nearly 75% of Earth's ice-free land area directly and indirectly affecting the rest of the globe through pollution and climate change. Tallied together, global agricultural systems, land use, and forestry contribute close to 20% of all human-caused greenhouse gas emissions [22].

The impact of humans on the environment takes many forms:

1. Consumption of resources such as land, food, water, air, fossil fuels, and minerals.
2. Waste products resulting from consumption, such as air and water pollutants, toxic materials, and greenhouse gases [1].
3. Economic growth and population growth drive climate change, according to the IPCC, with economic growth taking on outsized importance since the turn of the twenty-first century. The largest growth in greenhouse gas emissions comes as economies industrialize. From a historical perspective, early industrializing countries, specifically the United States, Russia, Germany, the United Kingdom, and Japan, have added the most CO_2 into the atmosphere and thus are most responsible for climate change [14]. In recent decades, the world's two most populous countries, China and India, have joined the top carbon emitters. Overall, just ten countries account for over two-thirds of current annual energy-related greenhouse gas emissions [42, 43].
4. Carbon emissions per person are greatest in countries where energy use is high and consumption is relatively inexpensive, namely in the United States, Australia, and Canada, as well as in smaller oil and gas-producing countries such as Qatar, Trinidad and Tobago, Kuwait, and the United Arab Emirates [14]. On average, each American, Australian, and Canadian emits close to 16 tons of CO_2 each year, more than twice as much as the average Chinese and over eight times more than the average Indian [14]. Per person emissions in the least developed countries are negligible, even though these countries are the least prepared and most vulnerable to the effects of climate change.

Impacts of Climate Change on Global Economics

1. Climate change could cut crop yields, especially in the world's most food-insecure regions. At the same time, changes in agriculture, forestry, and land use are responsible for about 25% of greenhouse gas emissions. The agriculture sector is at the core of addressing the climate challenge.
2. The Swiss Re Institute warns that the largest impact of climate change is that if global temperatures rise by 3.2 °C, it could wipe out up to 18% of GDP from the worldwide economy by 2050.
3. Climate change could cause the global economy to lose 10% of its total economic value by 2050.
4. According to U.N. Sustainability Report 2022, 1.6 billion people will lack of safely managed drinking water, 2.8 billion people will lack safely managed sanitation, and 1.9 billion people will lack basic hand hygiene facilities (U.N. The Sustainable Development Goals Report, Department of Economic and Social Affairs [5]).
5. Climate variability and extremes, conflict, economic shocks, and growing inequalities keep the world from achieving zero hunger by 2030. Since 2014, the number of people going hungry and suffering from food insecurity has increased. Additionally, the COVID-19 pandemic exacerbated an already deteriorating situation, with about 150 million more people facing hunger in 2021 than in 2019. In other words, an estimated 1 in 10 people worldwide are suffering from hunger. In addition, nearly 1 in 3 (a staggering 2.3 billion people) were moderately or severely food insecure in 2021, meaning they lacked regular access to adequate food. This represents an increase of almost 350 million people since the beginning of the pandemic. The most alarming increases were seen in sub-Saharan Africa, Central and Southern Asia, Latin America, and the Caribbean. The unfolding crisis in Ukraine is yet another threat to food security. Ukraine and the Russian Federation are large producers and exporters of essential food commodities, fertilizer, minerals, and energy. Together they are considered the world's breadbasket, supplying 30% and 20% of global wheat and maize exports, respectively, and 80% of global exports of sunflower seed products. At least 50 countries import 30 percent or more of their grain from these two countries, with many African and Least Developed Countries (LDCs) importing more than 50%. Ukraine and the Russian Federation are also leading exporters of fertilizers. The conflict has caused a steep and sudden reduction in grain exports, sunflower seeds, and fertilizers. As a result, import-dependent countries are vulnerable to rising food costs and supply chain disruptions. Joint, coordinated activities and policy solutions are urgently needed to avert food shortages for the world's poorest people and reduce the impact of the conflict and lingering consequences of the pandemic on global food insecurity.
6. Unsustainable consumption and production patterns are the root causes of the triple planetary crises of climate change, biodiversity loss, and pollution. These crises, and related environmental degradation, threaten human well-being and the achievement of the Sustainable Development Goals (SDGs). If we continue on the prevailing development pathway, the Earth's finite capacity will be unable to sustain the livelihoods of current and future generations. Transforming our

relationship with nature is critical to a sustainable future. As the world develops strategies for sustainable recovery from the pandemic, governments and all citizens should seize the opportunity to work together to improve resource efficiency, reduce waste and pollution, and shape a new circular economy (SDG Indicators, U.N. Goals 12).

Questions for Discussion About Climate Change, Economy, and the Role of Governments in Solving These Problems

The global human population has reached an alarming level, challenging the availability of natural resources needed to ensure a decent quality of life, equality, and justice while preserving global ecosystems and the climate from disastrous events. The following discussion aims to analyze these aspects:

1. **Resource Demand and Environmental Impact**: As the human population increases, the demand for environmental resources to produce goods and services has surged. This heightened demand leads to greater production, generating more waste products that pollute the environment and emit greenhouse gases, contributing to climate change. Furthermore, human overpopulation results in habitat loss and deforestation as more land is cleared for agriculture, housing, and other human activities. This leads to a loss of biodiversity and mass species extinction as more species are displaced from their habitats. Overpopulation also causes land, water, and air pollution due to increased waste production and resource consumption. It contributes to soil degradation and desertification as more land is used for agriculture. The depletion of finite resources such as fresh water, arable land, and fossil fuels occurs at speeds faster than their rate of regeneration, while renewable resources are used at unsustainable rates. Climate change is exacerbated by excessive greenhouse gas emissions, contributing to global warming. Additionally, increased carbon dioxide emissions dissolve in seawater, leading to ocean acidification.
2. **Impacts of Climate Change**: Climate change causes numerous impacts, such as poverty, environmental pollution, health hazards, water stress, severe ecological events, and economic problems. What measures can governments take? Can they support their citizens' needs, or will they be unable to support the growing population? How can these problems be solved?
3. **Funding of Solutions**: Another question is where governments can generate funding to save the planet and support their citizens. The answer could come from the productivity of its citizens, aid from other countries, or taxing the rich and shifting the burden from poorer to wealthier people. Is this a viable solution? Let us discuss this in detail. If the rich, hypothetically equal to 10% or 20% of the global population, own most of the world's wealth, can governments confiscate their wealth to distribute it and solve environmental and climate change problems? There are doubts this can happen for many reasons. The human population's needs are enormous, requiring a lot of goods and services to support everyone.

4. **Food Security**: As an example, discussing food security problems caused by climate change and greenhouse gases, if we calculate the needed calories to support all humans currently surviving on Earth, we assume each person needs 2000 cal per day. The total daily calorie requirement would be 2000 × 8,000,000,000, resulting in 16 trillion calories per day, or 5840 trillion calories per year. Where can we obtain these calories from the productive lands or waters of the Earth to provide a secure food supply for all humanity [20]? Is this feasible? Can governments support their citizens with food from crops, animals, and other green vegetation to meet the essential needs for human survival?
5. **Biological Resources and Efficiency**: Additionally, the storage of seeds or other biological resources for human and animal survival needs to be sufficient. Further considerations include the efficiency of these biological materials in doubling production for crops, vegetation feeds, and animal products. Are there high-quality soil properties to grow good crops, vegetation, and other genetic resources to support food security? Are there sufficient water resources to support crop production and other biological materials for food security as the global population reaches 8 billion and continues to grow?
6. **Agricultural Challenges**: Another concern is that higher temperatures, floods, and increasing CO_2 levels in the atmosphere negatively affect essential crops such as corn and wheat, which are declining. Additionally, plant diseases are increasing, and so are crop prices due to higher demand.

Climate Model Analysis and Characterization

Results of the utilized model showed the relationship between human population growth, CO_2 emissions, and rising air temperatures. Under the relaxed growth assumption, CO_2 levels are expected to reach 478 PPM (parts per million) by 2050. With a regular population growth rate, CO_2 levels are forecasted to be 450 PPM by the same year (Tables 1 and 2). Correspondingly, air surface temperatures are projected to rise significantly. Specifically, temperatures are expected to increase by more than two degrees Celsius by the year 2050 and by five degrees Celsius or more by 2100 if the trend of the human population growth rate increases above the regular rate.

Table 1 Global population in billion, air surface temperature predicted from global CO_2 and air-surface temperature of our planet earth from the year 1960 to the year 2050—data are presented in 10 years intervals prediction at regular growth (less than 1%) rate of human population

Years	Population Predicted	CO_2 Prediction from collected data	Prediction of Air Surface Temperature
1960	3.22	314.39	-0.09
1970	3.99	329.53	0.03
1980	4.76	344.68	0.15
1990	5.53	359.82	0.27
2000	6.29	374.97	0.39
2010	7.06	390.11	0.51
2020	7.83	405.26	0.63
2030	8.6	420.4	0.90
2040	9.36	435.55	1.05
2050	10.1	450.69	1.20

Table 2 Global Population in Billion, Air Surface Temperature Predicted From Global CO_2 and Air-Surface Temperature of Our Planet Earth From The Year 1960 To The Year 2050—Data Are Presented In 10 Years Intervals Prediction at Relaxed Growth Rate of Human Population At 1.7%

Years	Population Predicted	CO_2 Prediction from collected data	Prediction of Air Surface Temperature
1960	3.25	314.99	-0.09
1970	4.18	333.16	0.03
1980	5.10	351.34	0.15
1990	6.02	369.51	0.27
2000	6.94	387.69	0.39
2010	7.86	405.86	0.51
2020	8.78	424.04	1.07
2030	9.70	442.21	1.27
2040	10.62	460.38	1.47
2050	11.54	478.56	2.20

4 Conclusion and Recommendations

The most important findings extracted from this chapter are as follows:

1. Climate change is an imminent issue facing global nations and humanity, caused by the increasing human population and their demands from the environment that exceed the balance with the natural resources available on Earth.

2. Governments and non-governmental organizations (NGOs) should promote education on the impacts of increasing human populations and its consequences for climate change problems. As a result of the increasing human population, the demand from the environment and different ecosystems has become enormous. This will increase the degradation of the ecosystems that provide products and services that all humans depend on.
3. Individuals and communities should work together to take steps towards population reduction and control by establishing family planning. It can be done with the will of the people. Furthermore, family planning allows people to manage their economic aspects because reducing the number of individuals in a family will reduce the burden of expenses and consequently provide better living standards.
4. The impacts of climate change include increasing droughts and reduction of rainfalls that feed lakes and rivers, which impacts crop production and causes economic loss. Furthermore, climate change and increasing hurricanes will displace populations and increase migration from one place to another.
5. Governments and NGOs should promote family planning education and the well-being of people to control population growth. This can lead to a better life and the standard of living everyone intends to obtain.
6. Suppose we are to develop more sustainably in the future. In that case, we need to ensure that an adequate stock of natural resources is available by reducing its demands to meet future generations' needs and by addressing irreversible environmental problems such as global climate change. To fulfill these aims, Sayer and Campbell [18] indicated that an integrated natural resource management approach is adaptive, interdisciplinary, and involves diverse stakeholders.

References

1. Australian Academy of Science (2015) Population and environment: a global challenge. Earth & Environment. Retrieved 14 July 2024 from https://www.science.org.au/curious/earth-environment/population-environment
2. CDC (2012) Diarrhea; common illness, global killer. (Accessed on May 5, 2023) Centers for Disease Control and prevention (U.S.)
3. Concern Worldwide (2021). Why water is a women's issue. Concern Worldwide. https://concernusa.org/news/water-is-a-womens-issue/
4. Concern Worldwide U (2021) Why water is a women's issue. Concerned Worldwide U.S. Retrieved 5 May 2023. https://www.concern.net/
5. DESA, U.N. (2022) World economic situation prospects. UN Department of Economic and Social Affairs (DESA), 232
6. DESA, U.N (2019 and 2023) Global sustainable development reports 2019 and 2023. The 17 GOALS | sustainable development
7. Earth Eclipse (2024) Problems of overpopulation. Retrieved 14 July 2024 from https://eartheclipse.com/environment/problems-of-overpopulation.html
8. FAO (2008) Data series. Food and Agriculture Organization, U.N., Rome, Italy
9. FAO (1960–2008) Statistical database. Data series 1960–2008. Food and Agriculture Organization, U.N., Rome, Italy. Retrieved from www.fao.org

10. Giovetti O (2021) With nearly 75% of Bangladesh underwater, is the country facing a humanitarian crisis? Concern Worldwide U.S. Retrieved 5 May 2023 from https://www.concernusa.org/story/bangladesh-underwater-humanitarian-crisis/
11. Mekonnen MM, Hoekstra AY (2016) Four billion people facing severe water scarcity. Sci Adv 2(2):e1500323. https://doi.org/10.1126/sciadv.1500323
12. NOAA (2023) Climate change. Retrieved from http://www.noaa.gov/climate.html
13. Pettinger T (2020) Population growth—pros and cons. Economics Help. https://www.economicshelp.org/blog/167320/economics/population-growth-pros-cons/
14. Ritchie H, Roser M (2019) CO_2 and greenhouse gas emissions. Our World in Data. Retrieved from https://ourworldindata.org/co2-and-other-greenhouse-gas-emissions
15. SAS (2010) SAS statistical package version 9.2 for P.C. Base SAS 9.2 procedures guide: statistical procedure, 3rd ed
16. SPSSSCIENCE (2009–2010) SigmaPlot 11.2. user's guide part 2 statistics. System Software
17. STELLA (2001) An introduction to system thinking by Barry Richmond. High-Performance Systems Inc
18. Sayer J, Campbell B (2004) The science of sustainable development: local livelihood and the global environment. Cambridge University Press
19. Shakir Hanna SH, Harris KT, Osborne-Lee IW, Cesaretti GP, Misso RA, Andreopoulou ZS (2014) Global ecological human imprint, sustainable development, and environment: assessment and impacts. Eur J Sustain Dev 3(1):1–24
20. Shakir Hanna SH, Osborne-Lee IW, Khalil MT (2013) Sustainable economy of ecological footprint in Africa: an economic analysis and impacts. World Environ 3(1):9–17
21. Shakir Hanna SH, Osborne-Lee IW (2011) Sustainable economy of the ecological footprint: economic analysis and impacts. In: Villacampa Y, Brebbia CA (eds) Ecosystems and sustainable development VIII. WIT Press, South Hampton, UK, pp 313–326
22. Shukla PR, Skea J, Calvo Buendia E, Masson-Delmotte V, Pörtner HO, Roberts DC, Malley J et al (2020) Climate change and land: an IPCC special report on climate change, desertification, land degradation, sustainable land management, food security, and greenhouse gas fluxes in terrestrial ecosystems. Technical summary. IPCC
23. UNDP (2013) The rise of the south: human progress in a diverse world. Human Development Report 2013. United Nations Development Programme
24. UNEP (2023) About climate change. Retrieved from https://www.unep.org/explore-topics/climate-change/about-climate-change
25. UNICF (2021) Reimaging Wash Water Security for All. United Nation Children's Funds. 24pp
26. USDA (2012) Retrieved from http://ers.usda.gov/data-products.aspx#.UnuTTbrnbIV
27. Vörösmarty CJ, Green P, Salisbury J, Lammers RB (2000) Global water resources: vulnerability from climate change and population growth. Sci Adv 289(5477):284–288
28. WHO (2005) Ecosystems and human well-being: health synthesis: a report of the millennium ecosystem assessment
29. WWF (2002) Living planet report 2002. Jenkins M, Jakubowska J, Gaillard V, Groombridge B, Wackernagel M, Monfreda C, Deumling D, Gurarie E, Friedman S, Linares AC, Sánchez MAV, Falfán ISL, Loh J, Randers J, Monfreda C (eds) World Wildlife Fund (WWF), International. Avenue du Mont-Blanc, CH-1196 Gland, Switzerland. Retrieved from http://www.panda.org
30. WWF (2002) Living planet report 2002. World Wide Fund for Nature (WWF). Retrieved from http://www.panda.org/livingplanet
31. WWF (2002) The global conservation organization. WWF, The Global Conservation Organization, Living Planet Report/Footprint, 2002
32. WWF (2004) Living planet report 2004. Worldwide Fund for Nature International (WWF), Global Footprint Network, UNEP World Conservation Monitoring Centre. WWF, Gland, Switzerland. Retrieved from http://www.panda.org/livingplanet
33. WWF (2006) Living planet report 2006. World Wide Fund (WWF) for Nature, Gland, Switzerland. Retrieved from http://www.panda.org/livingplanet

34. WWF (2008) Living planet report 2008. Humphrey S, Chapagain A, Bourne G, Mott R, Oglethorpe J, Gonzales A, Atkin M, Loh J, Collen B, McRae L, Carranza TT, Pamplin FA, Amin R, Baillie JEM, Goldfinger S, Wackernagel M, Stechbart M, Rizk S, Reed A, Kitzes J, Peller A, Niazi S, Ewing B, Galli A, Wada Y, Moran D, Williams R, Backer WD, Hoekstra AY, Mekonnen M (eds) World Wide Fund (WWF), International Avenue du Mont-Blanc 1196 Gland, Switzerland. Retrieved from http://www.panda.org
35. WWF (2010) Living planet report. World Wide Fund for Nature, Gland, Switzerland. Yale Center for Environmental Law & Policy/Center for International Earth Science Information Network at Columbia University. 2010 Environmental Performance Index. Retrieved from http://epi.yale.edu/Home
36. WWF (2012) Living planet report 2012: biodiversity, biocapacity, and better choices. Editor in chief: Grooten M. Lead editors: Almond R, McLellan R. Editorial team: Dudley N, Duncan E, Oerlemans N, Stolton S
37. World Bank (1960–2008) Data series and research. Retrieved from http://data.worldbank.org/topic/agriculture-and-rural-development
38. World Bank (1960–2012) Data series and research. Retrieved from http://data.worldbank.org/topic/agriculture-and-rural-development
39. World Resources Institute (1960–2005) Earth trends environmental information. World Resources Institute. Retrieved from http://Earthtrends.wri.org/
40. World Resources Institute (2000–2001) People and ecosystems: the fraying web of life. World Resources Institute
41. World Resources Institute (2012) U.S. drought demonstrates complexity, severity of water risk by Robert Kimball. Retrieved from http://www.wri.org/search/site/Robert%2520Kimball%2520and%2520drought
42. World Resources Institute (2020) Climate watch. https://www.climatewatchdata.org/ghg-emissions
43. World Resources Institute (2020) Historical GHG Emissions. Retrieved 5 May 2023 from https://www.climatewatchdata.org/ghg-emissions?end_year=2019&start_year=1990

Climate Change and Public Health

Hanan Ali Sayed Ibrahim, Amal Saad-Hussein, and Nahed Mohamed Mohamed Ismail

Abstract Climate change is introduced within the context of public health, providing a comprehensive and updated resource for epidemiologists, public health, and environmental health professionals. Published studies link the impacts of climate change on public health with increases in respiratory illnesses and changes in the patterns of vector-borne and infectious diseases, including food-borne and water-borne illnesses. Climate change may affect the pattern of schistosomiasis infection, transmission, and the distribution of their snail intermediate hosts. Additionally, the impacts of climate change on environmental pollutants and their public health risks are defined. Public health nutrition is discussed considering upcoming climate changes. This chapter incorporates epidemiological tools, such as surveillance, risk estimation, modeling, and artificial intelligence, in studying and managing climate change's impact on public health. Strategies for mitigation and adaptation for sustainable global food systems are discussed. Furthermore, the public mental health impacts due to climate change and natural disasters are considered, with a specific focus on women's health. Public health strategies and priority actions for mitigation, adaptation, and resilience are addressed. Research gaps are identified and highlighted.

H. A. S. Ibrahim
Public Health and Community Medicine, Department of Public Health, Theodor Bilharz Research Institute, Giza, Egypt

Department of Community, Occupational and Environmental Medicine, Faculty of Medicine, Helwan University, Helwan, Egypt

H. A. S. Ibrahim
e-mail: hanan.ali@med.helwan.edu.eg

A. Saad-Hussein
Environmental Health and Preventive Medicine, Department of Environmental and Occupational Medicine, Environment and Climate Change Research Institute, National Research Centre, Cairo, Egypt
e-mail: al.hussein@nrc.sci.eg

N. M. M. Ismail (✉)
Aquatic Ecology, Department of Environmental Research, Theodor Bilharz Research Institute, Giza, Egypt
e-mail: dnahed2000@yahoo.com

© The Author(s), under exclusive license to Springer Nature Switzerland AG 2025
M. T. Khalil et al. (eds.), *Climate Changes Impacts on Aquatic Environment*, Earth and Environmental Sciences Library, https://doi.org/10.1007/978-3-031-74897-4_2

Keywords Vector-borne diseases · Schistosomiasis · Environmental pollutants · Non-communicable diseases · Women's health · Mental health · Surveillance · Artificial intelligence · Resilience · Mitigation · Adaptation strategies

1 Introduction

Human-caused climate change is widely recognized as a serious international concern with significant effects on human health. Between 2030 and 2050, heat stress, as well as Malaria, diarrhea, and malnutrition, are expected to account for over 250,000 fatalities per year due to climate change [1–5]. The annual direct costs for medication and healthcare are projected to be between USD 2 and 4 billion by 2030, excluding indirect expenses in health-determining areas such as agriculture, water, and sanitation [1–5]. Deaths and illnesses from more frequent severe weather events, such as heat waves, floods, and storms, along with food system instability, increased prevalence of infectious diseases (including zoonotic, food-borne, waterborne, and vector-borne diseases), and mental health problems, are some of the impacts of climate change on human health (Fig. 1) [1–5].

According to the Intergovernmental Panel on Climate Change's Fifth Assessment Report (IPCC AR5), there is high to very high confidence that climate change will increase risks of injuries, diseases, and deaths due to more intense heat waves and

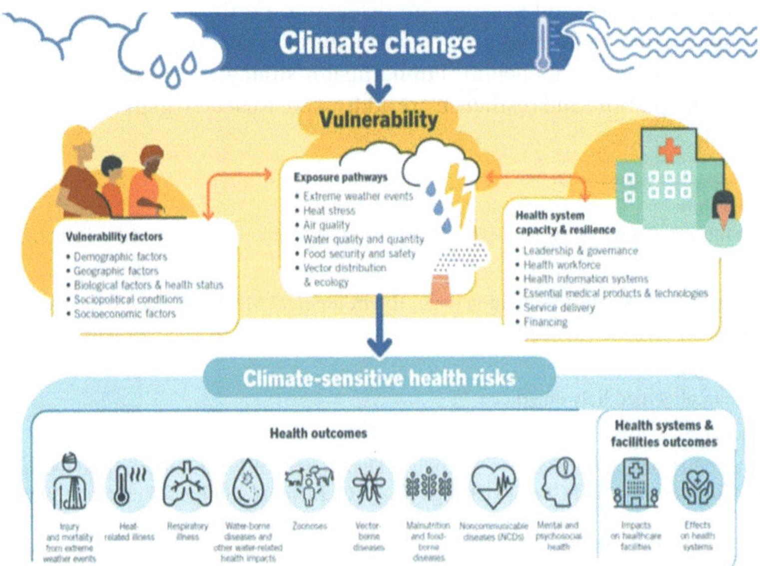

Fig. 1 An overview of climate-sensitive health risks, their exposure pathways, and vulnerability factors. Climate change impacts health directly and indirectly and is strongly mediated by environmental, social, and public health determinants. *Source* WHO [1–5]

fires, increased risks of undernutrition, and reduced labor productivity in vulnerable populations [1]. Early studies by Kalkstein and Greene [3], Diaz et al. [5], and Xu et al. [7] established that populations, particularly the elderly and the young, are more susceptible to the hazardous impacts of severe temperatures. Multiple studies indicate that infants, children, and toddlers have an increased risk of elevated temperatures, leading to higher rates of infectious and allergic disorders [7]. This vulnerability is linked to children's unique physiology, metabolism, and behavioral characteristics. Additionally, women bear a disproportionate share of the burden of the hazardous impacts of climate change [8]. Climate-related events and gradual shifts will also impact communities' mental health [9].

In Egypt, the incidence of human parasitic infestations, physiological problems, cancers (especially skin cancer), eye opacity, fungal infections (such as fungal keratitis), respiratory illnesses, heat strokes, and heat-related health problems may increase due to direct climate change impacts. Indirect impacts may arise from variables such as population migrations and changes in the social and economic order [10].

The WHO recommends improving infectious disease monitoring to create a reliable and timely early warning system [1–5]. As a rapidly expanding field, applying artificial intelligence (AI) in infectious disease prediction models related to climate change could be beneficial [10]. Preventing injuries and diseases, improving public health readiness, and reducing risks depend on a robust public health response to climate change. Public health strategies can be effectively planned and executed based on essential public health services [12]. Engaging public health in climate policies and planning is crucial [13].

The primary objective of this study is to highlight the growing scientific and practical responses to the effects of climate change on public health. Key areas covered include respiratory illnesses, waterborne illnesses, food-borne illnesses, and major health concerns related to climate change. Additionally, climate change may impact vector-borne illnesses such as schistosomiasis and Malaria. Air and water pollution caused by global warming can also affect health. The prevalence of noncommunicable illnesses, nutrition, women's health, and mental health in the context of climate change are discussed. Effective public health techniques, including monitoring infectious diseases, using models and AI for illness prediction, and risk assessment, are essential for addressing health issues climate change brings. By emphasizing these public health implications, policymakers, public health, and environmental health professionals will be better equipped to adopt, mitigate, reduce, and build resilience against the negative effects of climate change on human health.

2 Effect of Increasing Global Temperature on Public Health

Climate change poses catastrophic health consequences, with the Intergovernmental Panel on Climate Change (IPCC) stating that the world must restrict temperature increases to 1.5 °C. Past emissions have already committed the world to a certain amount of warming. An increase of 1.5 °C is dangerous, and every additional tenth of a degree would devastate human health [1–5].

Ragettli et al. [13] conducted a national case-crossover study with distributed lag non-linear models (DLNMs) to estimate the non-linear relationship between temperature and mortality in Switzerland from 2003 to 2016. They found warm-season temperatures above the 90th percentile significantly increased mortality risk, particularly affecting the older population. Temperatures below the 98th percentile did not significantly impact mortality for those under 75. The study concluded that high temperatures threatened human life in Switzerland and suggested that a single threshold temperature for heat advisories could be used nationwide. The intensity of heat waves had a more significant impact on mortality than their duration.

Africa, including Egypt, is highly susceptible to climate change. Research on eight Egyptian governorates showed that maximum and minimum temperatures have risen by approximately 1.3 °C since 1960. Under the RCP4.5 scenario, temperatures are expected to rise from 2010 to 2040 and then decrease. However, under the RCP8.5 scenario, warming rates are projected to increase significantly from 2050 to 2100 [15].

Each degree of warming over 1.5 °C increases health hazards, including heat-related illness and death. Adaptation can mitigate these effects to some extent. The transmission of infectious diseases such as Malaria, dengue fever, West Nile virus, and Lyme disease can increase or decrease depending on the disease, location, and temperature changes. There is high confidence that ozone-related mortality could increase if precursor emissions remain constant [16].

Hot days and nights are linked to negative health effects, especially for older populations who cannot recover from daytime heat. Warm evenings contribute significantly to heat-related mortality [17, 18, 19]. High daytime temperatures are particularly concerning as they often occur during peak outdoor activity hours. Therefore, it may be reasonable to determine heat warning thresholds based on mean temperatures over 24 h, considering both daytime and nighttime temperatures [20].

3 Climate Change Impacts on Respiratory Illnesses

Children under one year are vulnerable to extreme temperatures, which can exacerbate respiratory and gastrointestinal diseases [7]. Weather conditions, particularly cold and dry conditions, influence the transmission dynamics of viruses like influenza

[21]. High humidity can increase the airborne transmission of pathogens, while low relative humidity can increase susceptibility to respiratory infections [22].

Chest infections, including pneumonia, are sensitive to climate change. Hospital admissions for pneumonia show seasonal variations linked to air pollution, rainfall, humidity, and temperature [23]. Severe rainfall and flooding can increase rodent diseases, such as hantavirus and leptospirosis, due to increased contact between humans and rodents in slums and damaged houses. Additionally, climate change impacts on agriculture can lead to crop failure and starvation, driving rodents into homes in search of food and shelter.

By addressing these impacts, public health professionals can better prepare for and mitigate the negative effects of climate change on human health.

4 Climate Change Impacts on Food-Borne or Waterborne Infectious Diseases

Over two million deaths and four billion cases of diarrhea are attributed to bacteria, protozoa, and viruses spread by contaminated water each year [24]. Climate change contributes to an increase in natural disasters, including floods, which are major causes of mortality, injury, and infectious diseases like cholera and dengue fever, as well as non-communicable disorders such as mental illness and malnutrition [25].

Research by Liu et al. [26] indicates that low-income cities in China are more likely to experience outbreaks of infectious diarrhea following floods. In Egypt, an area's geography, socioeconomic status, and infrastructure influence the predictive meteorological characteristics for diarrhea morbidity rates [27]. Waterborne infectious diarrhea is a serious health concern, particularly in economically vulnerable communities. Public control techniques during floods can mitigate this risk [26]. Moreover, early warning systems based on meteorological data should be developed for better disease management [27].

In Vietnam, integrating early warning systems into healthcare programs to predict diarrheal diseases due to climate change has facilitated timely interventions. These interventions include enhancing treatment protocols, promoting breastfeeding, and immunizing children against rotavirus [28].

5 Climate Change Impacts on Endemic Vector-Borne Diseases

The ecosystems of vector-borne illnesses are highly sensitive to changes in temperature and precipitation. High temperatures and low humidity can limit the survival of ticks and fleas. At the same time, low humidity can also limit the survival of adult A. aegypti mosquitoes, thereby affecting the spread of diseases like rickettsia and dengue fever [29, 30]. Strong winds can reduce mosquito biting rates, extend their flight range, and disperse them around water reservoirs [31]. Understanding these effects relies heavily on mathematical models, though there is direct evidence for some vector-borne illnesses [32].

Climate change affects the spread of vector-borne diseases by impacting pathogens, vectors, hosts, and disease transmission pathways [22]. The pace of change and development of vector-borne illnesses and their transmission dynamics in the next decades will significantly depend on temperature and geographical dispersion [33]. Significant regional changes in the distribution of vector-borne diseases have been observed in temperate, peri-Arctic, Arctic, and tropical highland areas over the last few decades [34]. Failure to act against or adapt to climate change will lead to more drastic developments in the future.

Parasitic illnesses that infect intermediate hosts may respond differently to climate changes. Many trematodes of human and animal health concern have freshwater snails as intermediate hosts. Understanding the ecology of these snails is crucial for understanding how the parasites spread. Climate change affects newly developing illnesses and impacts the life cycles of both intermediate hosts and parasites.

For instance, *Ribeiroia ondatra*, a frog-mutating flatworm, is responsible for amphibian limb malformations. Climate change affects the life stages of this multi-host trematode parasite, impacting the growth, egg production, and mortality rate of snails. Interacting infection and temperature can also affect growth and fecundity in infected snails at 26 °C. Climate change may alter host-parasite dynamics, leading to “phenological mismatches” between hosts and parasites, which could result in increased infestations in snail and amphibian hosts, making them more vulnerable [35].

By addressing these impacts, public health professionals can better prepare for and mitigate the negative effects of climate change on public health.

6 Impact of Climate Change on Schistosomiasis and Their Intermediate Host Snails

6.1 Schistosomiasis

The blood fluke that causes schistosomiasis and bilharzia has infected about 250 million individuals, mostly in tropical and subtropical regions. As the second most common neglected tropical illness in Sub-Saharan Africa (SSA), behind hookworm infections, this parasitic infectious disease ranks high on the list of public health concerns in the region [36, 37, 38, 39]. Over 220 million individuals worldwide are afflicted with the parasitic worm that causes schistosomiasis [40]. There are 78 nations where schistosomiasis is known to be transmitted, and more than 800 million people in Africa, Latin America, the Middle East, and Southeast Asia reside in endemic regions [41]. The four schistosome species found in Africa are *Schistosoma mansoni* (intestinal), *Schistosoma haematobium* (urogenital), *Schistosoma intercalatum* (intestinal), and *Schistosoma guineensis* (intestinal). The first two are widespread, but the latter are uncommon outside central African nations. The levels of Schistosoma japonicum are high in a few other places, such as China. *Schistosoma mekongi* is unique to the Mekong River and is very uncommon. All Schistosoma species have a common but intricate life cycle in which the parasite moves back and forth between the intermediate hosts, as snails and a definitive host, as humans, bovines, and domestic cattle [33, 42]. The water temperature must be just right to support the parasite and the aquatic snail.

In addition, Caminade et al. [34] reviewed the literature and found that five different species of Schistosoma cause schistosomiasis and utilize aquatic intermediate hosts (snails). The growth of irrigation systems in hot climates, where the parasite in the snails may infect humans, has contributed significantly to the disease's rising worldwide incidence since the 1950s. The risk of infection is anticipated to rise dramatically due to climate change, and it may spread to formerly unaffected regions of northern China by the 2050s. However, the sickness has been much reduced because of the recent expansion of praziquantel distribution to adults and children in Africa, where most cases occur.

McCreesh et al. [43] observed that rising temperatures are anticipated to become favorable for enhanced transmission of S. mansoni throughout most of Eastern Africa, adding to concerns about the impact of global warming on disease transmission. They analyzed a climate change model that may be responsive to temperature variations in the snail host used by S. mansoni throughout its intermediate stages in East Africa. The model was tested with three scenarios predicting either a low, modest, or large increase in regional temperatures. Predictions were tested to see how they would fare if the air and water temperature relationships were changed and the snail death rate was altered. Their research concluded that much of eastern Africa might see a 20 percent rise in infection risk during the next 20 to 50 years. Additionally, S. mansoni may spread to uncontrolled regions. S. mansoni can become a new endemic in eastern Zambia, Burundi, South-Western Kenya, and Rwanda.

The first incidence of schistosomiasis on the French island of Corsica was reported in 2015 [44]. Several members of one family were sick while swimming in a river due to the presence of competent snail hosts, the warm summer weather, and an infected traveler's introduction of the parasite. Furthermore, Stensgaard et al. [38] found that the geographic ranges of schistosomiasis are more likely to vary than to grow due to climate change. Further clarification was provided by contrasting the existing regional distributions of the two most common African schistosome species with their thermo-physiological niche borders, which revealed that both species are present near the thermo-physiological niche boundaries.

Meanwhile, S. haematobium is more likely to suffer from less favorable climatic conditions. Both African species may migrate significantly from their "thermal comfort zone" to a warmer Africa. The capacity of parasites and snails to adapt or relocate in response to climate warming will thus affect schistosomiasis transmission.

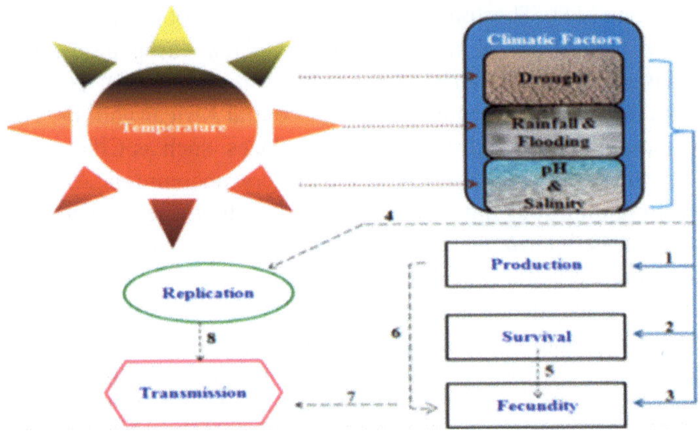

Fig. 2 Proposed model eliciting effects of change in climatic factors on Schistosomiasis transmission. (1) Changes in climatic factors are an essential determinant in the production and development of snails, as well as the production and development time of miracidia and cercaria in the intermediate host (snails) and freshwater depends on climate variability, (2) The snails, miracidia, and cercariae in freshwater and intermediate hosts depend on a change in climatic factors to survive; (3) Climate changes seriously influence the fecundity of the snails and the hatching of schistosome eggs into miracidia; (4) Replication of miracidia in the intermediate host to form sporocytes, which in turn produce cercaria, (5) Increase in survival rate leads to an increase in fecundity rate, (6) Climate change enhances the rapid reproduction of snails and the rapid metamorphosis of miracidia into cercaria in the intermediate host, (7) An increase in the fecundity rate of snails enhances schistosomiasis transmission by increasing the production number of cercaria within snails, (8) The cercaria penetrates the definitive human host, thereby metamorphosing into schistosomula that develop into adult worms that lay eggs responsible for the morbidity and mortality resulting from this disease. *Source* Adekiya et al. [33]

Climate variation has been suggested to be a possible factor affecting schistosomiasis transmission, according to a review of the literature on the impact of climate change on the transmission of schistosomiasis in Sub-Saharan Africa. Climate change factors, such as temperature, precipitation, flood, drought, and pH on both snails and Schistosomes, are depicted in Fig. 2. These factors are known to have significant impacts on the mortality and fecundity rate of the snails and the parasite during the transmission of the schistosomal life cycle [33, 45, 46].

6.2 *Freshwater Intermediate Host Snails of Schistosomiasis*

Some helminth trematodes, such as Schistosoma spp., rely on freshwater intermediate host snails (family: Planorbidae) for transmission. Thus, these snails drive the widespread spread of schistosomiasis [47]. S. haematobium was responsible for about 112 million urogenital schistosomal infected cases, or over 50% of the total incidence of schistosomal infections in the Sub-Sahara area [48, 42]. This might be because the Bulinus spp. (intermediate host: snails) are found throughout the area despite being native to countries like Cameroon, Egypt, and Senegal [36].

The snails' impact on the local human population was the subject of several modeling investigations. Multi-component integrated methods for eradicating schistosomiasis have been evaluated using the findings from this research and the accompanying modeling in the People's Republic of China. At the same time, researchers in rural Kenya used a model that included information from both the snail and human populations to understand the spread of the Schistosoma parasite better. The model results showed that the adaptive method with or without snail control was more successful when adjusted [49].

To examine how the intermediate host snail and the parasitic stages inside the snail fare at varying atmospheric temperatures, Yang and Bergquist [41] used a mix of Coupled Model Inter-comparison Projects, CMIPs, and biological modeling as two meteorological models. As revealed in their research, all three Schistosome species (S. mansoni, S. haematobium, and S. japonicum) would have a rise in transmission areas between 2021 and 2050 and between 2071 and 2100. However, the model projected that schistosomiasis transmission may be reduced in certain locations.

Snail habitat appropriateness varies in Zimbabwe, with separate high- and low-suitability zones, and temperature may be the primary determinant [50]. In a biologically based model for freshwater snails, the main potential climatic and environmental factors expected to be suited for snail habitat for Bulinus globosus, Biomphalaria Pfeifferi, and Lymnaea natalensis were integrated into the model. With the possible exception of B. pfeifferi, an intermediate host for intestinal schistosomiasis, it may increase around 2055 and then decline towards 2100. They concluded that future warming in Zimbabwe may cause a decline in the geographical distribution of appropriate snails' habitats.

However, Kalinda et al. [51] constructed a deterministic compartment simulation model of the snail B. globosus's life cycle using data from laboratory and field trials. Their model's snail reproduction and survival rates were comparable to those seen in controlled laboratory settings. The model further generated realistic dynamics of the snail population in response to a shift in climate. Both snails and cercariae were shown to decrease in abundance when ambient temperatures were raised, with a maximum fall in snail abundance of 14% and 27% and a decrease in maximum cercariae by 8% and 17%, when the temperatures were increased by 1 °C and 2 °C, respectively. Their results showed that future temperature increases owing to climate change might affect B. globosus abundance and, by extension, the incidence of schistosomiasis.

7 Impact of Climate Change on Malaria

Climate change is a key contributor to vector-borne illnesses like Malaria and dengue fever worldwide. According to the World Health Organization [52, 53], Malaria infects over 200 million people yearly, while dengue fever infects about 50 million. Extreme temperatures were found to reduce mosquito survival rates, while increasing rainfall that leads to open water collections are critical for mosquito breeding [54, 55], suggesting that climate has a significant impact on the life cycles of mosquito vectors transmitting these diseases.

Climate changes are among the drivers of the geographical range in predictions of global impacts on the intensity of transmission of parasitic diseases, such as Malaria, and on the seasonality of the disease; furthermore, these relationships are not always linear and may lead to complex patterns of change in risk as the planet warms [56, 57, 58]. A huge load is predicted with higher degrees of warming. However, regionally diverse patterns exist, suggesting that the burden of Malaria might grow with climatic changes due to the broader geographic range of the Anopheles vector. There are expectations that climate change may cause changes in vector populations, such as increases or decreases depending on the level of local warming, the mosquito vector's ecology, and other variables [56].

7.1 Aedes (Mosquito Vector for Dengue Fever, Chikungunya, Yellow Fever and Zika Virus)

Many studies have investigated "the projections of the geographic distribution of *Aedes aegypti* and *Aedes albopictus* (principal vectors) or the prevalence of dengue fever," they have all come to the same conclusion. There will be more mosquitoes and a wider geographic range at an increase of 2 °C compared to 1.5 °C. Consequently, more people will be at risk of dengue fever. Projections also indicate that Chikungunya's geographic distribution will extend due to climate change, with larger expansions predicted at higher degrees of warming [59].

7.1.1 Other Vector-Borne Diseases

Depending on the location and the extent of warming, West Nile virus transmission zones in North America and Europe might expand (both latitudinally and altitudinally), especially along the present borders of its transmission territories, and seasonal transmission could be extended [60]. According to most forecasts, climate change would likely increase the distribution and seasonality of Lyme disease and other tick-borne illnesses in North America and Europe [61, 62]. Greater temperatures and higher routes of greenhouse gas emissions result in bigger expected changes. Climate change projections of effects on leishmaniosis and Chagas disease suggested that future health burdens might grow or decrease depending on the level of increasing temperature [63, 64].

8 Impact of Climate Change on Environmental Pollutants:

8.1 Climate Change Impacts on Environmental Chemical Pollutants

Balbus et al. [65] showed that climate change stressors influence the responses, fate, and bioaccumulation of environmental contaminants and the persistence and movement of chemical pollutants in the environment [66]. Toxic chemical pollutants may be released, degraded, transported, and mobilized at higher rates due to rising temperatures, which might increase their environmental concentrations or degradations and human exposure [67]. Therefore, air quality will be impacted by the rate at which atmospheric chemical reactions occur due to global warming, humidity, or acidic precipitation [66].

Stagnation of wind speed promotes the buildup and deposition of air pollutants, while fluctuations in wind speeds may also impact the dispersion and transit of pollutants from place to place. Pollution-related diseases and death rates are so affected by climate change. Thus, in Morocco, PM10 levels rose throughout the summer due to the lack of change in the weather compared to the winter, whereas PM2.5 showed no seasonal fluctuation [68].

In addition, the re-appearance of organochlorine pesticides (OCPs) in the atmosphere of residential areas in India, for example, was determined to be attributable to the dispersion of its contents from the previously utilized sources before the rigorous prohibition of POPs used for agricultural purposes [69].

8.2 Climate Change Impacts on Environmental and Biological Pollutants

Climate change impacts on fungus

During 1997–2007, the relative frequency (RF) of keratomycosis (fungal keratitis) increased significantly in unanticipated regions, proving that invasive fungal infections may be related to global climate warming. The rise in RF was statistically associated with the elevation of low temperatures and the increase in the average humidity levels in the air [70].

As a result, climatic change may influence fungal development, particularly in poorly ventilated areas, and the creation of mycotoxins, as it is known that fungal growth is enhanced by warmth and humidity. Natural occurrences of mycotoxins were exacerbated by climate change [71]. One of the most dangerous carcinogenic fungal mycotoxins is aflatoxin B1 (AFB1). According to research by Meijer et al. [72], the mean AFB1 levels in African maize are higher than the legal limit set by the European Union, and its concentrations in food may reach extremely high levels, resulting in acute aflatoxicosis. AFM1 is produced from AFB1 by hydroxylation in the liver and then excreted in the milk of lactating females and the urine of those exposed to the toxin [73]. Exposure of African people is mostly related to milk consumption and nursing, as shown by Zinedine et al. [73]. In addition, it has been shown that high mycotoxin levels were detected in the biological fluids of workers who have been exposed occupationally to high fungal concentrations in their workplace due to the increase of the indoor air temperature and humidity [74, 75]. Aflatoxin B1 was discovered in the sera of 95% of individuals with HBsAg and 90% of those with Anti-HCV Ab, but it was present in the sera of only 76.5% of those without hepatitis B or C infection. Aflatoxin B1 was present in all cases with dual infection [76]. Liver damage from a combination of chronic hepatitis infection and aflatoxin B1 was predicted to be severe.

Climate change impacts on cyanobacterial toxins

Freshwater hazardous algal blooms (cyanobacteria species) have been shown to increase in number due to climate change [77]. Most often found in nutrient-rich lakes, rivers, streams, and reservoirs, these cyanobacteria contribute to water dangers by making toxins [78].

Recent studies have shown that climate change effects and the difficulty of restoring water quality and biological health would exacerbate the symptoms of cultural eutrophication in lakes and estuaries. Warmer water temperatures in lakes and estuaries, as expected by climate change in many parts of the globe, will exacerbate eutrophication concerns. The rise of cyanobacteria in freshwater systems is a direct global warming impact on eutrophication [79, 80]. A rise in cyanobacteria and the toxins they produce may have devastating impacts on humans, fish, and other members of freshwater ecosystems if certain conditions are met [81, 82].

According to research by Moss et al. [83], blue-green algae, which cause unpleasant blooms in lakes and estuaries, thrive in environments with an abundance of nutrients and warm temperatures. In addition, a rise in water temperature accelerates the release of nutrients already present in the bottom sediments and depletes the water of oxygen.

Researchers and resource managers have a formidable task in slowing the spread of cyanobacterial hazardous blooms (CyanoHABs). Climate change has proved to affect watershed hydrologic and nutrient loading dynamics, internal nutrient dynamics, mixing regime, lake and estuary temperatures, and other parameters, which presents new challenges for management. These alterations benefit CyanoHABs over other phytoplankton and may affect the success of control efforts. Adapting to climate change may include revising reduction objectives for nutrient inputs and determining nutrient-bloom thresholds for at-risk waterways. Flushing and artificial mixing are examples of physical-forcing mitigation measures that will need tweaks to the effects of climate change [84].

In their research, Saleh et al. [82] considered that cyanobacteria may have an impact on water quality metrics and the fish Oreochromis niloticus in the fish ponds at the Al-Abbassa Fish Hatchery in Sharkia Governorate of Egypt. Anabaena, Gleotrichia, Lyngbya, Oscillatoria, and Phormidium were the five genera of cyanobacteria discovered in the research. The major genus in the chosen ponds was Oscillatoria sp. Significant seasonal differences were found in the physicochemical properties of collected water samples. After 72 h, the survival rate of O. niloticus was lowest when exposed to an extract from Anabaena sp. The collected O. niloticus fish showed increased biochemical markers compared to the control group. The cyanobacterial genera discovered in the fishponds negatively impacted water quality and O. niloticus fish populations.

9 The Burden of Climate Change on Non-Communicable Diseases

Children experiencing intense heat events had much higher rates of kidney illness, fever, and electrolyte imbalance [7]. In addition, the human body's inability to properly battle for thermoregulation increases mortality rates when exposed to intense heat or cold [85]. This includes serious cardiovascular, pulmonary, and cerebrovascular repercussions that may lead to death. High and low daily temperature exposure were equally associated with increased hospital admissions for individuals suffering from respiratory and cardiovascular problems [86, 87].

Variation in climate change-related cancer incidence rates has also been observed. The RF of bilharzial bladder cancer appeared to be declining in most Egyptian governorates with the increase in air temperature, except in Frontier governorates; the time series trend of RF of bilharzial bladder cancer in different Egyptian governorates was found to be related to climate change during the period 1995–2005, with different variations. Increases in the RF of bilharzial bladder cancer among women in Upper and Lower Egypt governorates and the discovery of positive cases among men in unexpected governorates (Sinai and the Red Sea) led to a shift in the gender ratio [88]. Farmers in the Nile Valley and Delta migrated to the urban and frontier governorates for higher incomes due to the destruction of farmland caused by rising sea levels.

9.1 The Burden of Climate Change on Nutrition

9.1.1 Effect of Climate Change on Food Systems and Nutrition

The interplay between climate change and unsustainable agricultural systems compounds the negative effects on food and nutrition security. Several aspects of climate change—increasing temperatures, unpredictable precipitation, and severe weather, to name a few—are already impacting dietary habits and nutritional status. Bioavailability, water availability, soil fertility, decreased food output, decreased food nutrient concentration, increased food anti-nutrient content, and increasing incidences of infections are ways climate change may affect food systems [89].

Climate change effects on people's ability to eat well have been more pronounced in certain places of the globe than others. Malnutrition has been linked to climate change in many regions, including South Asia, where the devastation of rice crops due to high flooding occurrences is a major contributor. During drought, reduced grain output, especially maize, was also a powerful predictor of malnutrition in sub-Saharan Africa [90]. Within the same framework, it was shown that LMICs in Africa and Southeast Asia would have the greatest declines in food availability, resulting in both fewer deaths from overweight and obesity and more from undernourishment [91]. Several factors mean that the Eastern Mediterranean Region (EMR) will be particularly vulnerable to the effects of climate change on its food systems [92].

The Eastern Mediterranean Region is one of the most water stressful worldwide, and it is already afflicted by dramatic temperature and precipitation swings. Many nations in the region are also prone to drought, which reduces food production and availability. Agricultural self-sufficiency is low among the region's countries. The region is highly reliant on imports, especially staple foods, which makes the region vulnerable to global market shocks accompanied by climate change and threatens the population's access to adequate, safe, and nutritious food. Furthermore, the region is home to nations that are endemic for vector-borne diseases like Malaria, which are likely to worsen dramatically as average temperatures rise. A significant population increase is being seen in the area. High rates of food insecurity and malnutrition in all its manifestations are pervasive across the area. Many refugees and people have been uprooted living in the EMR.

Malnutrition may be caused by an abundance of nutrient(s) or a deficiency of one or many nutritional elements. In the following material, obesity and over-nutrition will be discussed; under-nutrition and/or nutritional deficiencies will be referred to as malnutrition(s).

9.1.2 Climate Change and Obesity

Climate change/global warming, greenhouse gas emissions, and obesity all interact with one another in complex ways. The rise in global temperatures makes individuals less likely to engage in physical activity and less likely to engage in adaptive thermogenesis, which may increase their carbon footprint. Increased consumption of unhealthy foods (such as meats), reduced production of fruits and vegetables in some regions, decreased energy expenditure (due to a lack of exercise), endocrine dysregulation, and economic disruption due to storms, drought, and flood all play a role in the epidemic of obesity that has been linked to climate change [93].

There is a link between obesity and global warming. A single obese person can produce an additional 81 kg of carbon dioxide equivalent (CO_{2eq}) per year due to a higher metabolic rate (7% of total), 593 kg of CO_{2eq} due to increased food and drink consumption (52% of total), and 476 kg of CO_{2eq} due to increased use of automobiles and airplanes (41% of total). Therefore, a single obese person may be responsible for 1.149 tons/y of CO_{2eq} in excess GHG emissions, which is almost 20% more than the emissions attributable to a lean person. Obesity contributes an extra 1.6% of world emissions [94].

9.1.3 Undernutrition and Stunting

Changes in weather patterns have been linked to an increase in malnutrition [90]. Child malnutrition, including anemia, underweight, wasting, and stunting, was shown to be more likely due to the susceptibility of agriculture to climate change, according to large-scale observational research conducted in India [95].

Climate/weather variables and individual vulnerabilities were found to be factors most often linked to anthropometric measurements (especially stunting) in children less than five years old [96]. The authors argued that environmental factors, such as temperature and precipitation, are just as important as socioeconomic ones in explaining why some children go undernourished.

9.1.4 Micronutrient Malnutrition

Vulnerable people are particularly in danger of micronutrient malnutrition (a lack of Vitamin A, zinc, and iron) due to climate change. Instead of affecting the micronutrient content of food, the interaction of rising temperatures and growing levels of carbon dioxide in the atmosphere is expected to diminish the total production of key staple crops, fruits, vegetables, and nuts [97].

Carbon dioxide-induced decreases in crop zinc and iron contents are predicted to cause around 125.8 million disability-adjusted life years worldwide between 2015 and 2050, with Southeast Asian and sub-Saharan African nations bearing the most burden. Infections, diarrhea, and anemia may all develop as a risk of zinc and iron deficiencies [98]. Beach et al. [99] provided similar forecasts on the impact of elevated atmospheric carbon dioxide on the availability of iron, zinc, and protein (macronutrient). The presently impacted nations will bear the brunt of the consequences. Adaptation options to compensate for micronutrient insufficiency include fortification of staple foods, micronutrient supplementation, bio-fortification, and the development of crops that are resistant to abiotic stresses such as greater temperature, carbon dioxide, and increased soil salinity [97].

9.1.5 Vulnerability of Malnutrition Due to Climate Change

Previous research on the susceptible populations adversely impacted by malnutrition was summarized by Lieber et al. [90]. Younger children and the elderly were shown to be the most susceptible to weather and climatic changes. Adults over 70 were shown to be more susceptible to drought than those between the ages of 60 and 69. In contrast, children between the ages of 1 and 2 were found to be the most sensitive owing to changes in infantile feeding habits during this time. The physiological changes, limiting financial and social position, and functional deterioration that come with aging are regarded to put older persons at a greater risk of malnutrition. During and after natural disasters, older people are often abandoned at home by their offspring, who have migrated to nearby cities in search of seasonal jobs. It was also discovered that gender had a significant moderating role. The impacts of climate change on malnutrition were felt more acutely by girls compared to boys. This finding highlights the heightened susceptibility of girls to extreme weather events caused by various social factors, including food allocation to boys in some cultures. During droughts, men aged 15–45 were more likely to experience wasting than women, which was thought to be due to increased seasonal migration among men searching for work and food [90].

9.1.6 Strategies to Mitigate the Effect of Climate Change on Nutrition.

The Global Syndemic (obesity, undernutrition, and climate change) was identified, and solutions were proposed by the Lancet Commission [100]. Dietz and Pryor [101] expanded on these measures by proposing a sustainable food and agriculture system and active transport system. Sustainable diets were described by Burlingame and Dernini [102] as ones that contribute to food security and healthy lives for the current and future generations while also having little effect on the environment. Sustainable diets minimize negative effects on biodiversity and ecosystems while being socially and environmentally acceptable, easily available, economically fair, reasonably priced, and, last, nutritionally sufficient, safe, and healthful. Nearly 10 billion people will need to eat healthy diets for the planet by 2050, and the EAT-Lancet Commission's summary report "Healthy Diets from Sustainable Food Systems, Food Planet Health" aims to accomplish this goal. The goals of the report are to promote both a healthy diet and environmentally friendly food production. In order to meet these two objectives, it was suggested that the following five strategies be implemented in line with the United Nations' Sustainable Development Goals: "seek international and national commitment to shift towards healthy diets; reorient agricultural priorities from producing high quantities of food to producing healthy food; sustainably intensify food production in order to increase high-quality output; implement strong and coordinated governance of land and oceans; and reduce food losses and waste by at least half" [103].

Dietz and Pryor [101] recommend implementing sustainable active transport systems as the second step. The characteristics that characterize a sustainable diet also apply to sustainable transportation systems. Eliminating fossil fuel sector subsidies, raising taxes, and investing more in public transportation are all viable options for promoting more active modes of transportation. Urban planning and housing placement that encourage walking, biking, and other active transportation are integral to this community infrastructure [101].

Changes in human behavior contributing to the greenhouse effect will be challenging to implement. They included personal and institutional levels of community policymaking and, finally, at the state and federal levels [101]. Therefore, it is crucial to establish monitoring methods to evaluate development and guarantee accountability [101]. The Lancet Countdown on Health and Climate Change generated the corresponding indicators. Some primary indicators are health hazards and their effects; adaptation, planning, and resilience for health; mitigation activities and health co-benefits; financial resources; and public and political engagement. Indicators include things like the cost of heat-related deaths, the number of people who die prematurely due to exposure to ambient air pollution in their industries, the amount of green space in cities, and the amount of attention given to health and climate change in the media [104].

10 Climate Change and Women's Health

Several facets of climate change may negatively impact women's health. Low physiologic adaptation to increased temperature has a bigger influence on the health of the elderly and pregnant women than it does on males. Some nations are more susceptible to cultural risks due to inadequate medical and cooling infrastructure, bulky clothes, and a lack of accessible public transportation [105, 8].

10.1 Mechanism of Climate Change Impact on Women's Health

Numerous research demonstrating the negative impacts of climate change on women's health were highlighted by Sorensen et al. [8] in their comprehensive analysis of the topic.

Exposure to high temperatures during pregnancy is harmful. Premature birth, birth abnormalities, and stillbirth are all linked to it. Furthermore, preeclampsia, high blood pressure during pregnancy, and a negative prognosis for the baby are all associated with high ambient temperatures.

The health of women is negatively impacted by poor air quality. Because of their physiological makeup and higher rates of anemia, women are at a greater risk of cardiac illness and the toxicologic consequences of airborne pollution than males. Placental hypoxia may result from the use of biomass and/or waste plastics for cooking and heating at home, which cause the deposition of inhaled particles in lung tissue and systemic hypoxia. This has been related to fetal malformations and intrauterine growth retardation.

The effects of disasters burden more and more women. When natural disasters strike, women are disproportionately affected. Ninety percent of the casualties of the

1991 cyclones in Bangladesh were women. There is an increased risk of problems such as preeclampsia, uterine hemorrhage, and low birth weight children for pregnant women giving delivery following disasters. Women and girls are disproportionately affected by physical, sexual, and domestic abuse in the wake of climate-driven catastrophes. Mental health issues, including depression and anxiety, are quite widespread. Unemployment and economic uncertainty hit them harder than others [8].

Bryson et al. [106] studied the effect of food insecurity and malnutrition on women as a result of climate change. They are more likely to have adverse effects from dietary deficits during menstruation, pregnancy, and lactation, as has been noted. Therefore, the negative health effects of climate change are more likely to be felt by women in low-resource communities. Due to pregnancy-related illnesses and unique care requirements, pregnant women are more vulnerable. Deficiencies of the maternal micronutrient, anxiety, depression, gestational diabetes, hypertension, and mortality could be due to food insecurity and undernutrition during pregnancy. Pregnant women in low-resource communities often struggle to get the nutrition they need because of a lack of food availability and access, particularly during the hunger seasons when food is scarce (usually the dry season), and climate change is only expected to make things worse. Women are undernourished for a variety of cultural and social reasons. As the principal agricultural producers, women have less power as the climate changes. It has also been discovered that women, with the right kind of assistance and partnerships, may be resilient and adapt to environmental exposures that threaten their food security and health [106, 8].

Water security and waterborne diseases affect women more than others. Women often take on the responsibility of bringing water into the home, but those who do so regularly are at a higher risk of contracting water-related illnesses. Most of a woman's day in India during a water shortage is spent transporting water. Women and girls of all ages have more cumulative harm to their spines and necks because of water gathering. Heat stress, heat stroke, and the danger of violence are all exacerbated by long-distance travel. When women (especially pregnant women) do not have access to safe water and toilets, it may have disastrous consequences for their health [8].

Vector-borne illnesses are connected to climate change. That could be due to the physiological changes and decreased immune function during pregnancy; pregnant women are more vulnerable to vector-borne illnesses. Intrauterine growth retardation and increased susceptibility to bleeding are two negative outcomes of malaria infection during pregnancy due to anemia and impaired trans-placental nutrition transfer. Malaria is a known cause of maternal mortality. Increased likelihood of cesarean birth and intrauterine development restriction have both been linked to Dengue virus infection in pregnant women. Microcephaly, central nervous system abnormalities, and mental retardation have all been linked to the Zika virus [8].

Ahmed et al. [88] discovered that the male-to-female ratio for bilharzial bladder cancer has shifted. Females in some of these places were suspected of replacing their husbands in agriculture. So, the burden of agriculture on women might expose them to higher rates of schistosomal infection than in the past. This trend was linked to the increased movement of male farmers from agricultural areas to the new governorates.

Pregnancy outcomes could be affected by the impact of climate change. Researchers showed that exposure to tropical storms induced by climate change and high temperatures caused a wide range of delivery problems, including low birth weight or fetal losses in the womb [107, 108]. Climate shocks, such as extreme heat waves [108] and droughts, might be to blame because they reduce the availability of vital nutrients, leading to stunted development in children [109].

11 International Policy Framework

Sorensen et al. [110] argued that social, cultural, and physiological variables modulate health effects and gender disparities in health effects. Reducing unfavorable health outcomes requires policy action directed at these determinants, which are typically adjustable.

Better data collection, sector-to-sector coordination, monitoring of gender-specific objectives, and fair stakeholder involvement are needed if climate, development, and disaster risk reduction policy frameworks are to be updated to include a gendered viewpoint.

Mitigation and adaptation policy actions may be strengthened by recognizing women's strengths as teachers, caretakers, knowledge keepers, and catalysts for social change [110].

11.1 Role of Health Care Providers, Especially Obstetricians and Gynecologists

FIGO (International Federation of Gynecology and Obstetrics) has highlighted advocacy, capacity development, education, and research interpretation as four foundations to address the climate problem. Healthcare practitioners should take the lead in these areas. To educate professional healthcare providers, the lay public, patients, ministers of health, and other leaders to make the changes necessary to identify these crises, a strong emphasis must be placed on research, education, and advocacy in response to shifting health impacts and global awareness.

Women's sexual and reproductive health and rights, as well as the health of newborns and children, are in greater danger due to the climate catastrophe. Our patients and their families are feeling the effects of climate change, and obstetricians and gynecologists have the opportunity to educate the public and advocate for action. For the well-being of present and future generations, climate change was framed in the context of women's reproductive health as a public health problem, a human rights issue, a social justice issue, a political issue, an economic issue, and a gender issue. In recognizing the need for government policies, societal solutions, and global cooperation to address and reduce contributors to climate change, including the production of fossil fuels, FIGO adds its voice to the chorus of international scientists and medical professionals who have warned of the dire consequences of the current climate crisis for pregnant women, developing fetuses, and reproductive health [111]

12 Public Health Surveillance, Modeling, and Artificial Intelligence

Notifiable disease reporting monitoring systems continue to play an important role in public health management since they allow for the early detection of outbreaks, the tracking of illness development, and the informing of preventative and mitigation programs. However, conventional surveillance systems must catch up in data reporting, analysis, and dissemination. The scientific community came up with additional cutting-edge methods of operation. The fast development and invention of early warning for disease outbreaks may be attributed to the World Health Organization's efforts to expand current monitoring systems for infectious diseases. A climate-informed early warning system (EWS) consists of four main components: (i) environmental monitoring, (ii) high-risk condition forecasting and active surveillance, (iii) warnings and communication, and (iv) a mechanism for early action. In order to better plan for and respond to climate-sensitive illnesses, health systems may benefit substantially from the development of integrated surveillance. To better use information for identifying, investigating, and reacting to public health hazards, integrated surveillance includes integrating several surveillance systems (such as disease monitoring and weather surveillance). As a result, the healthcare system benefits from increased efficiency with which surveillance data is shared. Early warning systems and climate-informed monitoring may improve health system readiness. The purpose of an early warning system is to provide advance notice of potential dangers in order to mitigate their potential effects and be ready for a rapid reaction. Health systems may benefit from increased adaptive capacity and climate resilience if they have access to early warning systems in the face of a rapidly shifting environmental and risk scenario. When evaluating climate-informed early warning systems for infectious illnesses, WHO emphasizes developing quality standards for verifying prediction models [1–5].

A web-based system, Early Warning, Alert, and Response (EWAR) was established by the World Health Organization to alert authorities of impending public health crises. It is a crucial and immediate part of any surveillance setup. The following are all parts and steps involved in EWAR. First, "early warning" is the timely identification of signs that may foretell possible severe public health catastrophes. Notifications from health facilities, community members, and other organizations are potential early warning data sources that feed into IBS and EBS systems. (ii) Alert management is the process of systematically handling all incoming data, from signal verification through risk assessment and characterization, to determine whether a reaction is necessary to lessen the threat to public health. For maximum effectiveness, it is recommended that all signals be fed into a single system where they can be studied and controlled methodically. (iii) Response: When an alarm is detected, public health measures are taken in order to better prepare for and respond to public health crises; WHO improved the ability of nations to utilize this system and released an implementation and strengthening of Early Warning Alert and Response (EWAR) handbook [111].

Rees et al. [113] commented on various scientific techniques to close the gap between real-time monitoring of emergent concerns and early understanding of possible health implications. To detect the elevated risks of infectious disease outbreaks anticipated with climate change, two risk assessment methodologies, event-based surveillance systems (EBS) and risk modeling, were created. They are also used to guide efforts to avoid, diagnose, and lessen the impact of infectious disease outbreaks brought on by climate change. The EBS systems may be used with traditional surveillance systems to improve early warning of public health concerns by analyzing open-source internet data, including media stories, government reports, and social media (like Twitter).

In order to better filter, categorize, and analyze health-related internet data, EBS systems have lately included artificial intelligence (AI) technologies, including machine learning and natural language processing. Disease risk may be evaluated by statistical and mathematical approaches through the consideration of host (such as the number of reported cases), pathogen (such as pathogenicity), and environmental variables through risk modeling (e.g., climate suitability for reservoir populations). Open-source internet data on health and human and commodity movement are two examples of the growing sorts of data used in these models. This data is useful for locating vulnerable groups and tracing potential transmission routes across borders [113].

One such example is the use of AI in epidemiological disease monitoring. Another use of data mining is the identification of cholera hotspots. Field data was used with satellite data on the environment, climate, and health to derive and explain the origins of disease evolution [114].

Moulton and Schramm [115] propose comparable ideas, stressing the need to evaluate the United States' ability to conduct public health monitoring in light of climate change. Indicators and data, systems (electronic or otherwise), personnel, and policies are all areas where surveillance might be strengthened. Their method can be replicated in other nations.

12.1 Artificial Intelligence (AI) and Modeling's Role in Disease Prediction and Risk Evaluation

The public health sector is increasingly using AI and machine learning. Prediction and forecasting of diseases and the epidemiology of diseases are the two primary areas of study. Artificial intelligence might establish infectious illness prediction models in relation to climate change. Dengue fever has rapidly spread to more nations than ever before, and this tool was used to anticipate where it would appear in the future. Infectious diarrhea outbreaks may be predicted based on environmental and weather conditions [10].

West Nile virus (WNV) cases, intensity, and geographic spread peaked in 2018 compared to earlier trends in 2010. Positive summer-spring temperature anomalies, a lower water availability index, and drier winter conditions were identified as predictors of WNV outbreaks in Europe, utilizing AI with a high-performance machine learning classifier. To prevent further West Nile virus (WNV) outbreaks in Europe, an artificial intelligence framework may assist in providing early warnings for active monitoring and vector management. The model's findings may be used to increase risk communication, secure enough laboratory and blood bank capacity, support longer-term research to fill in knowledge gaps and coordinate One Health surveillance and response throughout WNV transmission seasons. Public health response may be improved with the help of a road plan toward an AI-based WNV early warning system. Suppose the European Climate and Health Observatory will succeed in its mission. In that case, a WNV climate early-warning system will be needed to account for and explain the complex interplay between climate and other causes. Using projected climatic data, the model may help researchers locate, analyze, and plan for future WNV transmission hotspots throughout Europe [116].

Xu et al. [117], created an ecologically based model for the dengue system. They accurately forecast the dynamics of dengue. Dengue fever's cyclical occurrence in human populations may be partially explained by weather patterns, namely rainfall and temperature's impact on mosquito populations and the disease's transmission efficiency.

To keep tabs on the spread of major infectious illnesses, researchers are turning to cutting-edge machine-learning algorithms for early or real-time verification. Regarding public health and preventative measures, machine learning is a cutting-edge instrument with enormous potential. Machine-learning models provide a chance to keep tabs on introducing and spreading infectious illnesses in light of the current global epidemics over the last several decades. They will also become more commonplace in the healthcare industry and scientific study. By combining many machine-learning models, we can anticipate where and when infectious disease outbreaks will occur; further study will enable the development of even more precise and believable models. When many data sets are used, better conclusions may be drawn. The most likely ones are found when the data source is not unique, but the accuracy of the findings is improved when many data sets are utilized. Future studies should use machine-learning techniques to enhance the accuracy of traditional epidemiological models [118].

To maximize the effectiveness of territorial resilience action management, the Artificial Neural Network (ANN) is now the most useful tool at hand. To reduce the devastation caused by climate change, severe or extreme weather events, and air pollution, ANN was created to select, manage, maintain, and make the greatest use of resilience initiatives. ANN is the culmination of years of collaboration amongst specialists in fields as diverse as computer science, meteorology, atmospheric physics, medicine, mathematics, geology, environmental engineering, and many more. Analytical maps of urban areas must be dynamically linked to local climate data and weather predictions via ANN. A variety of acceptable steps to be undertaken with resilience actions are suggested by ANN after they discover those components in the region to be conserved that are sensitive to any major weather event or consequences of climate change that may harm human health or the urban environment. Since ANN can predict which areas are most at risk, it may help with health interventions by alerting relevant health systems and giving local operators a head start on preventative measures. When applied to urban areas that need to be preserved, ANN can monitor and evaluate the positive effects and effectiveness of resilience actions implemented to select the most effective actions on the territory for both the environment and human health, optimizing future responses of the ANN. The "training function" plays a crucial role in artificial neural networks. The harder ANNs work, the better they become, and eventually, they'll be able to recommend the best preventative activities to be taken by remembering the choices made and the outcomes attained by the resilience acts that have already been taken. The city of Phoenix is used as a case study for a study on health resilience action (Arizona, USA). This novel strategy employing the ANN may greatly increase a city's resilience by proactively and dynamically addressing climate and health catastrophes. ENVINNET is an ANN designed to make Phoenix's hospitals and other medical institutions more resilient to natural disasters.

To strengthen health resilience in times of extreme stress, such as when dust storms blow in from the desert, the ENVINNET is based on an analysis of the metropolitan area and its weak spots as a function of health resilience. It is anticipated that ENVINNET's computing capacity and model design will make future resilience activities and human health warnings credible and sustainable. Using ENVINNET, automated spatiotemporal projections for the Phoenix region can be developed, which can then be used to give urban health alerts. The capability of self-correction over time is crucial to its responsiveness. When a dust storm rolls into town and causes a spike in air pollution, ENVINNET's mission is to help those in danger of losing their health (extreme weather events). Extreme stress is put on the populace, leading to asthma-like respiratory crises in youngsters and the worsening of other preexisting disorders. This highlights the importance of the unique ENVINNET's ability to provide 24–48–72-h warning to Phoenix's healthcare institutions so that they may better prepare for the arrival of the disaster and increase their resilience [119].

Modeling using AI and machine learning is a rapidly expanding field of study. The proposed models and/or systems must have sufficient sensitivity, specificity, predictive values, and reliability to discover early instances and promptly disseminate the findings.

12.2 Quantitative Risk Assessment of Climate Change's 2030s and 2050s Impacts on Certain Causes of Mortality

The World Health Organization [52, 53] paper demonstrated the use of several models to forecast cause-specific mortality in 2030 and 2050. Global climate-health models were developed for several climate-sensitive health outcomes, including heat-related mortality in the elderly, coastal flooding mortality, diarrheal disease mortality in children under the age of 15, malaria population at risk and mortality, dengue population at risk and mortality, under-nutrition (stunting) and associated mortality, and under-nutrition (stunting) and associated mortality.

Due to climate change, there will be an estimated 38 thousand fatalities in elders from heat exposure, 48 thousand from diarrhea, 60 thousand from Malaria, and 95 thousand from infant under-nutrition in 2030 compared to a world without climate change. Between 2030 and 2050, it is predicted that climate change will cause an average of 250 thousand more fatalities annually. This estimate is not meant to reflect the full extent to which climate change is expected to affect human health.

According to projections from the World Health Organization, climate change effects from child malnutrition and diarrheal illness are expected to decrease between 2030 and 2050. However, it is predicted that by the 2050s, the fatalities caused by heat exposure would rise to nearly 100 thousand annually. Because of expected increases in mortality in low- and middle-income nations, the effects will be most severe under a low economic development scenario. South Asia is expected to be hit worst by the mortality effects of climate change by the year 2050. These findings suggest that by the 2030s, climate change will have a major effect on children's health.

Even under optimistic scenarios of future socioeconomic growth and with the measures of adaptation, climate change is likely to have major unfavorable implications on future mortality. This suggests that in addition to the immediate health advantages predicted to accrue from actions to decrease climate pollutants, such as reduced particle air pollution levels, avoiding climate-sensitive health hazards is another incentive to mitigate climate change. It also bolsters the argument for considering climatic variability and changes when designing programs to address health concerns such as malnutrition, diarrhea, vector-borne illness, and excessive heat. It is crucial to guarantee that the poorest and most vulnerable communities benefit most from economic growth, climate policy, and health initiatives due to the significant impact of socioeconomic development on future risk estimates [52, 53].

12.3 Climate Change and Mental Health

Natural catastrophes, severe weather occurrences, gradual shifts in climate change, and the public's perception of these factors might all impact mental health. Depression, post-traumatic stress disorder (PTSD), and major depressive disorder (MDD) are the most frequent mental health issues in the aftermath of catastrophic weather disasters. Substance abuse, home violence, complicated grief, survivor guilt, vicarious trauma, recovery fatigue, and thoughts of suicide are among other results [9, 120]. Twenty to thirty percent of people who survived natural disasters like hurricanes and floods also suffered from depression and/or post-traumatic stress disorder (PTSD). Mental health was also negatively impacted by the wildfire. Suicide rates among farmers were shown to be higher during droughts, even though droughts tend to be more gradual. Potential factors include monetary losses, sadness over altered landscapes, and the dissolution of vocational and/or gender-based identities. The effects on mental health might last for weeks, months, or even years. When it comes to mental health, those most at risk are women, children, people with low incomes, and the indigent population [9].

Stress, post-traumatic stress disorder, anxiety, and trauma are all examples of psychosocial effects that have been related to armed conflict and forced migration. Forced migration and displacement are the results of civil wars. Migrant populations may experience psychological distress due to their exposure to new cultural, linguistic, and lifestyle norms. When refugees are accepted, protected, and provided with improved living circumstances in host nations, this may strengthen their psychological resilience [120].

As people in the community face several stresses due to climate change, the chance of criminal conduct, violence, and hostility rises, posing a threat to community health [120].

Although gradual changes are harder to spot than sudden ones, they will have far-reaching consequences for many communities. The strongest link between heat and psychological well-being is unmistakable. Aggression levels seem to rise in tandem with this phenomenon. Aggression may have severe consequences, both when directed outward (violence, murder) and inside (suicide). Higher temperatures were linked to an increase in psychiatric hospitalizations. The frustration-aggression theory suggests that exposure to such settings increases stress and frustration. At the same time, a lack of opportunity to engage in regular physical activity or poor sleep quality is another possible contributor [9]. Hospitalizations for mood and behavioral disorders such as schizophrenia, mania, and neurotic disorders rise during periods of extreme heat and humidity. People with preexisting mental health disorders and issues, those on prescription medicines (particularly lithium, neuroleptic, and anticholinergic drugs), and those with substance abuse (alcohol, narcotics) problems are more likely to have heat-related mental health morbidity [120].

Increased levels of ozone close to the ground and other changes in air quality caused by the combustion of fossil fuels have been linked to increased psychological stress and psychotic episodes. Damage to cognitive abilities caused by air pollution is both immediate and cumulative. As a result, individuals are less likely to spend time outside, leading to a corresponding drop in exercise, friendships, and social relations and a general increase in stress levels [9].

Economic instability due to changes in occupational structure and agricultural circumstances may be a secondary pathway via which climate change impacts mental health. This causes unnecessary strain on the families involved. Climate-related forced migration has been linked to psychological distress. A rise in local and global conflict has been linked to climate change [9].

Anxiety may result from one's interpretation and worry about climate change. Solastalgia, or the emotional reaction to environmental deterioration, is a new concept in the field of mental health, along with ecological grief and eco-anxiety. Worry grew as people mourned the disappearance of familiar locations and ways of life and fretted about the future consequences of climate change [9].

One's social environment moderates physical and mental health. The worry and anxiety caused by climate change might be exaggerated or downplayed on social media. Mental health issues may be alleviated with the help of community resources. Those with a large group of friends and family to lean on are better able to deal with stress than their lonelier counterparts. Treatment for mental health issues should be included within the scope of available resources [9].

Psychologists and therapists need to be ready to handle climate-related psychological distress. The availability of mental health services grew, and they morphed to accommodate new therapies. Positive social experiences have been linked to decreased stress and increased well-being, so it stands to reason that social participation might help those with perceptual anxiety [9].

12.3.1 Priority Actions to Manage Mental Health Related to Climate Change

There must be international cooperation and a firm commitment to action. To effectively compel governments to act against climate change, the public must be aware of its health implications' severity, size, and breadth. According to [120], the following psychological adaptation methods would best promote the mental health of a community in a world with climate change:

•"Policy responses: increasing access and funding to mental health care; • Surveillance and monitoring: conducting epidemiological surveys after extreme weather events and monitoring emergency department visits during heat waves and in the aftermath of extreme weather events; • Practice: the application of a stepped-care approach to mental health that is often used in disaster mental health to support different levels of interventions depending on the timing of the disaster and the level of distress; • Preparation and response: climate change adaptation/resilience planning in the mental health system;• Community-based interventions: climate change resilience plans that address psychosocial well-being; and,• Special training for care providers and first responders: e.g., psychological first aid."

12.3.2 World Health Organization Recommendations

The World Health Organization [121] suggests the following five strategies for mitigating the psychological effects of climate change:

In order to be better prepared for and able to react to the climate disaster, mental health policies and services, such as Mental Health and Psychological Support (MHPSS) should take climate change into account; include MHPSS in health and climate change policies and initiatives; expand upon international pledges; use community- and cross-sector-based techniques to mitigate climate change's psychological and emotional toll; and fill the massive financial holes in mental health care and in adapting to the health effects of climate change.

13 Gaps and Future Directions

Hwong et al.'s [122] scoping assessment proposed the following gaps and future objectives regarding climate change and mental health.

13.1 Gaps

Research questions and findings on climate change and mental health were affected by various factors, including definitions, study design, data-collecting techniques, and analytical methodologies. Consequently, it is important to remember that these findings should be seen as preliminary.

The indirect consequences of climate change on mental health and accompanying inequities have received little research attention, especially for those who already suffer from mental health issues.

Few studies have looked at the impact of climate change on child mental health or drug use, and most of those have tended to concentrate on adults rather than communities.

13.2 Suggestions for the Future

More study is required to investigate the amplification impacts of climate change on mental health, which contributes to inequities. There is a need for uniform, rigorous measurements of climatic events, geographical units of analysis, and mental health outcomes across research.

Studying the relationship between climate change and community-level mental health outcomes can help shape public mental health interventions, systems planning, and policy. More research is needed to understand how climate change could affect developmental trajectories and related mental health outcomes [122].

More study is required to determine the extent to which climate change is already affecting people's mental health, which demographics are most at risk, and which treatments are most successful. Another topic of interest is the strengths that individuals rely on to keep going even when their surroundings change [9].

13.3 *Public Health Response to Climate Change*

The health impacts of climate change are inevitable. Thus, public health measures are urgently needed to prepare for, manage, and reduce them. The prevention of accidents and diseases, as well as improving public health readiness and reducing risk, all depend on an efficient public health response to climate change. The 10 Essential Services of Public Health, created in 1994 by the American Public Health Association and many other federal, state, and local organizations and partners, serve as the standard framework for public health activity. Climate change is associated with the following ten services [12]:

1. Monitor the health status of the community by recording the occurrence of illnesses and the spread of climate-related trends.
2. Investigate and diagnose community health issues and threats, such as the spread of illness via contaminated water, food, or insects.
3. Communicate the health effects of climate change to the general public and policymakers to raise awareness, promote understanding, and encourage action.
4. Mobilize public health partnerships with businesses, other professional organizations, the religious community, and others to identify and address health issues and implement those ideas.
5. Create municipal heat-wave preparedness plans that will aid in the health of individuals and communities.
6. Maintain a safe and healthy environment by strictly enforcing relevant legislation (Little role for public health).
7. Provide health care services to connect individuals with vital personal health services and guarantee their availability in times of need.
8. Teaching the public and private healthcare staff about climate change will prepare them to deal with its effects.
9. Assessing preparedness initiatives, such as heat-wave plans, may provide light on the efficacy, accessibility, and quality of personal and population-based health services.
10. Investigate the health impacts of climate change using cutting-edge methods like modeling and investigate the best ways to adapt to these changes for fresh insights and effective solutions to pressing health issues.

13.4 *Integrating Public Health into Climate Change Policy and Planning*

Some scholars evaluated the literature documenting the development of public health's involvement in climate change action, expanding on the work of [12], who identified ten basic roles and vital public health services and their link to climate change. Public health has the potential to be a proactive partner fully integrated into climate policy planning and implementation in the future decade, but the model still has room for improvement [13].

13.4.1 Public Health Adaptation Strategies

To prepare communities for future, present, and predicted climate hazards to public health, the Climate Change Adaptation Resource Center (ARC-X) develops adaptation methods. To better prepare communities for the health impacts of climate change, these methods follow the five-step Building Resilience Against Climate Effects (BRACE) program developed by the Centers for Disease Control and Prevention (CDC). Forecasting climate impacts and assessing vulnerabilities, projecting the disease burden, evaluating public health interventions, creating and implementing a climate and health adaptation plan, assessing the plan's impact and improving the quality of activities, and finally, evaluating the plan's success are the five steps that make up the program. The BRACE mentioned above five-step approach is used in public health adaptation strategies for high heat, water, and air quality [123].

Adaptation solutions for excessive heat include public education and outreach, financial incentives, new tree planting and landscaping initiatives, public building retrofitting, revisions to relevant policies, plans, designs, and regulations, and the incorporation of air quality improvement measures.

Adaptation plans for water quality and public health should focus on predicting climate effects and analyzing vulnerabilities. The national climate assessment may be used to understand regional climate risk forecasts better, allowing for anticipating climate consequences. The major climate hazards are outlined. Changing water temperatures may increase the danger of waterborne diseases such as Vibrio cholerae and toxic algal blooms during times of the year and in locations where these pathogens were not previously prevalent. Increased runoff, higher temperatures, and discharges from point sources of pollution may all raise the exposure risk of waterborne pathogens (bacteria, viruses, and parasites like Cryptosporidium and Giardia) caused by extreme precipitation events.

Extreme weather also causes severe damage to water systems. Weather events and storm surges increase the chance of failure in water, sewage, and storm-water systems. This raises the danger of exposure to water-related infections, chemicals, and algal toxins in receiving waters, and when these contaminants make their way into source waters, they may impede attempts to purify drinking water.

Anticipating climate effects and analyzing vulnerabilities are recommended adaptation techniques for air quality and public health. Similar to how water quality may be predicted by examining regional climate risk forecasts, the national climate assessment can help us anticipate climate consequences. Increased ozone's negative health effects are a major climate danger. Increases in ozone layer due to climate change will lead to premature deaths, hospitalizations, missed school days, and acute respiratory problems. The increased risk of mortality, severe chronic and acute cardiovascular and respiratory health effects, and exacerbated allergy and asthma disorders are all directly attributable to wildfires. Specifically, rising temperatures, altered precipitation patterns, and rising atmospheric carbon dioxide concentrations are predicted to contribute to rising levels of some airborne allergens, leading to an increase in asthma attacks and other allergic illnesses. This will exacerbate existing indoor air quality issues and lead to the emergence of new ones due to the changes mentioned above in outdoor conditions that affect indoor conditions. Alterations in the outdoor-to-interior air ratio may also result from climate change. However, since interior pollutants are less likely to be diluted by outside air, reduced outdoor and indoor air mixing leads to greater quantities of pollutants created within.

Populations and communities that may be more vulnerable to these impacts include those who use vulnerable locations for fishing and swimming, those who spend extensive time outdoors as a profession or trade, and those who have preexisting health concerns or are at a particularly vulnerable life stage. To better analyze public health requirements and vulnerabilities, public health professionals may benefit from collaborating with water utilities, water resource managers, transportation officials, air quality managers, state officials, and industry.

13.4.2 Centers for Disease Control and Prevention (CDC) Policy on Climate Change and Public Health [124]

The Centers for Disease Control and Prevention (CDC) has highlighted the following priority health initiatives related to climate change, building on current programs and the Essential Public Health Services.

1. Be a reliable resource for knowledge on the effects of climate change on health in the United States and beyond.
2. Monitor information on climate-related changes in the environment, illness risks, and the actual incidence of diseases.
3. Increase its ability to estimate and predict the health consequences of climate change.
4. Increase knowledge of the connection between climate change and health impacts by strengthening its scientific foundation.
5. Determine the geographic areas and demographic subsets most vulnerable to health hazards like heat waves.
6. Advise the general public, policymakers, and medical professionals on mitigating climate change's health impacts.

7. Collaborate with other government agencies, the commercial sector, nonprofit groups, universities, and international organizations to better address the health implications of climate change in the United States and across the world.
8. Serve as a role model in protecting public health from the impacts of climate change by influencing local, state, and federal governments, community leaders, healthcare providers, NGOs, religious groups, businesses, and the general public at large.
9. Practice contingency plans for potential health crises such as heat waves, natural disasters, and contagious illnesses.
10. Help state and municipal health authorities, the commercial sector, and others prepare for the health implications of climate change on a national and global scale by providing technical guidance and assistance.
11. Boost workforce growth by ensuring the next generation of public health workers is trained to deal with the health risks presented by climate change.

In light of [22] research, it is reasonable to infer that individuals may play important and active roles in adopting the negative health implications of climate change via proactive adaptation methods. As such, they stressed the need to identify vulnerable groups and develop region-specific projections of climate change's health implications to assign the appropriate control measures. This might be accomplished by redistributing financial and healthcare resources and enhancing public health initiatives in light of scientific predictions of climate change's catastrophic occurrences. Additionally, early warning systems based on climate change estimates successfully assisted policymakers and various communities in developing active protective strategies to avoid or mitigate the potential health implications of climate change [22].

13.5 Climate Change Resilience of Health Systems and Healthcare Facilities

The health system infrastructures might be damaged by climate change-related severe weather events and catastrophes, further exacerbating populations' vulnerability. A lot is riding on the public health systems, and they are struggling under the weight of rising health issues attributed to climate change and the precarious state of the economy [125]. There are financial and societal costs associated with the rise in new and reemerging infectious illnesses and the rise in weather-related accidents and fatalities. Ministry of Health policies worldwide, particularly in at-risk nations and areas, must account for these costs.

Furthermore, healthcare systems' high greenhouse gas (GHG) emissions were shown to add significantly to the global warming crisis [126]. About 4.4% of all GHGs are emissions from healthcare facilities (HCFs) [1–5]. That is why it is crucial to strengthen climate change resilience in ways that contribute to environmental sustainability [126]. The healthcare system, including its infrastructure and emergency preparation plans, must be strengthened by identifying existing and future climate hazards and following such evidence-based guidelines [128].

Climate change resilience is defined as "the capacity of social, economic, and environmental systems to cope with a hazardous event, trend, or disturbance, responding or re-organizing in ways that maintain their essential function, identity, and structure while also maintaining the capacity for adaptation, learning, and transformation," [129]. The capacity to foresee, react to, cope with, recover from, and adapt to climate-related shocks and stressors in order to deliver long-term benefits in population health despite climate change is what the World Health Organization (WHO) calls "climate resilience." That is why it is crucial to have measures of health system resilience, which may shed light on how well the system is adapting to the risks and difficulties posed by climate change now and in the future [121].

Several programs and comparative toolkits were developed to assist healthcare facilities (HCFs) introduce resilience and sustainability practices. The WHO's framework for healthcare facilities that are both climate-resilient and ecologically sustainable is helping these facilities develop steadily over time. Key strategies and actions for bolstering resilience and enhancing environmental sustainability are outlined in this advice for health professionals and HCFs management [130]. This advice aims to equip environmentally sustainable healthcare professionals and strengthen the ability of HCFs to safeguard and promote the health of specific populations in the face of a warming planet [121]. To do this, we need to create a comprehensive list of actions that would boost the climate resilience and environmental sustainability of HCFs in the medium and long term, with consideration given to each HCF's individual requirements and priorities. The personnel at HCF might utilize this guideline to their advantage by incorporating data from this framework and the interventions into their routine health facility planning activities [130].

Therefore, it is important to strengthen HCFs' role to ensure that they are ready to react to the challenges induced by climate change, such as extreme weather events that may lead to natural disasters, disease epidemics, and long-term stresses. This is part of a preventive approach to public health that provides basic health services to cope with climate-sensitive health hazards.

As outlined by WHO [130, 121], HCFs must be resilient in four key areas to continue delivering safe and high-quality health care in the face of climate change.

A healthy workforce consists of sufficient numbers of trained workers with fair pay and benefits who are equipped with knowledge of environmental hazards and encouraged to take action to mitigate them.

Sustainable and secure management of water, sanitation, hygiene, and healthcare waste; Reliable and environmentally friendly power generation, distribution, and use.

The facility's infrastructure, technology, products, and all of the processes and procedures that make it run smoothly are essential to providing quality medical treatment.

The World Health Organization's strategy for developing healthcare facilities that are both climate-resilient and ecologically sustainable is also a guideline for creating a sustainable healthcare system. To ensure the health and well-being of current and future generations, this section of the guideline adopts a national environmental sustainability policy for health systems. It directs HCF to improve, maintain, or restore health while minimizing negative environmental impacts and maximizing opportunities to restore and improve it. Disease prevention, health promotion, and public health services; health workforce engagement as a driver of sustainability; increasing community resilience and promoting local assets; creating incentives for change; and fostering innovative practices are all part of this [131].

Cost savings and reductions in greenhouse gas emissions can result from implementing energy efficiency measures, using alternative energy sources, reducing water use and waste, and improving waste management and environmental sustainability at healthcare facilities that adopt the green hospital concept around the world [132, 133]. Several pieces of evidence [131] attest to the seriousness of the direct and indirect effects on the environment. Three main benefits of environmental sustainability are highlighted: (1) it can help reduce costs and increase health systems' resilience; (2) it can benefit patients, providers, the health workforce, and health systems' core functions; and (3) it may help reduce environmental health risks.

14 Conclusion

Addressing the complex relationship between climate change and mental health requires targeted research, standardized methods, and a robust public health response. Future research should address identified gaps, with a focus on vulnerable populations and community-level impacts. Public health systems must integrate climate change considerations into their planning and operations, enhancing resilience and sustainability to safeguard health in a warming world. Implementing effective adaptation strategies and green practices will be crucial for mitigating the health impacts of climate change and ensuring the continued effectiveness of health systems.

References

1. Smith KR et al (2014) Human health: impacts, adaptation, and co-benefits. In: Field CB, Barros VR, Dokken DJ, Mach KJ, Mastrandrea MD, Bilir TE et al (eds) Climate change 2014: impacts, adaptation, and vulnerability. Part A: global and sectoral aspects. Contribution of working group II to the fifth assessment report of the intergovernmental panel on climate change. Cambridge University Press, Cambridge, United Kingdom and New York, NY, USA, pp 709–754
2. WHO (World Health Organization) (2021) Health and climate change global survey report. Geneva: World Health Organization Licence: CC BY-NC-SA 3.0 IGO
3. Kalkstein LS, Greene JS (1997) An evaluation of climate/mortality relationships in large U.S. cities and the possible impacts of a climate change. Environ Health Perspect 105:84–93
4. WHO (World health organization) (2021) Newsroom, fact sheets, climate change and health. https://www.who.int/news-room/fact-sheets/detail/climate-change-and-health

5. Díaz J, Linares C, García-Herrera R, López C, Trigo R (2004) Impact of temperature and air pollution on the mortality of children in Madrid. J Occup Environ Med 46:768–774
6. WHO (World Health Organization) (2021) Quality criteria for the evaluation of climate-informed early warning systems for infectious diseases. https://www.who.int/publications/i/item/9789240036147. Accessed 24 May 2023
7. Xu Z, Etzel RA, Su H, Huang C, Guo Y, Tong S (2012) Impact of ambient temperature on children's health: a systematic review. Environ Res 117:120–131. https://doi.org/10.1016/j.envres.2012.07.002
8. Sorensen C, Saunik S, Sehgal M, Tewary A, Govindan M, Lemery J, Balbus J (2018b) Climate change and women's health: impacts and opportunities in India. Geohealth 2(10):283–297. https://doi.org/10.1029/2018GH000163
9. Clayton S (2021) Climate change and mental health. Curr Environ Health Reports 8:1–6. https://doi.org/10.1007/s40572-020-00303-3
10. Lotfy WM (2014) Climate change and epidemiology of human parasitosis in Egypt: a review. J Adv Res 5(6):607–613
11. Rodríguez-González A, Zanin M, Menasalvas-Ruiz E (2019) Public health and epidemiology informatics: can artificial intelligence help future global challenges? An overview of antimicrobial resistance and impact of climate change in disease epidemiology. Yearb Med Inform 28(1):224–231. https://doi.org/10.1055/s-0039-1677910
12. Frumkin H, Hess J, Luber G, Malilay J, McGeehin M (2008) Climate change: the public health response. Am J Public Health 98(3):435–445. https://doi.org/10.2105/AJPH.2007.119362
13. Fox M, Zuidema C, Bauman B, Burke T, Sheehan M (2019) Integrating public health into climate change policy and planning: State of practice update. Int J Environ Res Public Health 16:3232. https://doi.org/10.3390/ijerph16183232
14. Ragettli MS, Saucy A, Flückiger B, Vienneau D, de Hoogh K, Vicedo-Cabrera AM, Schindler C, Röösli M (2023) Explorative assessment of the temperature–mortality association to support health-based heat-warning thresholds: a national case-crossover study in Switzerland. Int J Environ Res Public Healt 20:4958. https://doi.org/10.3390/ijerph20064958
15. Mostafa AN, Wheida A, El Nazer M, Adel M, El Leithy L, Siour G, Coman A, Borbon A, Abdel Wahab M, Omar M, Saad-Hussein A, Alfaro SC (2019) Past (1950–2017) and future (−2100) temperature and precipitation trends in Egypt. Weather Clim Extremes 26:100225. https://doi.org/10.1016/j.wace.2019.100225
16. Hoegh-Guldberg O, Jacob D, Taylor M, Bindi M, Brown S, Camilloni I et al (2018) Impacts of 1.5 °C global warming on natural and human systems. In Masson-Delmotte V, Zhai P, Portner H-O, Roberts D, Skea J, Shukla PR et al (eds) Global warming of 1.5 °C. An IPCC special report on the impacts of global warming of 1.5 °C above pre-industrial levels and related global greenhouse gas emission pathways, in the context of strengthening the global response to the threat of climate change, sustainable development, and efforts to eradicate poverty. Cambridge University Press, pp 175–312. https://doi.org/10.1017/9781009157940.005
17. Murage P, Hajat S, Kovats RS (2017) Effect of night-time temperatures on cause and age-specific mortality in London. Environ Epidemiol 1:e005
18. Ragettli MS, Vicedo-Cabrera AM, Schindler C, Röösli M (2017) Exploring the association between heat and mortality in Switzerland between 1995 and 2013. Environ Res 158C:703–709
19. Royé D, Sera F, Tobías A, Lowe R, Gasparrini A, Pascal M et al (2021) Effects of hot nights on mortality in Southern Europe. Epidemiology 32:487–498
20. Xu Z, Cheng J, Hu W, Tong S (2018) Heatwave and health events: a systematic evaluation of different temperature indicators, heatwave intensities and durations. Sci Total Environ 630:679–689
21. Lowen AC, Mubareka S, Steel J, Palese P (2007) Influenza virus transmission is dependent on relative humidity and temperature. PLoS Pathog 3(10):e151. https://doi.org/10.1371/journal.ppat.0030151
22. Wu X, Lu Y, Zhou S, Chen L, Xu B (2016) Impact of climate change on human infectious diseases: empirical evidence and human adaptation. Environ Int 86:14–23. https://doi.org/10.1016/j.envint.2015.09.007

23. Oloyede I, Ijezie E (2020) Epidemiological and seasonal variations of pneumonia in children admitted in the University of Uyo Teaching Hospital, Uyo, Akwa Ibom State, Nigeria: a retrospective 5-year study (2013–2017). Nigerian J Paediatrics 47:42–47
24. El-Kowrany SI, El-Zamarany EA, El-Nouby KA, El-Mehy DA, Abo Ali EA, Othman AA, Salah W, El-Ebiary AA (2016) Water pollution in the Middle Nile Delta, Egypt: an environmental study. J Adv Res 7:781–794. https://doi.org/10.1016/j.jare.2015.11.005
25. Alderman K, Turner LR, Tong S (2012) Floods and human health: a systematic review. Environ Int 47:37–47
26. Liu Z, Zhang F, Zhang Y, Li J, Liu X, Ding G, Zhang C, Liu Q-Y, Jiang B (2018) Association between foods and infectious diarrhea and their effect modifiers in Hunan province, China: a two-stage model. Sci Total Environ 626:630–637. https://doi.org/10.1016/j.scitotenv.2018.01.130
27. Saad-Hussein A, Helmy AM, El Leithy L, Wheida A, El Nazer M, Alfaro SC et al (2023) Temporal trend of diarrhea morbidity rate with climate change: Egypt as a case study. Environ Sci Pollut Res 30:5059–5075. https://doi.org/10.1007/s11356-022-22431-z
28. Thompson CN, Zelner JL, Nhu TDH, Phan MVT, Phuc HL, Hung NT et al (2015) The impact of environmental and climatic variation on the spatiotemporal trends of hospitalized pediatric diarrhea in Ho Chi Minh City, Vietnam. Health Place 35:147–154. https://doi.org/10.1016/j.healthplace.2015.08.001
29. Requena-García F, Cabrero-Sañudo F, Olmeda-García S, Gonzalez J, Valcarcel F (2017) Influence of environmental temperature and humidity on questing ticks in central Spain. Exp Appl Acarol 71:277–290
30. Rodrigues J, Catão AML, Dos Santos AS et al (2021) Relative humidity impacts development and activity against Aedes aegypti adults by granular formulations of Metarhizium humberi microsclerotia. Appl Microbiol Biotechnol 105:2725–2736
31. Endo N, Eltahir EA (2018) Modelling and observing the role of wind in Anopheles population dynamics around a reservoir. Malar J 17:1–9
32. Fouque F, Reeder JC (2019) Impact of past and on-going changes on climate and weather on vector-borne diseases transmission: a look at the evidence. Infect Dis Poverty 8:51
33. Adekiya TA, Aruleba RT, Oyinloye BE, Okosun KO, Kappo AP (2020) The effect of climate change and the snail-schistosome cycle in transmission and biocontrol of schistosomiasis in Sub-Saharan Africa. Int J Environ Res Public Health 17(1):181. https://doi.org/10.3390/ijerph17010181
34. Caminade C, McIntyre KM, Jones AE (2019) Impact of recent and future climate change on vector-borne diseases. Ann New York Acad Sci Special Issue: Clim Sci:157–173. https://doi.org/10.1111/nyas.13950
35. Paull SH, Johnson PTJ (2011) High temperature enhances host pathology in a snail–trematode system: possible consequences of climate change for the emergence of disease. Freshw Biol 56:767–778. https://doi.org/10.1111/j.1365-2427.2010.02547.x_2010
36. Adekiya TA, Kappo AP, Okosun KO (2017) Temperature and rainfall impact on schistosomiasis. Glob J Pure Appl Math 13:8453–8469
37. Niu Y, Li R, Qiu J, Xu X, Huang D, Shao Q, Cui Y (2019) Identifying and predicting the geographical distribution patterns of Oncomelania hupensis. Int J Environ Res Public Health 16(12):2206
38. Stensgaard AS, Vounatsou P, Sengupta ME, Utzinger J (2019) Schistosomes, snails and climate change: current trends and future expectations. Acta Trop 190:257–268
39. Zein-Eddine R, Djuikwo-Teukeng FF, DarY DG, Van den Broeck F (2017) Population genetics of the Schistosoma snail host Bulinus truncates in Egypt. Acta Trop 172:36–43
40. WHO (World health organization) (2019) Neglected tropical diseases. Summary. https://www.who.int/neglected_diseases/diseases/en/externalicon
41. Yang GJ, Bergquist R (2018) Potential impact of climate change on schistosomiasis: A global assessment attempt. Trop Med Inf Dis 3:117
42. Oyinloye B, Adenowo F, Gxaba N, Kappo A (2014) The promise of antimicrobial peptides for treatment of human schistosomiasis. Curr Drug Targets 15:852–859

43. McCreesh N, Nikulin G, Booth M (2015) Predicting the effects of climate change on Schistosoma mansoni transmission in eastern Africa. Parasit Vectors 8:4. https://doi.org/10.1186/s13071-014-0617-0
44. Berry A, Fillaux J, Martin-Blondel G, Boissier J, Iriart X, Marchou B et al (2016) Evidence for a permanent presence of schistosomiasis in Corsica, France, 2015. Euro Surv 21(1). https://doi.org/10.2807/1560-7917.ES.2016.21.1.30100
45. Monde C, Syampungani S, van den Brink PJ (2016) Natural and human induced factors influencing the abundance of Schistosoma host snails in Zambia. Environ Monit Assess 188(1):1–14. https://doi.org/10.1007/s10661-016-5351-y
46. Stensgaard AS, Utzinger J, Vounatsou P, Hürlimann E, Schur N, Saarnak CF, Simoonga C (2013) Large-scale determinants of intestinal schistosomiasis and intermediate host snail distribution across Africa: does climate matter? Acta Trop 128:378–390. https://doi.org/10.1016/j.actatropica.2011.11.010
47. Dodangeh S, Daryani A, Sharif M, Gholami S, Kialashaki E, Moosazadeh M, Sarvi S (2019) Freshwater snails as the intermediate host of trematodes in Iran: a systematic review. Epidemiol Health 41:1–13. https://doi.org/10.1186/s13071-014-0617-0
48. Degarege A, Mekonnen Z, Levecke B, Legesse M, Negash Y, Vercruysse J, Erko B (2015) Prevalence of Schistosoma haematobium infection among school-age children in afar area, Northeastern Ethiopia. PLoS ONE 10:e0133142
49. Li EY, Gurarie D, Lo NC, Zhu X, King CH (2019) Improving public health control of schistosomiasis with a modified WHO strategy: a model-based comparison study. Lancet Global Health 7:e1414–e1422. https://doi.org/10.1016/S2214-109X(19)30325-3
50. Pedersen UB, Stendel M, Midzi N, Mduluza T, Soko W, Stensgaard AS et al (2014) Modelling climate change impact on the spatial distribution of fresh water snails hosting trematodes in Zimbabwe. Parasit Vectors 7:536. https://doi.org/10.1186/s13071-014-0536-0
51. Kalinda C, Chimbari MJ, Grant WE, Wang HH, Odhiambo JN, Mukaratirwa S (2018) Simulation of population dynamics of Bulinus globosus: effects of environmental temperature on production of Schistosoma haematobium cercariae. PLoS Negl Trop Dis 12:e0006651. https://doi.org/10.1371/journal.pntd.0006651
52. WHO (World Health Organization) (2014) Quantitative risk assessment of the effects of climate change on selected causes of death, 2030s and 2050s. https://apps.who.int/iris/bitstream/handle/10665/134014/9789241507691_eng.pdf. Accessed 24 May 2023
53. WHO: World Health Organization (2014) A global brief on vector-borne diseases. Tech Rep, World Health Organization
54. Barreca AI (2010) The long-term economic impact of in utero and postnatal exposure to malaria. J Hum Resour 45:865–892. https://doi.org/10.3368/jhr.45.4.865
55. Colón-González FJ, Fezzi C, Lake IR, Hunter PR (2013) The effects of weather and climate change on dengue. PLoS Negl Trop Dis 7:e2503. https://doi.org/10.1371/journal.pntd.0002503
56. Ren Z, Wang D, Ma1A, Hwang J, Bennett A, Sturrock HJW et al (2016) Predicting malaria vector distribution under climate change scenarios in China: challenges for malaria elimination. Sci Rep 6:20604. https://doi.org/10.1038/srep20604
57. Semakula HM, Song G, Achuu SP, Shen M, Chen J, Mukwaya PI et al (2017) Prediction of future malaria hotspots under climate change in sub-Saharan Africa. Clim Change 143(3):415–428. https://doi.org/10.1007/s10584-017-1996-y
58. Song Y, Ge Y, Wang J, Ren Z, Liao Y, Peng J (2016) Spatial distribution estimation of malaria in northern China and its scenarios in 2020, 2030, 2040 and 2050. Malar J 15(1):345. https://doi.org/10.1186/s12936-016-1395-2
59. Tjaden NB, Suk JE, Fischer D, Thomas SM, Beierkuhnlein C (2017) Modelling the effects of global climate change on Chikungunya transmission in the 21st century. Sci Rep 7(1):3813. https://doi.org/10.1038/s41598-017-03566-3
60. Semenza JC, Tran A, Espinosa L, Sudre B, Domanovic D, Paz S (2016) Climate change projections of West Nile virus infections in Europe: implications for blood safety practices. Environ Health 15(S1):S28. https://doi.org/10.1186/s12940-016-0105-4

61. Levi TF, Keesing K, Oggenfuss RS, Ostfeld RS (2015) Accelerated phenology of blacklegged ticks under climate warming. Philos Trans R Soc B: Biol Sci 370(1665):20130556. https://doi.org/10.1098/rstb.2013.0556
62. Ogden NH, Radojevic M, Wu X, Duvvuri VR, Leighton PA, Wu J et al (2014) Estimated effects of projected climate change on the basic reproductive number of the Lyme disease vector Ixodes scapularis. Environ Health Perspect 122(6):631–638. https://doi.org/10.1289/ehp.1307799
63. Ceccarelli S, Rabinovich JE (2015) Global climate change effects on Venezuela's vulnerability to Chagas disease is linked to the geographic distribution of five triatomine species. J Med Entomol 52(6):1333–1343. https://doi.org/10.1093/jme/tjv119
64. Gonzalez C, Paz A, Ferro C (2014) Predicted altitudinal shifts and reduced spatial distribution of Leishmania infantum vector species under climate change scenarios in Colombia. Acta Trop 129:83–90. https://doi.org/10.1016/j.actatropica.2013.08.014
65. Balbus JM, Boxall AB, Fenske RA, McKone TE, Zeise L (2013) Implications of global climate change for the assessment and management of human health risks of chemicals in the natural environment. Environ Toxicol Chem 32:62–78
66. Gouin T, Armitage JM, Cousins IT, Muir DCG, Ng CA, Reid L, Tao S (2013) Influence of global climate change on chemical fate and bioaccumulation: the role of multimedia models. Environ Toxicol Chem 32:20–31
67. Kibria G, Nugegoda D, Rose G, Haroon AKY (2021) Climate change impacts on pollutants mobilization and interactive effects of climate change and pollutants on toxicity and bioaccumulation of pollutants in estuarine and marine biota. Mar Pollut Bull 167:112293. https://doi.org/10.1016/j.marpolbul.2021.112293
68. Tahri M, Benchrif A, Bounakhla M, Benyaich F, Noack Y (2017) Seasonal variation and risk assessment of PM2.5 and PM2.5–10 in the ambient air of Kenitra, Morocco. Environ Sci: Processes Impacts 19:1427–1436
69. Chakraborty P, Zhang G, Li J, Sampathkumar P, Balasubramanian T, Kathiresan K et al (2019) Seasonal variation of atmospheric organochlorine pesticides and polybrominated diphenyl ethers in Parangipettai, Tamil Nadu, India: implication for atmospheric transport. Sci Total Environ 649:1653–1660
70. Saad-Hussein A, El-Mofty HM, Hassanien MA (2011) Climate changes and fungal keratitis trend: in Egypt. East Mediterr Health J (EMHJ) 17(6):468–473
71. Redzwan SM, Abd Mutalib MS, Wang JS, Ahmad Z, Kang MS, Adeul Rahman NA et al (2016) Effect of supplementation of fermented milk drink containing probiotic Lactobacillus casei Shirota on the concentrations of aflatoxin biomarkers among employees of Universiti Putra Malaysia: a randomised, double-blind, cross-over, placebo-controlled study. Br J Nutr 115:39–54
72. Meijer N, Kleter G, de Nijs M, Rau M-L, Derbx R, Fels-Klerx HJ (2021) The aflatoxin situation in Africa: systematic literature review. Comprehen Rev Food Sci Food Saf 20:2286–2304
73. Zinedine A, Ben Salah-Abbes J, Abbès S, Tantaoui-Elaraki A (2021) Aflatoxin M1 in Africa: exposure assessment, regulations, and prevention strategies–a review. Rev Environ Contam Toxicol 258:73–108
74. Saad-Hussein A, Taha M, Fadl N, Awad A-H, Mahdy-Abdallah H, Moubarz G et al (2016) Effects of airborne Aspergillus on serum aflatoxin B1 and liver enzymes in workers handling wheat flour. Hum Exp Toxicol 35:3–9
75. Saad-Hussein A, Elserougy S, Beshir S, Ibrahim MM, Awad A-H, Abdel-Wahhab MA (2012) Work-related airborne fungi and the biological levels of mycotoxin in textile workers. J Appl Sci Res 8:719–726
76. Sayed HA, El Ayyat A, El Dusoki H, Zoheiry M, Mohamed S, Hassan A et al (2005) A cross sectional study of Hepatitis B, C, some trace elements, heavy metals, Aflatoxin B1 and schistosomiasis in a rural population, Egypt. J Egypt Public Health Assoc (JEPHAss) 80(3 and 4):355–388
77. Paerl HW, Huisman J (2009) Climate change: a catalyst for global expansion of harmful cyanobacterial blooms. Environ Microbiol Reports 1:27–37

78. Howard MDA, Nagoda C, Kudela RM, Hayashi K, Tatters A, Caron DA et al (2017). Microcystin prevalence throughout lentic waterbodies in coastal Southern California. Toxins 9:231. https://www.who.int/neglected_diseases/diseases/en/external_icon
79. Barruffa AS, Sposito V, Faggian R (2021) Climate change and cyanobacteria harmful algae blooms: adaptation practices for developing countries. Mar Freshw Res 72(12):1722–1734. https://doi.org/10.1071/MF21081
80. Rastogi RP, Madamwar D, Incharoensakdi A (2015) Bloom dynamics of cyanobacteria and their toxins: environmental health impacts and mitigation strategies. Front Microbiol 6:1–22. https://doi.org/10.3389/fmicb.2015.00001
81. Häder DP, Villafañe VE, Helbling EW (2014) Productivity of aquatic primary producers under global climate change. Photochem Photobiol Sci 13:1370–1392. https://doi.org/10.1039/C3PP50418B
82. Saleh HA, Sayed SSM, El-Gamal MAH, Ismail NMM (2022) Effect of some freshwater cyanobacteria on Oreochromis niloticus (L.) fish and water quality in Egyptian aquaculture ponds. Int J Environ Stud. https://doi.org/10.1080/00207233.2022.2059257
83. Moss B, Kosten S, Meerhoff M, Battarbee RW, Jeppesen E, Mazzeo N et al (2011) Allied attack: climate change and eutrophication. Inland Waters 1:101–105
84. Paerl HW, Gardner WS, Havens KE, Joyner AR, McCarthy MJ, Newell SE, Qin B, Scott JT (2016): Mitigating cyanobacterial harmful algal blooms in aquatic ecosystems impacted by climate change and anthropogenic nutrients. Harmful Algae 54:213–222. https://doi.org/10.1016/j.hal.2015.09.009
85. Deschênes O (2014) Temperature, human health, and adaptation: a review of the empirical literature. Energy Economics 46:606–619. https://doi.org/10.1016/j.eneco.2013.10.013
86. Kovats RS, Hajat S, Wilkinson P (2004) Contrasting patterns of mortality and hospital admissions during hot weather and heat waves in Greater London, UK. Occup Environ Med 61(11):893–898. https://doi.org/10.1136/oem.2003.012047
87. Ziebarth NR, Schmitt M, Karlsson M (2014) The short-term population health effects of weather and pollution, Working paper. http://papers.ssrn.com/sol3/papers.cfm?abstract_id=2377611
88. Ahmed SA, Saad-Hussein A, El Feel A, Hamed MA (2014) Time series trend of Bilharzial bladder cancer in Egypt and its relation to climate change: a study from 1995–2005. Int J Pharm Clin Res 6(1):46–53
89. Owino V, Kumwenda C, Ekesa B, Parker ME, Ewoldt L, Roos N, Lee WT, Tome D (2022) The impact of climate change on food systems, diet quality, nutrition, and health outcomes: a narrative review. Fron Clim 4:941842. https://doi.org/10.3389/fclim.2022.941842
90. Lieber M, Chin-Hong P, Kelly K, Dandu M, Weiser SD (2022) A systematic review and meta-analysis assessing the impact of droughts, flooding, and climate variability on malnutrition. Glob Public Health 17(1):68–82. https://doi.org/10.1080/17441692.2020.1860247
91. Fanzo JC, Downs SM (2021) Climate change and nutrition-associated diseases. Nat Rev Dis Primers 7:90. https://doi.org/10.1038/s41572-021-00329-3
92. Al-Jawaldeh A, Nabhani M, Taktouk M, Nasreddine L (2022) Climate change and nutrition: implications for the Eastern Mediterranean region. Int J Environ Res Public Health 19(24):17086. https://doi.org/10.3390/ijerph192417086
93. Koch CA, Sharda P, Patel J, Gubbi S, Bansal R, Bartel MJ (2021) Climate change and obesity. Horm Metab Res 53(9):575–587. https://doi.org/10.1055/a-1533-2861
94. Magkos F, Tetens I, Bügel SG, Felby C, Schacht SR, Hill JO, Ravussin E, Astrup A (2020) The environmental footprint of obesity. Obesity 28(1):73–79. https://doi.org/10.1002/oby.22657
95. Mahapatra B, Walia M, Rao CAR, Raju BMK, Saggurti N (2021) Vulnerability of agriculture to climate change increases the risk of child malnutrition: evidence from a large-scale observational study in India. PLoS ONE 16(6):e0253637. https://doi.org/10.1371/journal.pone.0253637
96. Phalkey RK, Aranda-Jan C, Marx S, Höfle B, Sauerborn R (2015) Systematic review of current efforts to quantify the impacts of climate change on undernutrition. Proc Natl Acad Sci USA 112(33):E4522–E4529. https://doi.org/10.1073/pnas.1409769112

97. Semba RD, Askari S, Gibson S, Bloem MW, Kraemer K (2022) The potential impact of climate change on the micronutrient-rich food supply. Adv Nutr 13(1):80–100. https://doi.org/10.1093/advances/nmab104
98. Weyant C, Brandeau ML, Burke M, Lobell DB, Bendavid E, Basu S (2018) Anticipated burden and mitigation of carbon-dioxide-induced nutritional deficiencies and related diseases: a simulation modeling study PLoS Med 15(7):e1002586. https://doi.org/10.1371/journal.pmed.1002586
99. Beach RH, Sulser TB, Crimmins A, Cenacchi N, Cole J, Fukagawa NK et al (2019) Combining the effects of increased atmospheric carbon dioxide on protein, iron, and zinc availability and projected climate change on global diets: a modelling study. Lancet Planet Health 3(7):e307–e317. https://doi.org/10.1016/S2542-5196(19)30094-4
100. Swinburn BA, Kraak VI, Allender S, Atkins VJ, Baker PI, Bogard JR, et al (2019) The global syndemic of obesity, undernutrition, and climate change: the Lancet commission report. The Lancet 393(10173):791–846. https://doi.org/10.1016/S0140-6736(18)32822-8
101. Dietz WH, Pryor S (2022) How can we act to mitigate the global syndemic of obesity, undernutrition, and climate change? Curr Obes Rep 11(3):61–69. https://doi.org/10.1007/s13679-022-00480-4
102. Burlingame B, Dernini S (2012) Sustainable diets and biodiversity: Directions and solutions for policy, research and action: proceedings of the international scientific symposium biodiversity and sustainable diets united against hunger 3–5 November 2010, FAO headquarters, FAO, Rome
103. EAT-Lancet Commission (2019) Food planet health, healthy diets from sustainable food systems. Summary report of the EAT-Lancet Commission. Retrieved from https://eatforum.org/content/uploads/2019/07/EAT-Lancet_Commission_Summary_Report.pdf. Accessed 24 May 2023
104. Romanello M, Di Napoli C, Drummond P, Green C, Kennard H, Lampard P et al (2022) The 2022 report of the Lancet Countdown on health and climate change: health at the mercy of fossil fuels. The Lancet 400(10363):1619–1654. https://doi.org/10.1016/S0140-6736(22)01540-9
105. Duncan K (2006) Global climate change, air pollution, and women's health. WIT Trans Ecol Environ 99:633–643. https://doi.org/10.2495/RAV060611
106. Bryson JM, Patterson K, Berrang-Ford L, Lwasa S, Namanya DB, Twesigomwe S et al (2021) Seasonality, climate change, and food security during pregnancy among indigenous and non-indigenous women in rural Uganda: Implications for maternal-infant health. PLOS ONE 16(3). https://doi.org/10.1371/journal.pone.0247198
107. Currie J, Rossin-Slater M (2013) Weathering the storm: hurricanes and birth outcomes. J Health Econ 32:487–503. https://doi.org/10.1016/j.jhealeco.2013.01.004
108. Wilde J, Apouey B, Jung T (2014) Heat waves at conception and later life outcomes. Working paper. http://economics.usf.edu/PDF/Wilde_Apouey_Jung_HeatWavesConception.pdf
109. Carleton TA, Hsiang SM (2016) Social and economic impacts of climate. Science 353(6304):aad9837-1–aad9837-15
110. Sorensen C, Murray V, Lemery J, Balbus J (2018a) Climate change and women's health: Impacts and policy directions. PLoS Med 15(7). https://doi.org/10.1371/journal.pmed.1002603
111. Giudice LC, Llamas-Clark EF, DeNicola N, Pandipati S, Zlatnik MG, Decena DCD et al (2021) Climate change, women's health, and the role of obstetricians and gynecologists in leadership. Int J Gynecol Obstet 155(3):345–356. https://doi.org/10.1002/ijgo.13958
112. WHO (World Health Organization) (2022a) Early warning alert and response in emergencies: an operational guide. https://apps.who.int/iris/handle/10665/365730. Accessed 24 May 2023
113. Rees E, Ng V, Gachon P, Mawudeku A, McKenney D, Pedlar J et al (2019) Risk assessment strategies for early detection and prediction of infectious disease outbreaks associated with climate change. Can Commun Dis Rep 45(5):119–126. https://doi.org/10.14745/ccdr.v45i05a02

114. Traore BB, Kamsu-Foguem B, Tangara F (2017) Data mining techniques on satellite images for discovery of risk areas. Expert Syst Appl 72:443–456. https://doi.org/10.1016/j.eswa.2016.10.010
115. Moulton AD, Schramm PJ (2017) Climate change and public health surveillance: toward a comprehensive strategy. J Public Health Manag Pract 23(6):618–626. https://doi.org/10.1097/PHH.0000000000000550
116. Farooq Z, Rocklöv J, Wallin J, Abiri N, Sewe MO, Sjödin H, Semenza JC (2022) Artificial intelligence to predict West Nile virus outbreaks with eco-climatic drivers. Lancet Region Health—Europe 17:100370. https://doi.org/10.1016/j.10.1016/j
117. Xu L, Stige LC, Chan KS, Zhou J, Yang J, Sang S et al (2017) Climate variation drives dengue dynamics. Proc Natl Acad Sci USA 114(1):113–118. https://doi.org/10.1073/pnas.1618558114
118. Santangelo OE, Gentile V, Pizzo S, Giordano D, Cedrone F (2023) Machine learning and prediction of infectious diseases: a systematic review. Mach Learn Knowl Extr 5(1):175–198. https://doi.org/10.3390/make5010013
119. Mammarella MC, Grandoni G (2019) Resilience actions to counteract the effects of climate change and health emergencies in cities: the role of artificial neural networks. Annali dell'Istituto Superiore di Sanità 55(4):392–397. https://doi.org/10.4415/ANN_19_04_14
120. Hayes K, Blashki G, Wiseman J, Burke S, Reifels L (2018) Climate change and mental health: Risks, impacts and priority actions. Int J Ment Heal Syst 12:28. https://doi.org/10.1186/s13033-018-0210-6
121. WHO (World Health Organization) (2022) Measuring the climate resilience of health systems. Licence: CC BY-NC-SA 3.0 IGO. https://apps.who.int/iris/bitstream/handle/10665/354542/9789240048102-eng.pdf?sequence=1&isAllowed=y
122. Hwong AR, Wang M, Khan H, Chagwedera DN, Grzenda A, Doty B et al (2022) Climate change and mental health research methods, gaps, and priorities: a scoping review. Lancet Planet Health 6(3):e281–e291. https://doi.org/10.1016/S2542-5196(22)00012-2
123. ARC-X Climate Change Adaptation Resource Center (2023) Public health adaptation strategies for climate change. Retrieved from https://www.epa.gov/arc-x/public-health-adaptation-strategies-climate-change
124. Centers for Disease Control and Prevention (CDC) (2023) CDC policy on climate change and public health. Retrieved from https://www.cdc.gov/climateandhealth/pubs/Climate_Change_Policy.pdf
125. Opoku SK, Filho WL, Hubert F, Adejumo O (2021) Climate change and health preparedness in Africa: analysing trends in six African countries. Int J Environ Res Public Health 18:4672. https://doi.org/10.3390/ijerph18094672
126. Balbus J, Berry P, Brettle M, Jagnarine S, Soares A, Ugarte C et al (2016) Enhancing the sustainability and climate resiliency of health care facilities: a comparison of initiatives and toolkits. Rev Panam Salud Publica 40(3):174–180
127. WHO (World Health Organization) (2015) Operational framework for building climate resilient health systems. https://apps.who.int/iris/bitstream/handle/10665/189951/9789241565073_eng.pdf
128. Watts N, Adger WN, Agnolucci P, Blackstock J, Byass P, Cai W et al (2015) Health and climate change: policy responses to protect public health. Lancet 7:386(10006):1861–1914. https://doi.org/10.1016/S0140-6736(15)60854-6
129. Intergovernmental Panel on Climate Change (IPCC) (2018) Global warming of 1.5 °C glossary. Geneva. Retrieved from https://www.ipcc.ch/sr15/chapter/glossary/
130. WHO (World Health Organization) (2020) Guidance for developing climate resilient and environmentally sustainable health facilities. Geneva. https://apps.who.int/iris/handle/10665/335909
131. WHO (World Health Organization) (2017) Environmentally sustainable health systems: a strategic document. https://www.euro.who.int/__data/assets/pdf_file/0004/341239/ESHS_Revised_WHO_web.pdf

132. Dhillon VS, Kaur D (2015) Green hospital and climate change: their interrelationship and the way forward. J Clin Diag Res 9:LE01–LE05
133. El Mitainy E, El-Haggar SM (2019) Developing sustainability rating system for health-care facilities: focus on Egypt. J Environ Prot 10:958–971. https://doi.org/10.4236/jep.2019.107057

Impact of Climate Change on Aquatic Biodiversity and Migration

Climatic Variation and the Aquatic Biodiversity in Egypt

Marwa M. El-Naggar, Mohamed R. Fishar, and Magdy T. Khalil

Abstract Biodiversity and ecosystems throughout the globe are increasingly threatened by climate change. The ecosystems' function and structure as well as their role in society are altered as a result of the change in species' interactions with one another and with their environments due to climatic variations. In addition, climate change has the potential to wipe out endemic species that can adapt to alterations to a limited extent. Thus, Egypt joined the Convention on Biological Diversity in 1992 and ratified it in 1994. The parties were obliged to develop national plans for biodiversity protection in reference to article 6 of the convention. Obviously, the climate change has already affected biodiversity. Species and ecosystems may relocate or disappear according to the predicted future changes in the environment. Organisms have different atmospheric tolerances and dispersal abilities; therefore, some may modify their phonology (for example, their mating date), while others may adapt to new food supplies and localities. As a result, it is difficult to foresee the way communities could shift or how present relationships among species might be altered.

Keywords Climate change · Biodiversity · Mitigation · Freshwater ecosystem · Marine ecosystem

1 Introduction

The word "climate" is used to refer to the typical weather patterns of a region over extended periods of time [24]. Whereas climate change refers to a shift in average temperatures and precipitation patterns that lasts for an extended period of time and is caused either by natural disturbances like solar activity and orbital variations or by human activities viz. the industrial revolution, which led to global warming and

M. M. El-Naggar (✉) · M. T. Khalil
Department of Zoology, Faculty of Science, Ain Shams University, Abassia, Cairo, Egypt
e-mail: marwaelnaggar@sci.asu.edu.eg

M. R. Fishar
National Institute of Oceanography and Fisheries, NIOF, Cairo, Egypt

© The Author(s), under exclusive license to Springer Nature Switzerland AG 2025
M. T. Khalil et al. (eds.), *Climate Changes Impacts on Aquatic Environment*, Earth and Environmental Sciences Library, https://doi.org/10.1007/978-3-031-74897-4_3

ozone depletion. These days, global citizens in addition to the national and regional governments are highly concerned with climatic fluctuations. Warming of the climate system due to human activity is now confirmed beyond reasonable doubt according to scientists throughout the world. Humanity's plight has noticeably worsened because of the global climate disorder, particularly in the world's least developed regions.

Ocean acidification, ecological stratification, and the increase in marine dead zones are just a few ways in which marine species may be impacted by climate change. By reducing a system's susceptibility or enhancing its resilience, adaptation efforts may help alleviate the influences of climatic variation or even reap some of its benefits. Reducing ecosystems' overall sensitivity to climate change might require organizing the current activities and embracing updated initiatives and targets.

Egypt joined the Convention on Biological Diversity in 1992 and ratified it in 1994. Article 6 of this treaty requires signatories to develop national policies for biodiversity protection.

Public attention and substantial resources are now focused on environmental management goals, but climate change is expected to greatly hinder their realization. The State of the Global Climate 2023 report from the World Meteorological Organization [25] shows that records were once again broken, and in some cases smashed, for greenhouse gas levels, surface temperatures, ocean heat and acidification, sea level rise, Antarctic sea ice cover and glacier retreat. Weather hazards continued to trigger displacement in 2023, showing how climate shocks undermine resilience and create new protection risks among the most vulnerable populations.

Heat waves, floods, droughts, wildfires, and rapidly intensifying tropical cyclones caused misery and mayhem, upending everyday life for millions and inflicting many billions of dollars in economic losses. The WMO [25] report confirmed that 2023 was the warmest year on record, with the global average near-surface temperature at 1.45 °C (with a margin of uncertainty of $\pm$ 0.12 °C) above the pre-industrial baseline. It was the warmest ten-year period on record.

Although the present climate change in this decade is very mild compared to what is predicted for the future, its harmful effect on ecosystems has already been recorded. Changes in rainfall and drought patterns, as well as the frequency and severity of harsh weather events, are likely to have far-reaching effects on biodiversity. It is possible that certain species might profit from these changes (such as proliferating pests and illnesses); however, the rapid occurrence of these alterations implies that most species would not find it helpful since they will not be able to accommodate.

In this chapter, the impact of climatic changes on marine and freshwater biodiversity will be addressed in detail.

2 What Are the Future Expected Changes?

By the year 2100, global temperatures are expected to rise with an average of 1.4 to 5.8 °C, according to computer simulations. The effects of such a temperature rise are expected to include:

- Additional global mean sea level increase of 9–88 cm;
- Increased likelihood of flooding due to increased precipitation in temperate zones and southeast Asia;
- The likelihood of droughts and the occurrence of more intense, drastic climatic events such as heat waves, storms and hurricanes that increase with decreased precipitation across Africa, the Mediterranean area, certain regions of New Zealand and Australia as well as Central Asia.
- The spread of malaria and other "vector-borne illnesses," and the continuing melting of Arctic and Antarctic ice seas till their total disappearance as a result of global warming [22].

The impact of climate variation on biodiversity is obvious. Species and ecosystems may relocate or disappear altogether as a result of the predicted future changes in the environment. Varying species have different temperature tolerances and dispersal potentials; therefore, some may modify their phonology (for example, their mating date), while others may adapt to new food supplies. Thus, it is hard to expect the way species could change or how present relationships among them might be shifted.

The speed and scope of ecosystem or species' reactions to climatic alterations have been the subject of several studies. Species on land are thought to follow rising or falling temperatures by making their way to more northerly or southern latitudes, respectively. Furthermore, ocean acidification makes weak marine creatures like coral reefs more vulnerable when sea temperatures rise, and ocean circulation patterns shift.

3 Climatic Changes and Their Effect on Universal Marine Ecosystems

The seas constitute one of the world's greatest food stores, although this fact is frequently overlooked. The FAO estimates that almost 200 million human individuals throughout the world depend on aquaculture and fisheries for the sake of their livelihood. As seas warm and storms become more often, they ruin habitat, injure marine life and jeopardize fishing as a viable human occupation.

Unfortunately, there is still a lack of information on how climate change would affect the seas, and the complexity of the marine ecosystem necessitates further study. The ocean's circulation and mixing patterns may be altered by global warming. Microalgae (phytoplankton) regulates the seas' capacity to obtain the sunlight needed for photosynthesis by circulation and mixing, and their role will be affected by climatic disturbances.

Ocean acidification, ecological stratification and the increase in maritime dead zones are three ways in which climate change may impact marine organisms.

3.1 Ocean Acidification

Anthropogenic CO_2's effect on ocean pH would alter the calcification process for certain marine species, making global climate change an important factor in influencing ocean biology. Upon the dissolution of CO_2 in water, carbonic acid is formed, which is a weak acid that alters the chemical composition of seawater.

3.2 Elevation in Ocean Stratification

On average, oceans are warming at a rate of roughly 0.2 °C/decade; this phenomenon is attributed to climate change, and since warmer water is light, it covers the cooler water layer below it. This, in turn, affects the tiny sea creatures that are called phytoplankton. Though these creatures are tiny, they play a great role in keeping Earth habitable. Several oceans have been exhibiting signs of stratification during the last decade. Scientists have discovered that when water temperatures rise, phytoplankton growth decreases everywhere in the globe.

3.3 Increasing Oceanic Dead Zones

Extremely low levels of dissolved oxygen in water have led to the rapid expansion of "dead zones" during the last 50 years. Plankton populations proliferate in response to fertilizers and sewage runoffs. While they die rapidly, the bacteria that live in oxygen-depleted waters eat them. Though forty years ago dead zones were uncommon, they are nowadays found in hundreds.

4 Climate Variations Affecting Aquatic Biodiversity in Egypt

When it comes to global warming, Egypt is among the most susceptible regions. Because of global warming, the low-lying land in the Nile Delta area will particularly be at risk of a rise in sea level [6]. In Egypt, agriculture, coastal zones, water resources, food supplies, freshwater, and marine biodiversity in addition to terrestrial ecosystems are all impacted by global warming in Egypt.

4.1 Marine Ecosystem

4.1.1 Coral Reefs

Sponges, crabs, jellyfish, reef fishes, worms, lobsters, shrimps, bivalves, starfish, gastropods, marine birds, marine turtles, sea urchins, marine animals, sea cucumbers and marine snakes are just some of the aquatic creatures that consider coral reef structures their home. In addition, the tourism, fisheries, and coastline protection provided by coral reefs are projected to worth $375 billion globally every year.

Over the last decade, widespread coral bleaching episodes have grown in both frequency and intensity throughout the world. Although by the year 2023, widespread coral bleaching has been documented in numerous locations of the world's most important coral reef sites, yet several reef systems have not suffered from the harsh bleaching consequences. The worldwide occurrence of coral bleaching may be traced back to 1998. Extreme bleaching has occurred everywhere, and in many places, it has caused substantial death [8, 9].

As sea temperatures rise and storms get more powerful, corals in many tropical places are dying at an alarming rate. Pollution, increasing ocean acidity, and unsustainable fishing in addition to a variety of other persistent problems are caused by development and tourism. One of the primary physicochemical factors of coral calcification is the aragonite saturation state, which is reduced when pH decreases. Extensive evidence now points to a connection between changes in sea surface temperature and coral bleaching, in which corals lose their color because their symbiotic zooxanthellae are expelled. When temperatures rise to at least 0.8–1 °C above the high levels' mean recorded in summer for a minimum of four weeks, bleaching often occurs (Fig. 1) [12].

To measure how much-rising temperatures affected the 2011 bleaching event on the Egyptian reefs in the Red Sea, a more in-depth assessment was initiated in Egypt [9]. To do this, Hurghada Environmental Protection and Conservation Association

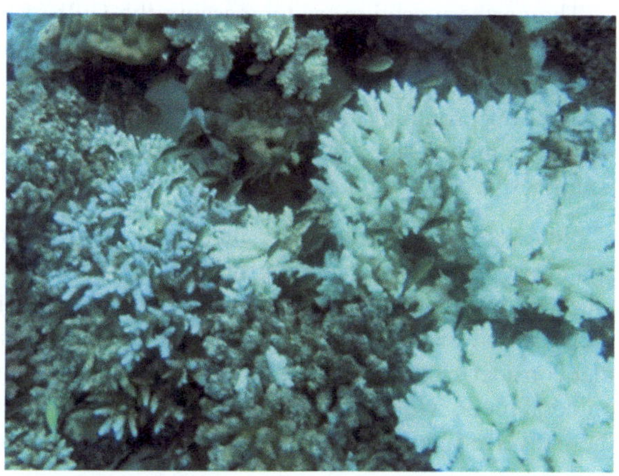

Fig. 1 Bleached coral reefs in Marsa Alam, Red Sea, Egypt

(HEPCA), in collaboration with the International Union for Conservation of Nature (IUCN), introduced Bleach Watch Egypt in 2010 as part of the Climate Change Project. They inspected 136 locations in the Red Sea for the absence or the presence of bleached coral colonies in the Suez and Aqaba Gulfs. In addition, quantitative surveys were conducted at 16 different locations. Along the Red Sea coast, the reefs were surveyed from the northern Gulf of Aqaba in Neweibaa to the southern Egyptian border in Shalatien. Careful consideration was given to selecting sites that would represent a cross-section of the bleaching event's geographic scope, including both protected and exposed reefs as well as offshore and inshore reefs.

Other reef-building corals, such as Pocilliopora, Montipora, Porites, Stylophora, Acropora, and some non-reef-building corals, such as sea anemones, Millipora and some soft corals were negatively impacted by the rise in water temperature, as inferred by the aforementioned authors. The widespread bleaching event was mostly confined to the top six meters of water, and then drastically decreased between six and ten meters in depth. Although coral bleaching was more severe in protected regions, it afflicted both types of locations during the major bleaching event. The widespread bleaching impacted both onshore and offshore locations.

In June 2023, Hanafy and Desoky [8] with HEPCA team surveyed coral reefs ecosystems of Gulfs of Suez and Aqaba, as well as the Egyptian coast of the Red Sea. The survey's overarching objective was to comprehensively assess coral bleaching and estimate recovery rates in bleached coral colonies. Also, for conducting an extensive inventory of coral bleaching in 2023 compared to the two bleaching events in 2012 and 2020. Moreover, to assess the rate of recovery in tagged bleached colonies, considering various species and genera and determining the sensitivity, tolerance, and resilience of coral species to heat stress induced by climate change. The main outcomes of the survey of 2023 were:

- The protracted duration of the 2023 heat wave exerts a more substantial influence on bleaching potential compared to the events of 2012 and 2020. This signals a potential trajectory of increased frequency, duration, and intensity of heat waves in the coming years.
- The northern section, encompassing the Gulf of Suez, the Gulf of Aqaba, and the Northern part of the Egyptian Red Sea, remains devoid of severe bleaching. Conversely, the potential for bleaching intensifies southward from Qusier City and peaks south of the Marsa Alam City area.
- The resilience demonstrated by the most sensitive species/genera, showcases the highest recovery and adaptability to heat stress.

Noteworthy that cnidarians including jellyfish and some coral types, fishes, sponges, crustaceans (including shrimp, spiny lobsters and crabs), worms, mollusks (such as cephalopods), echinoderms (including starfish, sea cucumbers and sea urchins), sea snakes, sea squirts and sea turtles are just some of the marine animals that consider reefs to be their home. Mammals, excluding humans, are uncommon on coral reefs, with whales and dolphins being the most common visitors. Some of these diverse species rely only on corals for sustenance, while others graze on algae and play important roles in intricating reef food webs. All these creatures will be affected by the effects of climate change on coral reef environments.

4.1.2 Marine Turtles

Loggerheads (*Caretta caretta*), green turtles (*Chelonia mydas*), leatherbacks (*Dermochelys coriacea*), hawksbills (*Eretmochelys imbricata*), and olive-ridleys (*Lepidochelys olivacea*) are the five species of marine turtles detected in the Red and the Mediterranean Seas of Egypt.

The Mediterranean is home for three different kinds of turtles: the resident loggerhead (*Caretta caretta*), resident green turtles (*Chelonia mydas*) and occasional visitor gigantic leatherback (*Dermochelys coriacea*). While several species of turtles call Egypt's Mediterranean and Red Seas home for hatching and eating, only green and hawksbill turtles are considered common [13]. Both the hawksbill turtle and the green turtle are now listed as endangered or critically endangered in the International Union for Conservation of Nature (IUCN) Red List. In addition, Convention on International Trade in Endangered Species of Wild Fauna and Flora (CITES) prohibits trading these species in nations that have ratified the convention since they are classified in Appendix I of the convention's Appendices [4].

The degradation of habitat and the unsustainability of coastal development due to erosion and rising sea level as a result of climate change are putting growing strain on nesting locations along the Egyptian Red Sea and Mediterranean coastlines. These are well-known dangers to turtle nesting areas [1], but their long-term effects on nesting populations are unknown. More research is required.

Rising temperatures pose a serious risk to sea turtles, which might lead to a decline in their numbers. The increasing temperatures would only produce one sex of sea turtle, since the sex is determined by the temperature of the sand in which the eggs mature. However, additional study is needed to determine how climate change can alter the gender distribution of sea turtles.

4.1.3 Sharks

In Egypt, we can see a lot of sharks from the coast because the reef walls rise so steeply and vertically from the water. If you wanted to see what you observed at Ras Muhammed, you'd have to spend at least two hours on a boat practically anywhere else in the world.

Most shark species found in the Indian Ocean are also present in the Red Sea since the two bodies of water are essentially one. Of the roughly 400 shark species estimated to exist today, 44 have been seen in the Red Sea [13]. The blue great hammerhead, scalloped hammerhead, sand tiger, angel, great white, nurse, leopard, grey reef, blacktip, oceanic whitetip, blacktip reef, silvertip, tiger, lemon, zebra and whale sharks are among the roughly 18 reef and pelagic shark species spotted in the waters of Ras Muhammed. At Ras Muhammed, you may see blacktip reef sharks not just in the deep water along the coral walls but also in shallow water near the coast and even in the mangrove swamps when the tide is high. Its diet consists mostly of reef and pelagic fish as well as shrimps and squid, as this diet befits a reef species. The bleaching of coral reefs is a major hazard to these sharks.

The oceanic whitetip shark (*Carcharinus longimanus*) may be found in all oceans except the Polar Regions, yet it is more comfortable in water that is warmer than 20 °C. Therefore, the northern part of the Red Sea is home to a very large population of these sharks.

Since variations in the water's temperature, salinity, and other physical characteristics might alter the electric impulses that sharks receive, it is possible that climate change over the past decade has contributed to behavioral shifts in sharks in the Egyptian Red Sea.

4.1.4 Dolphins

Dolphins are warm-blooded marine animals that are mostly found in the warm waters of the shallow spots of the Red Sea. In the IUCN Red List, most dolphin species are determined as endangered or severely endangered [13]. Because of their reliance on echolocation, changes to the physical properties of the water will affect their ability to locate food and evade predators.

4.1.5 Dugong

The sea cow, often known as a dugong, may grow up to 4 m in length. Coastal regions in the Red Sea, East Africa, and most of southern Asia are the habitats of this marine animal. Due to its sensitivity to temperature variations, this species is spotted in Egypt's southern Red Sea coastlines, while moving northward to Ras Muhammed in summer [21]. Due to centuries of hunting for its flesh and leather, the Dugong is on the verge of extinction.

4.1.6 Fisheries

The aquatic ecosystems and fishing resources are already feeling the effects of climate change. There are several published studies that show this to be the case for many different types of marine life, including tunas, cod, sardines, anchovies, krill, phyto- and zooplankton. Salmon, sturgeon and other fish that thrive in warmer waters have expanded their range northward, leading to local extinctions near the species' present range's periphery.

It is hard to forecast the effects of climatic changes on marine fish populations since they will vary greatly depending on the species, region and range. As a result, several species of salmonids will experience higher growth as a result of the warmer winters but will also be at greater risk of contracting infectious illnesses. Rising summer temperatures will have a devastating effect on human life expectancy. The effect on primary output will vary depending on location, but worldwide forecasts from most models indicate a mild rise of less than 10% [2].

However, significant shifts in the composition of the species of algae are to be anticipated, and this may have an impact on the development of higher trophic levels, especially in marine environments. Reduced upwelling of nutrients due to sluggish ocean currents [5] will also have a negative impact on primary production. Fish larvae's distribution and migratory routes may be affected by the dramatic shifts in ocean currents that are predicted.

4.1.7 Red Sea Fishes

Despite their location in nutrient-poor tropical seas, coral reefs are home to an outstanding variety of life. Reef fish or tropical, such as the butterflyfish, angelfish, the vivid parrotfish, and the damselfish consider these environments home. Many thousands of fish species may be found on coral reefs. Unfortunately, the loss of coral reef ecosystems will have a devastating effect on many species.

Over a thousand different kinds of fish are found in the Red Sea region of Egypt [16]. Compared to any other region on Earth, per square meter, the northern Red Sea includes more species of fish from the tiniest to the 6 m long. Throughout the year, the currents carry the nutrient-rich waters drawing them all to Ras Muhammed where these species congregate to benefit. Although the area of Ras Muhammed is impressive all the year round, the summer months draw an especially large number of gilled residents. Reef and pelagic fish are ecologically distinct groups of the Red Sea fish.

A. **Reef Fishes**

Colorful reef fishes are often seen in the icy blue waters of Ras Muhammed. The sheer number of options available renders the spectrum of hues nearly unfathomable. These bright colors serve a dual purpose of protecting the fish from predators and enticing potential mates. Blending in with many different shades of soft and hard corals is essential for survival in dangerous situations.

B. **Pelagic Fishes**

Pelagic fish are open-sea fish which are characterized by their large size. They are drawn to the Suez Gulf's rich nutrients and Ras Muhammed's reefs and walls, where they may feed on multitudes of smaller reef fish that have been drawn for the same reasons (nutrients and shelter). In Ras Muhammed, the reef rises rapidly from the depths, which is a major factor for the high abundance of these organisms. Large schools of pelagic fish often migrate together. They spend most of their time in the cooler, open ocean, but you may find them on the reefs again when it's feeding time. In addition, fishes that live in the open ocean are considered pelagic.

However, southern reefs such as Ras Muhammed have a wider variety of fish species than their northern counterparts. This southern reef was home to a total of

261 species. Because of the lesser concentration of divers and fishermen, exposed reefs supported a greater variety of fish species. There are 16 to 26 species of damselfishes (Pomacentridae) in all locations, forming the most abundant species, while 20 species of wrasses (Labridae) follow the formers in abundance. *Chromis dimidiata* is the most frequent damselfish, while *Labricus quadrilineatus* is the most common wrasse. The Scaridae (parrotfish) family consists of just nine species, with *Scarus ferrugineus* and *Hipposcarus harid* being the most frequent. The most frequent species of the family Acanthuridae (surgeonfishes) includes *Acanthurus negrifuscus*, *A. sohal* and *Naso literatus*. Remarkably, the butterflyfish family Chaetodintidae (*C. auriga*, *C. larvatus* and *C. fasciatus*) is more numerous in the North.

4.2 Freshwater Ecosystems

Freshwater environments have a lower species diversity than other ecosystems. While only making up around 1% of the Earth's surface, freshwater ecosystems are home to about 25% of all identified vertebrates, over 126,000 recognized animal species, and over 2600 described macrophyte plants.

IUCN and Conservation International chose to conduct a comprehensive assessment of the estimated 27,400 freshwater fish species, mollusks, plants, dragonflies and crabs as part of their Global Freshwater Biodiversity Assessment. There are now about 21,000 species that have not been evaluated on a worldwide scale; just 6000 of them are assessed in the 2023 IUCN Red List.

Freshwater ecosystems are already experiencing changes in their physical, chemical and biological features due to climate-induced changes in precipitation, air temperature and other stresses. The future will bring a worsening of many of these patterns. Thus, a focused attention is paid to the effects on habitat (transition and loss) and species (interactions with invasive species, range changes and phenology) in this chapter.

The River Nile and wetlands

The Nile Delta is one of the world's major river deltas and a winter habitat for a huge number of aquatic birds as well as other species of tiny animals and reptiles that are either endangered or have very limited ranges. Once home to vast papyrus (Cyperus papyrus) marshes, the Nile Delta is now mostly devoid of its namesake plant. The corridor is home to five internationally endangered species and many other important ecological hotspots. The Nile Delta has been inhabited by humans for at least 5000 years and actively cultivated for at least that long. Parts of the sand belt that are vulnerable to rising sea levels are crucial for safeguarding low-lying reclaimed agricultural fields, such as lagoons and wetlands. It would have a devastating effect. The lagoons are responsible for a significant proportion of Egypt's total fish harvest. Most freshwater fish would perish if water quality was altered by the rising sea levels.

Along the shore of the Nile Delta, you will find a vast network of freshwater and brackish wetlands. Algal blooms are caused by the combination of rising temperatures and eutrophication in our northern lakes [20]. In addition, confined bodies of water would be more vulnerable to the effects of climate change. Both precipitation and evaporation from the atmospheric water exchange contribute significantly to the water cycle in wetland ecosystems [19]. The salinity of inland lakes, viz. the level of salinity in the waters of Wady El-Rayan and Qarun may change resulting from the higher rate of evaporation.

Wetlands in low-lying coastal areas are particularly threatened by the rise in sea levels caused by climate change. They may be completely submerged if sea levels continue rising. On the other hand, the sea level decline may also have negative effect on these wetlands by drying them out since it reduces the standard level of the systems of the groundwater flow and streams. It is possible that wetlands may move landward or seaward in extremely wide, gently sloping coastal regions if sea level fluctuations were modest enough to allow wetland plant and soil communities to grow [19].

In the lines to follow, some influences of climatic fluctuations on species, populations and biological communities have been reported in grey and scientific literature:

1. Movement in the distribution of species.
2. Phylogenic shifts and developmental changes.
3. Variations in social make-up, competition and chances of survival.
4. Modified interactions with exotic and invasive species.
5. Implications on fisheries.
6. Impact on aquaculture.

5 Changes in Species Distribution and Range

Warming in the future will cause range shifts and expansions for warm-, cool and cold-water creatures although these changes will vary by area. Species at the southernmost edge of their range will move northward, becoming locally extinct at the southern edge of their range as they increase their northern range. A species' range and the potential pace of its response to changing circumstances are also heavily influenced by physical limits, including land-locked locations, drainage patterns and waterfalls.

– **Appearance of harmful algal blooms**

The thermal expansion of water, photosynthesis and the proliferation of plankton are all direct results of global warming. This is a fundamental mechanism for aquatic ecosystems, and the two rates often double for every 10 °C rise in temperature [3]. Based on their research on the impacts of climate changes on the aquatic environment, the danger of raphidophyte and dinoflagellate blooms would grow instead of decreasing.

– **Changes in community competition, survival and composition**

In addition to altering the survival and essential habitat needs of sensitive species, alterations in the basic characteristics of aquatic environments might affect the outcome of the competition among creatures with varying temperature endurance. Hard constraints on species occurrence are likely to be imposed by temperatures that routinely surpass physiological thresholds or lethal limits though soft constraints may be alleviated by the history of life and behavioral variation (including phenotypic plasticity) such as the increasing exploitation of thermal refugee. The rising temperatures in lakes and streams will have a negative impact on food supply and reproductive success of many fish and amphibian species (e.g. survival and prolific fitness).

– **Freshwater fisheries and aquaculture affected by climate variations**

Fluctuation in run-off and precipitation, occurring as a result of changes in atmospheric conditions, have major implications on the ecology of freshwater fisheries. Reduced lake levels and catches, for example, will have a significant effect on lake fisheries in southern Africa.

Due to the lack of seasonal turnover, the bottom layers of lakes and reservoirs may become more deoxygenated (i.e. hypoxic) as temperatures rise. Higher latitudes will witness a rise in river discharge; whereas, southern Latin America, southern Europe and West Africa will experience decreases. In general, a rise of 1 °C in global temperature is linked to an increase of 4% in river run-off. We may also anticipate changes in the frequency, severity and duration of flooding.

Climate change is predicted to negatively affect cold-water species, positively impact warm-water species, and neutrally influence cool-water species in the northern part of their range, while in the southern part, a negative effect is expected. In addition, a general movement of cold and warm water species is expected northward in rivers throughout the northern hemisphere. Lower water levels during the dry season may diminish the individuals that have the potential to spawn in a successful way, making riverine fisheries vulnerable to climate change. Fish use the time of flood episodes as a vital physiological trigger, migrating and spawning just before the flood begins so that their eggs and larvae may be carried to nursery locations on flood plains. Climate change, increased rainfall, and changes in animal and plant behavior are all factors that might reduce fishing output.

It is yet unclear what effects climate change will have on fisheries and aquaculture in the future. Understanding and promoting the vast variety of innovative acclimation assessments and activating their interactions with the current policy and legal administrative plans is the key to minimize negative repercussions and maximize possibilities. But, Mehrim and Refaey [15] concluded in their recent detailed study that climate change has already affected aquaculture and the impacts are likely to increase in all aspects of this vital sector. In order to reduce the possible dangers of climate change on fish productivity, it is very important to develop of new fish strains with increased salinity tolerance or increased temperature tolerance to cope with alterations caused by climate change.

Biodiversity safeguarded by protected areas

To prepare for potential climate change and rising temperatures, Leach et al. [14] investigated the function of the Egyptian protected areas in conserving biodiversity. To assess the expected consequences on the distribution of butterflies and animals in Egypt Maximum Entropy (MaxEnt), the researchers used one conservation science approach, and to gauge the efficacy of the Protected Area network of Egypt, they employed the other (Zonation). They hypothesized that the diversity of species and the conservation priority of different Egyptian sites will be profoundly impacted by the future climate. They reasoned that although biodiversity would rise in some places, it would fall sharply in others.

6 Socioeconomic Impact of Climate Change

- Many people in the Red Sea depend on tourism and other forms of recreation-related revenue, which would suffer if coral bleaching continues. Reef fishes, sponges, jellyfish, worms, shrimp, lobster, crab, bivalves, sea urchins, gastropods, marine turtles, starfish, sea cucumbers in addition to marine animals, birds and snakes are all inhabitants of coral reef structures. Many of these species are crucial to the economies of fishing and ecotourism. An annual global economic worth of $375 billion is attributed to coral reefs through tourism, fishing and coastal protection.
- Increases in both nutrient contents and water temperature are hypothesized to contribute to a rise in the frequency with which cyanobacterial blooms occur. There will be repercussions for Egypt's fisheries as a result of this.
- The coastal lakes, which are important to the national economy, might be negatively impacted by rising sea levels, increasing streamflow, higher temperatures, less summer winds and deeper waterbodies. The marshes of Egypt's Delta are a prime example of this.

7 Vulnerability

– **The River Nile**

There have been several reports on the vulnerability of the River Nile waters to global warming. It has been shown that certain Nile basins are very sensitive to even small shifts in precipitation. Water flow at Khartoum increases by 36% for every 10% rise in rainfall and decreases by 31% for every 10% drop in rainfall, making it abundantly evident that the Eastern Nile (The Blue Nile and Atbara) is particularly affected by rainfall fluctuations, both positively and negatively. Changes in evaporation and evapotranspiration as a result of temperature shifts have an impact on the Nile's water flow sensitivity and, subsequently, the diversity of species [17].

– **Egyptian inland lakes and coastal zones**

Their human settlements, tourism, agricultural resources and water supplies are all regarded as potentially susceptible to the effects of climate change and not only because of the direct impact of sea level rise. It is important to keep in mind that the low-lying Nile Delta area is very susceptible to the implications of climatic disturbances since it is the major agricultural territory of Egypt. This area hosts approximately half of all crops and more than one-third of the national residents [26].

– **Saltwater intrusion**

The potential effects of saltwater intrusion on groundwater quality and coastal wetlands cannot be ignored, particularly in low-lying locations along Egypt's Mediterranean coast. This, in turn, will cause freshwater biota to vanish and wetland diversity to decline. Thus, extensive research should be conducted on this issue to determine its significance.

– **Environmental extreme events**

Egypt's coastal regions, the whole nation, and even the Mediterranean Sea may feel the effects of the rise in severity and frequency of environmental catastrophic events. It's common knowledge that Saharan dust and heat waves have devastating effects on agricultural output, material longevity and public health. However, the dangers of transportation accidents and health issues will inevitably rise as the severity and frequency of maritime storms rise. Climate change will have far-reaching effects on marine life, including altering the typical pattern of winds and coastal currents. The costal locations in Egypt have witnessed some implications due to climatic alterations among which the following phenomena were recognized: decreases in rainfall along the Red Sea coast, shifts in the well-known Nawwat pattern of severe occurrences in Alexandria, dust storms at higher rates and frequencies in addition to predominating inversions in temperature.

– **Coral reefs and mangrove**

The changes in climate will have negative effects on fisheries and tourism in the Red Sea by bleaching coral in response to rising water temperatures, destroying ecosystems, and reducing biodiversity.

– **Diversity**

Elba and the South Sinai highlands have experienced a decline in plant and animal variety due to the extreme heat and drought conditions. Other delicate plant species (like Embet trees) disappeared from the lower sites of Elba Mountain as air temperature increased by roughly 3 °C during the 1960s, while some plant species migrated to the top areas of the mountains, searching for high humidity and low temperature.

8 Ongoing Studies and Exerted Efforts

- Research has been conducted to promote the continuous cultivation of mangroves and artificial corals, develop their protectorates and enhance preservation and administrative policies in South Sinai protected areas where these ecosystems already exist.
- The Natural Protection Sector in The Egyptian Environmental Affairs Agency (EEAA) has recommended guidelines for integrating anticipated climatic variations implications into biodiversity-related initiatives and programs. To identify the most susceptible regions to danger resulting from climate change, EEAA also offered a different strategy.
- In order to effectively manage coastal resources such as lakes and safeguard them against the effects of climate alterations, the Egyptian National Assembly has passed new legislation including the Integrated Coastal Zone Management (ICZM) in developmental plans. Therefore, reliable institutional monitoring is essential.

The following local adaptation measures are being considered:

- To mitigate the effects on low-lying deltas resulting from the rise of sea level via the creation of wetland zones. Such regions include Lake Manzala and Lake Burullus, which are qualified for the processes of adaptation via advancing maintenance and repairing the systems of natural sand dunes, which provide effective natural protection, as well as promoting the function of stakeholder engagement in assessing the trade-offs of adaptation solutions.
- Plans for development in Egypt's low-lying coastal zones in the Nile Delta should account for the possibility of flooding owing to the continuing rise of sea levels.
- Policies and necessary measures should be incorporated into land use plans, such as identifying the requirements of laws and regulations connected to coastal zone development to carefully account for climate dangers and evolving an adaptation policy for the sake of the lowland of the coastal zone regions.
- Finding ways to improve capabilities of individuals and organizations to carry out plans for integrated coastal zone management.
- In addition, many projects were outlined in the National Plan for Land Use to act upon the climatic alterations' impacts considering the following points:
- Since mountain ecosystems are a vital strategic resource for biodiversity in Egypt, it is important to develop an adaptation policy framework for their management.
- To account for the projected implications of climate variations on biodiversity, the Egyptian current and future network of protected areas should be reevaluated.
- Creating study plans for plants found in dry areas like mountains and deserts.
- It is recommended that people stay at least one kilometer inland from the shore.

9 Systematic Observation

– **Requirements of systematic observation**

The following methods are required for systematic observation:

In order to make informed decisions on how to respond to increasing sea levels, it is necessary to set up effective monitoring networks, systematic observation systems and institutional information systems. The key goals of the system should include the identification of susceptible regions, implementation and updating measures to protect resources, following up and enforcing planning requirements in addition to establishing databases. Furthermore, the use of remote sensing and non-traditional observing tactics should be improved in order to create institutional capacity for detecting the sea and coastal surface temperature fluctuations in the Red Sea and the Mediterranean as well as wetlands and lakes.

With regular monitoring of sea surface temperature, sea level oscillations and coastal land use, scientists and policymakers would have access to a wealth of information.

The Egyptian government delegated responsibility for national statistics to the Central Agency for Population, Mobilization and Statistics (CAPMAS). Its website provides statistics and information on a wide range of environmental and social variables. Several other groups are also conducting systematic climate observation to achieve certain goals. The following lines provide a brief summary of the systems and programs available for systematic observation:

– **Atmospheric and meteorological observation**

Since 1933, Egypt's weather forecasts and systematic observations have been overseen by the Egyptian Meteorological Authority (EMA). There are 112 stations spread around the country that are specified for monitoring air pollution, atmospheric conditions, global radiation and agrometeorological conditions.

– **Monitoring of air pollution**

The Egyptian Environmental Affairs Agency (EEAA) has awarded contracts for air pollution monitoring, measurement and laboratory analysis to the Environmental Hazards and Mitigation Center (EHMC) at Cairo University and the Institute for Graduate Studies and Research (IGSR) at Alexandria University. The National Institute of Standards (NIS) is the gold standard when it comes to quality control and assurance. Cairo, Alexandria, and other major cities in the Delta and Upper Egypt are all covered by a network of 47 stations.

– **Network for Coastal Water Quality Monitoring**

Egypt's Mediterranean coast is overseen by the Institute of Graduate Studies and Research (IGSR), Alexandria University, whereas Egypt's Red Sea coast is under the responsibility of the National Institute of Oceanography and Fisheries (NIOF).

Ain Shams University's Faculty of Science operates an independent reference laboratory that oversees a laboratory quality assurance program in which the monitoring institutions take part.

The EEAA has launched a webpage where this information may be found. In order to verify and supplement satellite observations of sea surface temperature (STT), this network keeps tabs on a variety of physical factors at strategic points along the coast.

10 Framework for Actions of Adaptation and Mitigation for Biodiversity Sustainability

Despite extensive documentation of species and habitats at risk, information gaps persist on the effects of rising temperatures on Egypt's biodiversity, particularly in the country's freshwater and dry terrestrial ecosystems. Yet, it is unclear what effects climate change will have on fisheries and aquaculture in the future. Scientific information is adequate to address implications of climate change for the time being and make strategies, notwithstanding uncertainties and gaps in understanding. Notably, taking early selective adaptation measures may lessen the severity of consequences and forestall the need for later, more expensive measures.

– **General approach to mitigation action**

Egypt understands that the only way to effectively combat global warming and climate change is to reduce greenhouse gas (GHG) emissions, especially by big manufacturers. The preventative strategies have been adapted from national programs and country studies. However, foreign donors' financial and technical assistance is necessary to fully execute these national strategies.

Reducing greenhouse gas emissions and furthering Egypt's long-term development objectives are both supported by enhancing the efficacy of energy and the use of renewable energy resources. Egypt has created several policies and strategies to improve the efficacy of energy, promote the usage of renewable energy sources and alleviate greenhouse gas emissions, all of which are goals of the United Nations Framework Convention on Climate Change.

Protecting the low-elevated coastal zones in the Nile Delta and the Mediterranean coast will necessitate ecologically friendly technology that will need to be transferred in the medium future in order to mitigate the consequences of climate change. There is an immediate need for both technical and financial backing to launch research initiatives using existing university and research center teams. As such, developing novel strains resistant to heat, salt and water stressors is a top concern across a variety of disciplines.

- Adaptational choices informed by the field of genetic engineering.
- Decrease in water lost via evaporation and transpiration.
- Techniques for marine aquaculture that are easy on the wallet.
- Exploiting unusual sources of water.

- Improved water usage efficiency and demand management are two areas where research has recently advanced as "no-regret" responses to climate change.
- Assessment of coastal area vulnerability and investigation of adaptation possibilities considering selected sea-level-rise scenarios.
- Impacts of saltwater intrusion on coastal wetlands: monitoring, modelling and evaluation.
- Socioeconomic factors associated with immigration of vulnerable people and job opportunities in secure places; climate change monitoring, modelling and evaluation and implications of climate change on coral reefs and tourism.

– **General approach to adaptation action**

By reducing a system's susceptibility or boosting its resilience, adaptation efforts help prevent or take advantage of the negative effects of climate change. Reducing ecosystems' overall sensitivity to climate change may require revising existing priorities and setting new goals and objectives.

Conservation efforts on the grassroots and in the courts, in government agencies, in the halls of power all count as adaptation acts. The restoration or protection of wetlands and riparian regions, for instance, may increase habitat quality and allow species migrations, lower stream temperatures, and mitigate scouring and flooding impacts of excessive rainfall or rapid melting of snow.

11 Conclusion

All aspects of Egypt's economic, social, and environmental growth are very susceptible to the effects of climate change, and a strong institutional framework for monitoring, integrating and modelling is essential for effective adaptation. The research conducted nowadays is meant to strengthen communities' ability to better manage their environment, land and crops, increase the effectiveness with which resources are used and safeguard sensitive coastal areas.

Recommendations

Policymakers should adapt early monitoring and rapid response policies to determine, control or abolish new and present intrusive species before reaching serious levels, as well as altering or determining policies, regulations and laws that focus on the implications of climatic fluctuations in the infrastructure planning to protect ecosystems. It is possible that severe consequences might be mitigated, and for the future, more expensive activities can be avoided if planned adaptation actions are implemented early. The measures are meant to (1) eliminate or lessen the impact of other, non-climate-related stresses that amplify the consequences of climate change; (2) create new or expand existing protected areas, buffer zones and connectivity corridors and (3) bolster efforts to keep an eye on things and make it easier to manage in uncertain situations, using methods like scenario planning and adaptive management.

References

1. Ahmed NHM, Hossam L, Ghallab A (2023) Treatment of Red Sea Hawksbill turtle, Eretmochelys imbricata suffered from floating syndrome using activated charcoal-simethicone combinat. J Adv Vet Res 13(2):292–294
2. Brander KM (2006) Assessment of possible impact of climate change on fisheries. WBGU, Materialien, Report of Wissenschaftlicher Beirat Der Bundesregierung Globale Umweltveränderungen
3. CIS (2023) Carnegie Institution for Science. "Climate is increasing risk of high toxin concentrations in Northern US lakes." ScienceDaily, 23 October 2023. www.sciencedaily.com/releases/2023/10/231023124427.htm
4. CITES (2023) CITES Secretariat Web site. Available at: https://cites.org/sites/default/files/eng/app/2023/E-Appendices-2023-05-21.pdf
5. Curry R, Mauritzen C (2005) Dilution of the northern north Atlantic ocean in recent decades. Science 308:1772–1774
6. El-Raie MS, Nasr O, Desouki FS, Dewidar Kh (1995) Potential impact of accelerated level rise on Alexandria governorate. Egypt J Cost Res Special Issue 14
7. El Said M (2024) Egyptian fisheries need urgent action to combat effects of overexploitation and climate change. Published online 20 February 2024, Springer Nature. https://doi.org/10.1038/nmiddleeast.2024.24
8. Hanafy MH, Desoky MYA (2023) HEPCA's periodic report on coral reefs status, coral bleaching event of 2023: exploring distribution, sensitivity, and recovery potential on the Egyptian coast of the Red Sea
9. Hanafy MH, Ismail M (2012) Climate change and its effect on the Egyptian coast of the Red Sea; the first recorded coral mass bleaching event. HEPCA
10. Hanafy MH, Sallam A (2003) Status of marine turtles nesting on the Egyptian beaches of the Red Sea. National Report to PERSGA, 45 pp
11. Hannah L, Midgley GF (2002) Conservation of biodiversity in changing climate. Conserv Biol 16(1):264–268
12. IPCC (2022) The intergovernmental panel on climate change sixth assessment report, working group III: mitigation of climate change. IPCC_AR6_WGIII_Full Report.pdf
13. IUCN (2023) IUCN Red list of threatened species. Available at: https://www.iucnredlist.org/resources/brochure
14. Leach K, Zalat S, Gilbert F (2013) Egypt's protected area network under future climate change. Biol Conserv 159:490–500
15. Mehrim AI, Refaey MM (2023) An overview of the implication of climate change on fish farming in Egypt. Sustainability 15:1679. https://doi.org/10.3390/su15021679
16. Osman YA, Samy-Kamal A (2023) Diversity and characteristics of commercial Red Sea fish species based on fish market survey: informing management to reduce the risk of overfishing. Fish Biol. https://doi.org/10.1111/jfb.15339
17. Pattnaik SR (2023) Impact of climate change on ecology and biodiversity of Africa—a review. Int J Agric Appl Sci 4(2):135–141. https://doi.org/10.52804/ijaas2023.4218
18. Penuelas J, Janssens IA, Ciais P, Obersteiner M, Sardans J (2020) Anthropogenic global shifts in biospheric N and P concentrations and ratios and their impacts on biodiversity, ecosystem productivity, food security, and human health. Glob Chang Biol 26:1962–1985
19. Salimi S, Almuktar SAAN, Scholz M (2021) Impact of climate change on wetland ecosystems: a critical review of experimental wetlands. J Environ Manage 286:112160. https://doi.org/10.1016/j.jenvman.2021.112160
20. Shalby A, Elshemy M, Zeidan BA (2021) Modeling of climate change impacts on Lake Burullus, coastal lagoon (Egypt). Int J Sedim Res 36(6):756–769
21. Shawky AM, Sallam WS, Mohamed SZ (2024) Assessing dugong distribution and overlapping threats along the northwestern Red Sea, Egypt. Egypt J Aq Biol Fish 28(1):1455–1488. https://doi.org/10.21608/EJABF.2024.341505

22. UNEP (2007) Convention on biological diversity. International day for biological diversity, biodiversity and climate change
23. UNEP (2023) Emissions gap report 2023: broken record, temperatures hit new highs, yet world fails to cut emissions (again), DEW/2589/NA. https://www.unep.org/resources/emissions-gap-report-2023
24. WMO (2006) WMO Glob Ozone Res Monit Proj Geneva
25. WMO (2024) World Meteorological Organization; State of global climate 2023 report, March 19, 2024, No. 1347, Geneva, 53pp. https://library.wmo.int/idurl/4/68835
26. World Research Institute (WRI) (2007) Ideas into actions. Annual report 2006–2007, 28 pp

Climate Change and Lessepsian Migration to the Mediterranean Sea

Magdy T. Khalil, Amr B. Mostafa, and Marwa M. El-Naggar

Abstract This chapter explores the intricate relationship between climate change and Lessepsian migration to the Mediterranean region, shedding light on the implications for biodiversity and ecosystem dynamics. The construction of the Suez Canal in 1869 initiated a significant transformation, facilitating the exchange of marine species between the Red Sea and the Mediterranean, a phenomenon known as Lessepsian migration. Climate change, characterized by escalating warming trends, further amplifies this migration process. Rising sea surface temperatures, attributed to climate change, create more hospitable conditions for thermophilic species originating from the Red Sea to migrate and establish themselves in the Mediterranean. Consequently, there is an increased likelihood of species introductions and range expansions, altering the composition and distribution of marine biodiversity in the region. Furthermore, climate-induced changes in ocean currents and circulation patterns play a crucial role in facilitating the dispersal of Lessepsian species, augmenting their colonization success in the Mediterranean. This dynamic interaction between climate change and Lessepsian migration poses significant challenges for ecosystem management, as invasive species introductions can disrupt native ecosystems and biodiversity. Understanding the complex interplay between climate change and Lessepsian migration is paramount for developing effective management strategies to mitigate the impacts of invasive species and safeguard the ecological integrity of the Mediterranean Sea. This chapter aims to provide insights into these interconnected processes, contributing to a comprehensive understanding of the implications of climate change for marine biodiversity and ecosystem dynamics in the Mediterranean.

M. T. Khalil (✉) · A. B. Mostafa · M. M. El-Naggar
Department of Zoology, Faculty of Science, Ain Shams University, Cairo, Egypt
e-mail: mtkhalil52@sci.asu.edu.eg

A. B. Mostafa
e-mail: amrbayoumy@sci.asu.edu.eg

M. M. El-Naggar
e-mail: marwaelnaggar@sci.asu.edu.eg

© The Author(s), under exclusive license to Springer Nature Switzerland AG 2025
M. T. Khalil et al. (eds.), *Climate Changes Impacts on Aquatic Environment*, Earth and Environmental Sciences Library, https://doi.org/10.1007/978-3-031-74897-4_4

Keywords Suez Canal · Marine biodiversity · Ecological dynamics · Environmental impact · Mediterranean ecosystem

1 Introduction

The Mediterranean Sea, with its rich biodiversity and intricate ecosystems, has long been a focal point for scientific inquiry and conservation efforts. However, the region is not immune to the far-reaching impacts of global climate change, which is increasingly reshaping its marine environments. One notable consequence of climate change in the Mediterranean is its influence on Lessepsian migration—named after Ferdinand de Lesseps, the French engineer behind the canal's construction. This migration involves the movement of marine species from the Red Sea to the Mediterranean through the Suez Canal.

The construction of the Suez Canal in 1869 facilitated the exchange of species between two distinct marine environments, leading to profound implications for Mediterranean biodiversity. With climate change exacerbating warming trends, the conditions are becoming more favourable for thermophilic species native to the Red Sea, adapted to warmer waters, to expand their ranges into the Mediterranean. This increases the frequency and success of Lessepsian migration events, causing shifts in species composition and distribution across the region. It's estimated that around 300 indigenous Red Sea species now inhabit the Mediterranean, with potentially more undiscovered species.

Climate change also influences ocean currents and circulation patterns, which play a crucial role in species dispersal. Changes in these processes may facilitate the transport of larvae and juveniles of Lessepsian species from the Red Sea into the Mediterranean, further enhancing the potential for establishment and colonization.

Against this backdrop of environmental change, understanding the mechanisms and implications of Lessepsian migration in the context of climate change is of paramount importance. Accordingly, this chapter seeks to comprehensively explore the ecological, environmental, and climatic factors driving Lessepsian migration through the Suez Canal. By delving into historical contexts, migration mechanisms, and ecological repercussions, we aim to unravel the complexities of this phenomenon and its far-reaching effects on marine biodiversity and ecosystem dynamics in the Mediterranean region.

1.1 Factors Contributing to Lessepsian Migration

The following environmental drivers promote the successful settlement and expansion of non-indigenous species from the Red Sea to the Mediterranean Sea:

1. **The salinity levels**. They are significantly impacted as the canal traverses Lake Temsah, located at Ismailia, intersecting with the Great and Small Bitter Lakes. The lakes in question were once arid salt basins, measuring approximately 13 km in length and 5 km in width, before their integration into the Suez Canal. De Lesseps estimated the thickness of the salt bed, approximating it to be 13.2 m, corresponding to an approximate weight of 970 million metric tons of salt.

Following the canal's inauguration, the gradual dissolution of the saline sediment at the bottom of the lakes transpired over six decades. The significant increase in salinity observed in different sections of the canal, particularly in hyper-saline Lake Bitter (68 ‰), coupled with the elevation in the temperature of the canal's water during the months of summer (with a temperature difference of approximately 10°C between the northern and southern ends), presents a considerable challenge for adult organisms attempting to navigate through the canal. Moreover, these conditions likely render the passage unfeasible for larvae, further exacerbating the ecological implications of this phenomenon. The salinity of the seabed has likely undergone a significant transformation over time, with a notable decrease observed from 52 ‰ in 1924 to an average of 49 ‰ during summer and 44 ‰ during winter in recent times. It is worth noting that despite these fluctuations, the evaporation rate appears to be adequate in maintaining these levels. The process of deepening lakes and reducing the concentrations of salt has been found to significantly impact the facilitation of water exchange and the migration of species [92, 95].

2. **Temperature**. The Mediterranean Sea is characterized by its temperate climate, hosting a diverse array of cold-water species. Conversely, the Red Sea boasts a tropical environment, maintaining winter temperatures above a minimum threshold of 18 °C. In order to facilitate the colonization of the Red Sea species beyond their customary range, tropical species must encounter summer temperatures that are sufficiently elevated to support their reproductive processes and egg development, adding to winter temperatures that surpass their lethal thresholds. The impact of global climate change and temperature fluctuations on the continued northward migration of tropical species remains a subject of considerable interest and investigation. The primary hindrance impeding the expansion of most Red Sea fish species into the Mediterranean Sea seems to be the prevailing lower winter temperatures. This phenomenon mirrors the effect observed in numerous tropical organisms, such as reef-building corals, which are also deterred from infiltrating these regions [38, 69].
3. **The hydrostatic pressure**. This phenomenon arises from the significant disparity in water levels separating the Red Sea from the Mediterranean, with the former currently measuring approximately 1.2 m higher. Due to the absence of channel gates in the canal, the unobstructed gravitational gradient propels water northwardly, particularly amplified during prevailing southeast winds. The enhanced locomotive patterns of animal migration are further influenced by the swift tidal currents of the Red Sea that propel into the Bitter Lakes, dispersing within the expansive basin. Consequently, the organisms propelled along this route are

compelled to endure a substantial portion of their canal transit under heightened salinity.

4. **The atmospheric effects**. Their role in facilitating species migration becomes crucial in the absence of prevailing currents for north or southbound movement on numerous days throughout the year. Indeed, the presence of southern winds facilitates the northbound migration of eggs and juveniles, offering a comparatively shorter route in contrast to the considerably lengthier southbound migration [92].

1.2 The Magnitude of Lessepsian Migration

The fact that the Red Sea species have colonized the east side of the Mediterranean can be viewed as a significant scientific endeavour, offering an opportunity to study the intricate dynamics of colonization and adaptation. This phenomenon allows for the observation and comparison of both the source populations and the populations that successfully establish themselves in the new environment [19, 27, 56].

The combined influence of elevated temperatures and salinities, coupled with reduced nutrient and oxygen levels, resulted in a significant decline in the biodiversity and ecological richness of the eastern Mediterranean ecosystems. According to existing literature, there is a notable disparity in species richness between the eastern and western basins of the Mediterranean, with the former reportedly harbouring approximately twice the number of species. The current mitigation of limited species diversity is achieved through the influx of the Red Sea biota, which possesses favourable adaptations for warm and saline aquatic environments facilitated by the Suez Canal. The biota in question, which has undergone evolutionary processes in response to dynamic environmental changes and variations originating from the richly diverse Indo-Pacific region, exhibits remarkable competitiveness [72].

During periods of elevated salinity levels, particularly in the Bitter Lakes, the canal waters assumed the role of a "filtrating funnel," impeding the migratory progress of numerous aquatic organisms, such as fish, corals, echinoderms and nearly all planktonic species.

The successful establishment of the Bitter Lakes in the Suez Canal by fish fauna, leading to their migration and subsequent expansion into the Mediterranean Sea, can be attributed to the salinity decline observed by Ibrahim et al. [45].

The phenomenon of Lessepsian migrants in the eastern Mediterranean has undergone a remarkable transformation, evolving from exotic species to assertive dominants. Certain fish and decapods have exhibited a propensity for robust population growth, further accentuating their prominence in the region. The coastal regions of numerous Mediterranean countries have witnessed substantial commercial hauls of migratory fish [8].

Consequently, the Suez Canal has been transformed into an unrestricted conduit, facilitating the ingress of the Red Sea water into the Mediterranean. Each year, numerous novel species originating from the Red Sea and occasionally the Indian

Ocean are unveiled within the Mediterranean region. A noteworthy proportion of the fauna discovered in the Levant basin can be attributed to their Indo-Pacific provenance, amounting to no less than 10%.

2 Fish Migration

A comprehensive analysis of the Mediterranean coast has revealed the presence of a remarkable diversity of marine fish species, with a staggering count of 430 or potentially more [5]. Notably, a significant portion of these species, precisely 146, can be traced back to their origins in the Indo-Pacific region. This noteworthy observation spans the period from 1896 to 2020, shedding light on the dynamic nature of fish populations in this region [8]. The prevailing direction of immigration, which predominantly moves in a northward trajectory, can be elucidated by considering the following factors:

(a) The comparative analysis reveals that the Red Sea boasts a significantly higher number of species, approximately 1000, in contrast to the eastern Mediterranean's comparatively modest count of 430. Furthermore, the Red Sea exhibits greater population densities across these species, further accentuating its ecological richness [28].
(b) The diverse array of fishes of the Red Sea in the fauna of the western Indo-Pacific is convincing evidence of their superior and flexible adaptation to a wide range of ecological niches, enabling them to compete effectively with species in the Mediterranean region.
(c) The facilitation of South-North passage, particularly for eggs and juveniles, is primarily attributed to the influence of prevailing winds and currents [23].

2.1 Coexistence with Indigenous Species

The successful establishment of numerous fish species in novel environments highlights the correlation between the dietary preferences of migrant species and their inclination towards non-selective feeding habits. The significance of this adaptation cannot be overstated for migrants as they navigate their unfamiliar surroundings. The establishment of successful colonization is contingent upon the congruence between the conditions of the environment in the target and source areas falling within the tolerable range of the colonizing species. Due to the inherent dissimilarities between these environments, it is anticipated that the invading population will exhibit a response to the novel stress, leading to a divergence from its progenitor population. Consequently, this divergence will facilitate enhanced adaptation to the newly encountered habitat [15, 19].

The presence of approximately 500 Lessepsian migrants in the Mediterranean, as currently estimated, has raised intriguing questions regarding their successful establishment. Interestingly, the limited productivity of the region does not hinder their colonization, possibly due to the availability of under-utilized ecological niches. Consequently, this phenomenon prompts further investigation into the intricate dynamics between these introduced species and the native flora and fauna, as highlighted by D'Amen and Azzurro [27]. The large quantity of these species primarily stems from the migrant's capacity to establish a specialized role in the novel ecosystem, thereby ensuring their persistence through effective reproductive processes during periods of favourable oceanographic circumstances conducive to the growth and maturation of juvenile stages.

2.2 Inter- and Intra-specific Competition

Examining the ecological process resulting from the convergence of spatial and temporal resource utilization is widely recognized as a significant determinant in structuring fish communities [45]. Competition is crucial in driving adaptations, such as habitat selection, resource allocation and extinction. However, it is important to note that competition is not prevalent in natural communities. This is primarily because resources, whether renewable or non-renewable, typically offer a greater number of ecological niches than specialized organisms to occupy them. In the context of ecological temporalities, it is noteworthy that numerous resources continue to be underutilized despite the presence of species that have evolved specialized adaptations for exploiting these resources [8]. Nevertheless, it is widely recognized that the impact of competition can be influenced by factors such as predation and environmental harshness/variability. The phenomenon of local extinction resulting from competitive interactions is likely constrained to fragmented habitats found in patchy landscapes and isolated islands [63].

When examining the ecological dynamics of fish species, it becomes evident that they have remarkable adaptability to switch habitats, which occurs frequently and can be reliably predicted. Fishes exhibit discernible modifications in their behavior when confronted with competitors, strategically aiming to minimize the overlap in resource utilization. The absence of documented instances wherein a Lessepsian migrant has completely displaced an indigenous species is notable. Local species that have been outcompeted would undergo vertical habitat displacement, typically by relocating to deeper and cooler waters. To date, there have been no documented instances of misplacement, a compelling indication of the underutilization of niches within the communities of the eastern Mediterranean [7, 56].

In certain instances, it appears increasingly likely that the introduction of novel competitors has resulted in a phenomenon of competitive interference, leading to a constricting of the trophic niche occupied by the native species. This plot suggests that the newly introduced species exhibit higher superiority than the native species. Furthermore, it is worth noting that various studies have corroborated that, as interspecific competition intensifies, such as by introducing a new competitor, individual species tends to exhibit a narrower dietary range. This phenomenon is often aligned with a decline in the native species aggregation's overall biomass, primarily attributable to a decrease in the individuals' number. Consequently, the invading competitor tends to supplant the displaced biomass. In contrast, it has been observed that a decrease in competition leads to a reduction in both the biomass of the initial species aggregation and their breadth of diet, as noted in the study of Mutlu et al. [63].

2.3 Trophic Characteristics of Migratory Fish Species

The feeding habits encompass four distinct categories: piscivorous, benthic invertebrate feeders, planktivorous, and herbivorous. Notably, the piscivorous and benthic invertebrate feeders each received an equal allocation of both benthic and pelagic feeders. The study revealed a notable resemblance in the trophic structure of the Red Sea's original ichthyofauna and the Levant's receiving ichthyofauna. However, a key distinction arises in the anticipated scarcity of herbivorous fish species in the Mediterranean, influenced by its temperate origins. The migratory species' notable prevalence of planktivorous individuals does not necessarily imply a susceptible and easily invaded location. Instead, it may be attributed to their transient nature and ability to adapt to diverse hydrographic conditions swiftly, facilitating rapid acclimation to novel environments [83].

Moreover, the presence of these species in schools with sizes medium to large mitigates the likelihood of stochastic extinction events, particularly throughout the critical start-up phase. The bathymetrical distribution of goatfishes (family Mullidae) is widely recognized as a crucial mechanism for facilitating coexistence between migrant and native species. For instance, *Upeneus moluccensis*, known for its migratory behavior, exhibits dominance within the range of 10–30 m. Conversely, *Upeneus pori*, a benthic invader, is most frequently observed at depths ranging from 40 to 55 m [75]. The bathymetrical allocation is indirectly substantiated by observing that the closer the demersal fish species are to the surface, the markedly higher average concentrations of Hg they exhibit. This correlation aligns with the depths that have experienced greater pollution due to human activities. The study examined the inter-specific relationships within a non-coevolved assemblage of estuarine fishes in California. The findings of this study indicate that, despite the vulnerability of the ecosystem to invasion, the recently encountered species exhibit a stable coexistence. These results suggest that the influence of co-evolution in determining the inter-specific relationships within this ecosystem is relatively minor [31].

- Bathymetric. The importance of bathymetry is to recognize that the observed exclusion is not attributable to the migration of certain species to different water depths but rather to the limitations of many researchers who have not been able to locate these species within their traditional fishing grounds. The observed bathymetrical partitioning phenomenon, specifically among lizardfishes belonging to the Synodontidae family, challenges the prevailing pattern observed in most native

Lessepsian-confamilial species. This pattern typically involves the invader species inhabiting shallow water, as observed in various crustaceans, Sphyraenidae, and Mullidae. It is intriguing to observe that various species employ distinct feeding strategies, such as chasing (caudal attack) or ambush (frontal attack), as well as engaging in diurnal or nocturnal activities. These adaptations enhance their likelihood of successfully occupying specific niches within the appropriate trophic level [70].

- Partitioning. Addressing the high tropic selectivity of herbivorous fish species *Siganus rivulatus* and *Siganus luridus*, which are Lessepsian migrants belonging to the Siganidae family, has been documented within the mother colony residing in the Gulf of Suez, while their offsprings migrate to the Mediterranean. Resource partitioning in the Gulf region was observed, but this pattern was disrupted upon the fish's arrival in the south-eastern Mediterranean. This disruption can be attributed to horizontal sea-level platforms, which exhibit minimal tidal motion and hinder grazing activities. The siganids exhibited a notable convergence in their dietary preferences since they both rely on a comparable array of algal species. Consequently, there was an increased degree of overlap in their diets, leading to diminished niche partitioning. The study revealed a notable increase in partitioning when there was a heightened presence of vegetation, indicating a correlation between vegetation diversity and abundance (specifically comparing rocky shore and sandy bottom habitats). A fascinating phenomenon emerges in the realm of siganids since these organisms exhibit a discerning inclination towards selecting a distinct dietary preference, often cantered around consuming one or a limited number of plant species. This predilection is particularly intriguing since it sets them apart from their counterparts, who exhibit a lesser inclination towards grazing upon these specific plant species, thereby establishing a unique dietary niche within their ecological community. Therefore, it can be inferred that the phenomenon leads to a decrease in competition and a simultaneous increase in resource partitioning [26].

Numerous scholars have assumed that the outstanding establishment of the Mediterranean region by the migrating Lessepsian was effectively facilitated by the presence of an unoccupied ecological niche in their newly adopted environment such as the case of the siganids. The temperate Atlantic is the primary source of the Mediterranean fish fauna's origins. The comparative analysis of herbivorous fish populations between temperate and tropical regions reveals a notable distinction in diversity and abundance. This disparity can primarily be attributed to the influence of temperature on the digestive physiology of these fish species in temperate regions. The presence of *Sarpa salpa*, a herbivorous indigenous fish species, in the subtropical ecosystem of the eastern Mediterranean region provides compelling evidence for a limited niche for herbivorous fish [89].

Hitherto, there has been a lack of comprehensive studies focusing on indigenous species and successful colonizers in the Levant basin, particularly in comparison to terrestrial ecology. However, it is widely believed that the substantial influx of the Red Sea species into this region does not appear to have a significant impact on the population levels of native species. This assumption is primarily based on observations derived from commercial fishing activities. Thus far, the influx of immigrant species has significantly enhanced the overall abundance of the catch. The impact of recent piscivore immigrants on the flourishing populations of earlier migrants has been observed and documented [53].

2.4 Anti-Lessepsian

The migration of species from the Mediterranean heading to the Red Sea is relatively rare. This movement is not solely due to the disparity in the sum of indigenous species between the Mediterranean and the Red Sea. The Red Sea exhibits a significantly higher biotic diversity than the Mediterranean, suggesting that the abundance of Lessepsian migrants may surpass that of anti-Lessepsian by three or more orders of magnitude [15].

As previously mentioned, a multitude of factors contribute to the facilitation of organism transportation within the canal, predominantly in a northward trajectory. The identification of *Sphaerodiscus placenta*, a Mediterranean species commonly known as a sea star, in El Belayim lagoon, located approximately 180 km south of the Suez Canal entrance, represents a compelling and unequivocal manifestation of the anti-Lessepsian migration phenomenon [78].

Considering the significant variations in environmental conditions between El Belayim and the Gulf proper is important. Notably, El Belayim experiences substantially higher salinity levels, reaching up to 60–60‰ and is likely subject to more pronounced seasonal and diurnal fluctuations than the surrounding waters. Consequently, it is reasonable to anticipate reduced competition within this specific biotope, compared to the open coastal waters.

2.5 What Constitutes a Fruitful Example of a Lessepsian Fish Migrant?

A notable disparity has been documented in numerous taxonomic groups wherein certain species exhibit a pronounced propensity for dispersal and colonization. In contrast, closely related species with comparable ecological demands do not display such characteristics. In the Red Sea, many fish families boasting numerous species can be observed, albeit with only a select few having successfully established populations in the Mediterranean region.

In the Red Sea, 14 distinct species of the Mullidae family, commonly known as goatfish were identified in the study of Echreshavi et al. [29] addressing the

Red Sea. However, among these species, only two have been specifically identified such as *Upeneus moluccensis* and *U. Pori*, the population of which has undergone migration to the Mediterranean region. In the Red Sea, a diverse assemblage of 15 distinct species belonging to the Holocentridae family, commonly known as squirrelfishes, can be observed [21]. Nevertheless, the colonization phenomenon in the Mediterranean is limited to a solitary representative, specifically *Sargocentron rubrum*.

The inquiry into the identification of a prospective colonizer was addressed by Echreshavi et al. [29], who were pioneers in conducting a multidisciplinary investigation on this matter. Their approach was utilized in the investigation of migratory mollusks in the Red Sea. Significant disparities have been observed in how invertebrates and fish react to environmental fluctuations. This study investigated the criteria differentiating successful colonizers across four crucial domains. The present study employed a multidisciplinary approach to investigate the Mullidae family, commonly known as goatfish. The present study selected four key factors to investigate their correlation with the achievement of successful colonization [63].

- The concept of genetic variability is a fundamental aspect in the field of genetics, playing a crucial role in shaping the diversity observed within and between species.
- The range of trophic niches.
- The concept of life history strategy is a fundamental aspect of academic inquiry.
- The relative significance of fish aggregation in the origin site (the Red Sea) possesses a significant academic interest.

2.5.1 Genetic Variability

Given the contrasting circumstances between the target and source areas, it becomes imperative for the colonizer to promptly adapt to encountered changes to grow a viable and enduring organism. To effectively address the novel selective pressures, it is imperative to consider the theoretical framework that underscores the significance of high genetic variability [24]. By possessing diverse genetic traits, organisms are better equipped to navigate the vast genetic landscape and identify the optimal genotype that can assert dominance, ultimately facilitating fruitful adaptation [41]. Five species that are non-colonizers belonging to the Mullidae family; namely, *Parupeneus rubescens*, *P. forsskali*, *P. macronema*, *Upeneus subvittatus*, and *Mulloides flavolineatus* were subjected to a comparative analysis with two mullid colonizers, *Upeneus pori* and *U. moluccensis*. The examination of allozymes through electrophoretic analysis was employed to investigate genetic variability. Surprisingly, the findings of O'Toole et al. [67] revealed a lack of correlation between genetic variability and the ability to colonize successfully. The investigation into distinct allozymes accountable for adapting to novel environmental circumstances and promoting triumph in colonization would unveil discernible disparities between individuals who successfully colonize and those who do not.

2.5.2 The Extensive Range of Trophic Niche

The trophic niche breadth refers to the range of resources that an organism utilizes in its ecological community. The theoretical underpinnings for analyzing this factor resemble the preceding factor, the genetic variability. Specifically, it posits that species exhibiting a broad dietary range, commonly called "generalist feeders," possess a higher propensity for successful colonization. Species exhibiting a limited trophic niche breadth, commonly called "specialist feeders," face a higher probability of encountering challenges in locating suitable food resources in a novel environment. A comparative analysis was conducted by Golani [39] to examine the feeding behavior of four mullid species, including the colonizer *Upeneus pori* in addition to *Parupeneus forsskali*, *Mulloides flavolineatus*, and *P. rubescens*. The investigation yielded no discernible correlation between the breadth of the trophic niche and the level of colonization success.

2.5.3 Life History Strategy.

Life history strategy refers to the adaptive patterns and trade-offs organisms employ to allocate their limited resources to maximize their reproductive success and survival in a given environment. The factor in question is commonly referred to as the cumulative amalgamation of demographic characteristics that ultimately govern a given species' overall reproductive success and survival. In their work, Koutsidi et al. [49] formulated a comprehensive model that elucidated the intricate dynamics underlying the determination of a continuity of life- history strategies. At one extreme of the continuum lies the archetype of the "r-strategist," distinguished by its remarkable capacity for rapid growth and pronounced reproductive potential. This is manifested through a heightened intrinsic rate of increase, early attainment of puberty, diminutive size of the body, abbreviated lifespan, and typically limited to a solitary breeding season. On the opposing spectrum lies the "K-strategist," distinguished by contrasting attributes.

According to the seminal work by Pilowsky et al. [71], it was postulated that r-strategists would exhibit superior colonization abilities. The underlying rationale behind their argument rested upon the hypothesis positing that populations of smaller size exhibit a heightened likelihood of experiencing random extinction events. Given the typically limited size of the initial cohort of invaders, typically consisting of only a handful of individuals, it becomes imperative for these invaders to possess the capacity for swift population expansion to circumvent the risk of extinction. Furthermore, it is worth noting that in the context of invasive species, there exists a tendency for these organisms to perceive their newly encountered environment as highly unpredictable when compared to the familiar source habitat to which they adapted themselves. This perception of unpredictability significantly increases the likelihood of ecological catastrophes befalling the invasive population, ultimately leading to a substantial decrease in their overall numbers, often resulting in a critically small remaining population size [49].

The investigation of the correlation between life history strategy and colonization success has also been conducted on the family Mullidae. Based on the data analysis, compared to the non-colonizers, the two colonizer species exhibit characteristics of "r-strategists". According to Golani's et al. [40] postulation, the colonization of the eastern basin of the Mediterranean, known for its heterogeneity in comparison with the Red Sea, was favoured by r-strategists due to their adaptability to the unpredictable nature of this ecosystem.

2.5.4 The Importance of Fish Assemblage in the Source Site

The success of colonization is contingent upon environmental congruity between the source and target habitats. The extent of this overlap must fall within the acceptable threshold determined by the colonizer. In their seminal study, Golani [39] demonstrated that the susceptibility to Lessepsian colonization within the eastern Mediterranean region is primarily observed in habitats characterized by shallow sandy or muddy substrates. The sandy shore emerges as the most analogous habitat to the Mediterranean ecosystem in the confines of the Red Sea. The investigation of the fish assemblage on the sandy shore of the Red Sea unveiled a noteworthy presence of Lessepsian migrants, which persistently occupied this habitat across all developmental phases [40]. Consequently, it can be inferred that establishing dominance in the comparable source habitat serves as a pre-existing adaptation for the prosperous establishment of the eastern Mediterranean region by migrating Lessepsian fish.

Considering the novel environmental circumstances, addressing, and analyzing the implications of this paradigm, a shift is imperative. Upon successfully establishing a population in the designated region, it can be inferred that the colonizers become geographically separated from their source population. Consequently, they become subjected to novel selective pressures, potentially leading to alterations in the newly formed population's phenotypic and genotypic characteristics [55]. To evaluate this assumption, a comparative analysis was conducted regarding the source population and the target. In the study of Golani [39], a comparative analysis was undertaken to examine specimens belonging to seven distinct species of Lessepsian migrants, originating from both the source population in the Red Sea and the target population in the eastern Mediterranean. Regrettably, the Mediterranean region exhibits a notable reduction in the spawning season across various species, which can be attributed to the inherent limitations imposed by the colder temperature regime. Certain species exhibited variations in meristic counts, specifically pertaining to the quantity of anal and dorsal rays, vertebrae and lateral line scales. The observed alterations are ascribed to the ambient temperature prevailing throughout the reproductive period, as documented by Golani [39].

In their seminal work, Echreshavi et al. [29] conducted a comprehensive analysis comparing the allozymes of both source and target populations of two Lessepsian fish migrants, namely *Upeneus moluccensis* and *U. pori* which hold a significant academic interest. No detectable genetic variations were observed. It is important to acknowledge that the employed approach of allozyme analysis exhibits limitations in terms of its sensitivity, rendering it less effective in detecting subtle modifications. Advances in scientific methodologies, exemplified by the remarkable capabilities of DNA sequencing, have paved the way for detecting subtle alterations. Consequently, research endeavors must continue to advance in this trajectory.

The investigation focused on exploring dietary adaptations within various species of Lessepsian migrants. As expected, the dietary patterns of colonizers exhibited a notable resemblance to those of the indigenous population. Several subtle distinctions were observed, one of which pertains to the feeding habits of *Upeneus pori* in the Mediterranean, where it exhibits a broader spectrum of prey size preferences. *Siganus rivulatus* and *Siganus luridus* were investigated in this study to gain insights into the feeding habits and ecological roles in their respective habitats considering these rabbitfish species. They both underwent modifications in the Mediterranean region. Nevertheless, in the origin and targeted environments, the trophic resources lack quantitative data, hindering the ability to ascertain whether these alterations are attributable to selectivity or availability.

2.6 The Profound Influence of Lessepsian Migrants on the Ecological Dynamics of the Eastern Mediterranean Region

The existence of Lessepsian fish species in the eastern Mediterranean accounts for approximately 13.2% of the overall ichthyofauna population in the region. The species in question exhibit a notable qualitative and quantitative significance beyond their mere representation in the local ichthyofauna. Notably, over fifty percent of these species have attained a prominent presence in the local fishery. The study conducted by Golani [39] revealed a noteworthy finding regarding the fishery using trawl on the Mediterranean coast of Israel. Specifically, it highlighted that a significant proportion, approximately half of the catch in this fishery comprises Lessepsian migrant species. The accurate quantification of Lessepsian migrants in the catch of alternative methods for fishing poses a challenge, yet their presence is believed to be significant.

In the Mediterranean, the allocation of Lessepsian emigrant species exhibits a discernible gradient from east to west. The Levantine coast harbours a noteworthy assemblage of 54 fish migrating species. The numerical value exhibits a gradual decline in a westerly direction, reaching its lowest point along the coastlines of Tunisia and Sicily. The southern coast of Turkey is home to a notable assemblage of thirty Lessepsian migrant fish species [22]. In contrast, Egypt's Mediterranean coast boasts an even more diverse community, with a total of thirty-two species. The southern coast of Italy has been documented to harbour a mere four Lessepsian species, while the western waterbody of the Mediterranean intriguingly remains devoid of any Lessepsian species.

Typically, the temporal emergence of species correlates positively with their current levels of abundance. Though the precise date of the initial documentation may not align precisely with the exact moment of a Lessepsian species' introduction to the Mediterranean, it is justifiable to posit that the likelihood of a species being observed and recorded rises in tandem with its population expansion following its arrival in the designated region. Hence, establishing a species' colonization can be traced back to its initial record, serving as a fundamental reference point. Multiple elucidations exist for this observed correlation.

The temporal duration following colonization positively correlates with the potential for establishing substantial and thriving populations. Furthermore, this extended period allows for additional opportunities for species to undergo further adaptation within the novel habitat. Furthermore, it is plausible to hypothesize that these particular species possessed a heightened capacity for colonization and competitive prowess, enabling their early arrival in the Mediterranean region, and subsequently establishing a thriving population. One plausible rationale could be attributed to the surge in ichthyological investigations witnessed in recent decades, which has unveiled a greater number of initial observations. Among these findings, certain instances may signify unsuccessful colonization endeavors, which would have remained undetected in the absence of meticulous research approaches. It is noteworthy to highlight that a significant proportion of species documented since 1970 exhibit a rarity status. Nevertheless, it is intriguing to observe that among these species, a select group consisting of *Sillago sihama*, *Lagocephalus suezensis*, *Herklotsichthys punctatus*, *Oxyurichthys papuensis* and *Pempheris vanicolensis*, which were registered in the late seventies, display a remarkably high prevalence in the eastern Mediterranean region. The absence of a discernible shared characteristic among these five species renders them a notable anomaly in the size progression of population D'Amen and Azzurro [27].

The successful colonization of Lessepsian migrant fish species in the eastern Mediterranean has frequently been attributed to their adept exploitation of underutilized ecological niches. The success of the two herbivore siganids, namely *Siganus rivulatus* and *Siganus luridus* is evidence. The entry of *Siganus rivulatus* into the temperate waters of the Mediterranean, characterized by a scarcity of herbivores, has been attributed to their behavior described in the study of Shapiro Goldberg et al. [79]. The absence of lucifugous fauna played a pivotal role in enabling the outstanding establishment of 3 light- avoiding Lessepsian migrating fish species, viz. *Pempheris vanicolensis*, *Apogon nigripinnis* and *Sargocentron rubrum*, as reported in the work of Yalgin and Türker [88]. It can be inferred that the process of diffusion and establishing colonies may be facilitated for species belonging to families with limited or no representation in the target area. Conversely, species from families well-represented in the target area would exhibit greater resistance to colonization by closely related species. Nevertheless, it is noteworthy that, thirteen Lessepsian migrant species have successfully infiltrated and established colonies in the Mediterranean region, even in the presence of numerous indigenous species from the same family that already inhabit this ecosystem.

The investigation of the influence of Lessepsian migrants on autochthonous species is a topic that only a limited number of studies have explored. The primary challenge stems from the need for more historical documentation preceding the onset of the invasion. Such a comprehensive study was undertaken by Mutlu et al. [62] to examine the migratory behavior of goatfishes (Mullidae), specifically focusing on two species, *Upeneus moluccensis* and *U. pori*. It delves into the ecological characteristics of two indigenous Mediterranean species, *Mullus barbatus* and *Mullus surmuletus*. In a previous investigation [61], an examination was carried out on lizardfishes (Synodontidae), encompassing the presence of a solitary Lessepsian migrant, *Saurida undosquamis*, alongside an autochthonous species, *Synodus saurus*.

The taxonomic group known as Sphyraenidae was also the subject of investigation, with findings yet to be published. The feeding behavior exhibited by both the colonizing and indigenous species within all three families demonstrated striking similarities, suggesting that niche partitioning may have been achieved based on variations in depth in the aquatic environment. In the Mullidae family, it was observed that the colonizer species predominantly inhabited a shallower sector, whereas an inverse pattern was noted among the Synodontidae family, specifically the lizardfish. The question arises as to whether the displacement of local species by colonizers can be definitively established, or if it is possible that the local species previously occupied the same bathymetric niche as their con-familial colonizers. The efficacy of investigating the bathymetric distribution of indigenous species in uncolonized regions to determine this inquiry is limited, as various additional environmental factors may concurrently influence the local species and impede the establishment of colonizer species.

It is imperative to acknowledge that since the investigation of Lessepsian migration, there has been no documented instance of local species extinction.

3 The Intricate Relationship Between Climate Change and Lessepsian Migration

The elevating temperature of the Mediterranean Sea is exhibiting a trend akin to the global warming phenomenon observed across the globe. Over the past three to four decades, a discernible upward trend has been detected in the temperature of the western Mediterranean Sea, affecting both its deep and surface waters. This notable phenomenon has been corroborated by the augmented occurrence of thermophilic marine species, as documented by Galil et al. [37]. Consequently, a multitude of fundamental inquiries emerges. Is there evidence of heightened incursions by species from the southern regions into the Mediterranean biota? To what extent is there a growing spatial convergence observed between exotic and endemic fish species in the Mediterranean region? In the realm of universal change, it is foreseeable that the Mediterranean Sea will witness a heightened pace in the introduction of Lessepsian species, alongside a rising trend in the settlement of species originating from the latitudes in the South. It is anticipated that a reversal in the equilibrium of species richness, specifically between endemic and exotic species, will occur after a certain time of climate variation.

Moreover, the Lessepsian species' progressive geographical expansion towards higher latitudes in the Mediterranean region may be attributed to the same underlying cause.

Hence, it becomes evident that Lessepsian migration represents an ongoing phenomenon characterized by a notable dearth of knowledge pertaining to the species involved in this migratory process.

Based on a comprehensive analysis of existing scholarly works, it becomes evident that the ongoing monitoring of pertinent environmental parameters and the natural environment's condition is imperative to enhance our comprehension of Lessepsian migration mechanisms and pathways. Furthermore, it is imperative to consider the prognostications regarding forthcoming alterations and the ramifications that non-indigenous organisms may have on the indigenous ecosystem.

Lessepsian migration is a multifaceted occurrence intricately linked to the interplay between environmental factors such as temperature and the biological characteristics of the species involved. Therefore, conducting a comprehensive investigation into the biology and ecology of Lessepsian species is imperative, as there is a substantial dearth of knowledge about these organisms. Upon careful examination of the provided information, it becomes evident that there exists a potential for enhanced comprehension regarding the dispersion models of these species in the Mediterranean region. Furthermore, a parallel consideration arises regarding the consequential effects exerted by these species on the indigenous populations and the local natural environment.

The equilibrium state of the exotic species' geographical dissemination is highly improbable. Menéndez-Guerrero et al. [60] conducted a study based on a hypothesis known as the "colonization lag" and anticipated that the climate variations monitored in the Mediterranean Sea will have a lasting impact on species compositions for several decades. This is due to the phenomenon of invasion lagging the pace of climate change. The potential linkage between global warming and the advancement of tropical Atlantic species along the African coast towards the latitude of the Strait of Gibraltar presents a plausible hypothesis. These species, even with intentional introduction, possess the inherent capacity to become invasive in the Mediterranean Sea.

Furthermore, it is worth noting that Lessepsian fishes, which constitute a mere 5.7% of the overall fish fauna in the Red Sea, pose a significant concern regarding potential future invasions. This apprehension is particularly heightened when considering the potential impact of rising sea surface temperatures, which are projected to increase by + 3.1 °C for the surface and + 1.5 °C for deeper layers by the year 2100, as indicated by the findings of Makris et al. [57]. The investigation into the anticipation of such phenomena and the discernment of fish species from the Red Sea that exhibit a higher propensity for encroaching upon the Mediterranean region represent pivotal domains warranting additional scholarly exploration. The comprehension of the worldwide spatial patterns of extinction risk poses a significant hurdle in conservation biology. The significance of adopting a global perspective in understanding the mechanisms behind the spatial models of annihilation threat and the pivotal role of climate warming in the ongoing extinction crisis is underscored by our findings. The limitations inherent in the monitoring method of our investigation preclude us from establishing a causal relationship between the rising prevalence of exotic fish species and the heightened vulnerability of endemic fish species to extinction. Numerous studies have illustrated the escalating influx of southern exotic species invasions in the Mediterranean Sea, a region renowned for its remarkable endemism. These invasions have been facilitated by global warming, which has enabled these species to expand their geographical distribution toward the northern regions.

4 The Phenomenon of Planktonic Migration: A Fascinating Ecological Process

The pivotal role of zooplankton in transferring energy from first producers to higher ecological niches in aquatic ecosystems is widely recognized. Moreover, these food items act as a radical source of sustenance for numerous animal species, notably economically significant fish species. The comprehensive examination of zooplankton species in marine environments is important in advancing our understanding of productivity and diversity in a specific ecosystem. Copepoda, a highly abundant and ecologically significant assemblage of marine zooplankton, typically constitutes a substantial proportion, ranging from 50 to 90% of the overall numerical composition in the zooplankton community. They play a crucial role in the marine food web as they function as a primary trophic level, serving as a vital nutritional resource for numerous carnivorous organisms. In a seminal study conducted by Mavruk et al. [59], it was discovered that the predominant dietary preference of fish larvae inhabiting the south-eastern Mediterranean region is the pelagic copepods.

The Mediterranean marine biota is predominantly sourced from the Atlantic Ocean. The contrasting temperature and nutrient levels between the North Atlantic and the Mediterranean have prompted significant adaptations in the marine life inhabiting the Mediterranean over the past five million years following the reflooding of the basin. An investigation into the currents and overall hydrography of the region may yield valuable insights into the prevailing distribution patterns. The composition of zooplankton in the studied environment has been found to predominantly consist of circum-tropical species and the Indo-Pacific species that have effectively established and thrived in this ecological setting. In their study, Bianchi et al. [14] elucidated that the distribution of Mediterranean species can be attributed to various origins. These include an Atlantic origin accounting for 50.2% of the species, followed by endemic species at 28.6%. Additionally, a significant proportion of species have an Atlantic-Pacific origin at 16.8%, while a smaller percentage can be traced back to an Indo-Pacific origin at 4.4%.

The Copepoda holds paramount significance in the composition of zooplankton, exhibiting unparalleled dominance in terms of biomass and species diversity. Isinibilir et al. [46] documented the presence of a diverse assemblage of forty Copepoda species in the eastern Mediterranean basin. It is worth considering *Clausocalanus furcatus*, *C. arcuicornis*, *Haloptilus longicornis*, and *Temora stylifera* as a potential choice among the various options available. The scholarly work on T. Furcatus is of great significance in the academic community [44]. *T. stylifera* and *Haloptilus longicornis* emerged as the predominant biomass constituents in the given context. The academic investigated the geographical distribution of a significant taxonomic group within the family Acartiidae in the province of Ponto-Mediterranean [10, 73].

The level of copepod diversity observed in both Lebanese and Egyptian waters is remarkably similar, indicating a substantial degree of biodiversity in these regions. Certain Indo-Pacific species, viz. *Calanopia media*, *Labidocera pavo*, *Calanopia elliptica* and *Labidocera madura* were addressed in previous studies [32, 51, 90]. These studies have revealed that the occurrence of these species is temporally restricted, with their presence being observed only during specific short periods of the year. Also, these explores revealed that the eastern basin exhibits a remarkable diversity of copepod species, with 173 species identified. Interestingly, this quantity closely coincides with the range of species recorded in the western waterbody (n = 70–176) [34, 50].

The study by Fernandez de Puelles et al. [33] revealed a noteworthy similarity in the zooplankton composition between the eastern and western Mediterranean Sea, as evidenced by comparing data obtained from the eastern basin. In the realm of coastal ecosystems, it has been observed that the level of specific diversity tends to be comparatively diminished in the inshore regions, particularly in cases where the continental shelf exhibits a narrower configuration in contrast to the offshore areas.

A comprehensive examination conducted prior to and after the construction of the Egyptian Aswan Dam revealed notable alterations in the copepod densities and composition in the Nile Delta and Abu Kir. The complexity of species migration from the Red Sea was highlighted [92]. The migration and distribution modalities of zooplankton are subjected to the influence of various biotic factors, such as predation and competition, as well as abiotic factors. Climatic variations exert a direct influence on hydrological parameters. The investigation into the impact of hydrological shifts in communities provides valuable insights into the ecological significance of climatic variation events in shaping the structure of zooplankton communities. The influence of anthropogenic activities and climatic change on the zooplankton community in the Egyptian Mediterranean waters is a subject of significant interest. It has been observed that elevated temperatures play a crucial role in facilitating the colonization of both indigenous species and tropical non-indigenous species, with a preference for environments of warm water [95].

4.1 The Phenomenon of Zooplankton Migration Through the Suez Canal

Compared to the Atlantic, the Red Sea exhibits a higher salinity and lower nutrient content, thereby endowing Red Sea species with distinct privileges over their Atlantic counterparts within the context of the saline and nutrient-deficient environment of the eastern basin of the Mediterranean. The phenomenon commonly referred to as the migration of Lessepsian species or Eritrean incursion pertains to the Red Sea species' invasion of the Mediterranean biota. The Suez Canal's circulation pattern and elevated salinity levels have provided favourable conditions for the infiltration and northward movement of erythrina species, as opposed to the migration of Mediterranean species in the adverse heading (known as anti-Lessepsian migration). The ongoing phenomenon of species infiltration, whereby various organisms effectively traverse the Suez Canal from the Red Sea to the Mediterranean Sea, appears to persist throughout the year, except for a brief period spanning two to three months in summer. During this time, the directional flow is reversed as the waters of the Mediterranean commence their journey heading to the Red Sea.

In the Suez Canal, Abdel-Rahman [2] documented a comprehensive inventory of copepod species, revealing 50 distinct species, with 35 species identified as migrant species and 15 species classified as Eritrean migrants engaging in northward or Red-Med migration. Additionally, seven species were identified as Med-Red migrants, signifying their migration from the Mediterranean Sea to the Red Sea. Furthermore, 13 species were found to migrate between both the Red and Mediterranean Seas.

In this study, we reported the discovery of five copepod species belonging to the Eritrean migrant's group. These newly identified species are *Centropages furcatus*, *Oncaea rufa*, *Acrocalanus gibber*, *Centropages gracilis*, and *Labidocera Pavo* [95]. In a study conducted by Abdel-Rahman [2], the presence of five copepod species belonging to the Med-Red migrants, including *Oncaea mediterranea*, *Acartia longiremis*, *Centropages ponticus*, *Calocalanus pavo* and *Aetideus armatus* were identified as newly migrated species. Velasquez et al. [86] stated that *Dioithona oculata* may have invaded the Eastern Mediterranean Sea through the Suez Canal and is now at the onset of its spread in the Mediterranean Sea, whereas Oithona davisae has been introduced via shipping, likely from the Northeast Atlantic, widely spreading and successfully establishing viable populations across the entire Mediterranean Sea, until the coastal Levantine Sea.

The present study documented the presence of eight distinct copepod species exhibiting migratory patterns between the Mediterranean Sea and the Red Sea. These newly identified migrant species included *Ctenocalanus vanus*, *Paracalanus crassirostris*, *Lubbockia squillimana*, *C. arcuicornis*, *Oithona plumifera*, *Oncaea venusta*, *Corycaeus ovalis* and *C. violaceus*, as mentioned by Uysal and Shmeleva []. The taxonomic analysis of two distinct copepod species; namely, *C. media* and *C. elliptica* was conducted in the study of El-Sherbiny, and Al-Harbi [30]. It is worthy to mention that the presence of these species, which is widely distributed in the Gulf of Suez and the Red Sea continued undiscovered in the Canal region until the comprehensive survey of Mansour et al. [58]. Subsequently, the distribution of both species became restricted solely to the canal's southern section. Remarkably, the successful inter-species migration across the canal has resulted in their expansion along the eastern coastline of the Levantine waters. The specimens were collected from the hyper-saline Bardawil lagoon **(Berdugo 1968)** [30] and the waters of Lebanon []. *Acartia centura*, a species found in the Indian and Atlantic oceans, exhibits notable abundance in the central Red Sea and the Gulf of Suez. The existence of this species had eluded detection along the canal until it was officially documented by Berumen et al. [13]. *Acartia centura* has demonstrated a notable expansion across various canal regions, and its distribution has further expanded to encompass the eastern Levantine waters [17]. *Acartia* (Acanthacartia) *fossae*, a species found in the Red Sea, has been documented along the coasts of Lebanon in the study of Lakkis [50] and in the Ponto-Mediterranean province as a Lessepsian migrant, as recorded in another study **(Belmonte and Potenza 2001)** [10]. In the Aegean Sea, Zenetos and Galanidi [94] documented the presence of *Arietellus pavoninus* as erythrean migrant, while *Labidocera detruncata*, *Arietellus aculeatus*, *L. madurae* were observed in the East Mediterranean in addition to *Euchaeta concinna*. According to Bariche et al. [9] observations, the occurrence of *Canthocalanus pauper*, a species typically found in the Mediterranean-Indo-Pacific region, and *Temora discaudata*, another Indo-Pacific species in Port Said provides compelling evidence for a migratory movement towards the North. In his seminal work, Gubanova et al. [42] examined *T. stylifera* comprehensively. The taxonomic classification of *Stylifera*, specifically the species *A. clause* and *A. latisetosa*, is of great interest in the academic community. The Latisetosa species is believed to have made its way into the canal through the Mediterranean; while *E. acutifrons*, *P. parvus* and *O. nana* headed to it from the two ends. Barroeta et al. [10] documented *Paracartia latisetosa* and *Acartia* (Acartiura) *clausi* as noteworthy examples of anti-Lessepsian immigrants.

The neritic species *Tintinnopsis beroidea* found along the coast of Syria [1] and *Tintinnopsis radix* recorded in the Delta of the River Nile have been extensively studied in the work of Kimor and Wood [48]. *Tintinnopsis beroidea*, a protozoan species, was documented as a common occurrence in the waters of Alexandria coast, as reported by Zakaria et al. [93].

The *Chelophyes appendiculata* is siphonophore species regarded as a migrant species heading to the Red Sea through the Mediterranean; this species was previously documented in the Levant basin of the Mediterranean Sea [64]. Several siphonophore species; namely, *Diphyes dispar*, *L. meteori*, *Apolemia uvaria*, *Sulcularia turgida*, *Lensia campanella* and *L. subtilis* regarded the Red Sea as their habitat. The presence of *Sulcularia turgida* and *L. subtilis* in the eastern Mediterranean basin was documented by Kimor and Wood [48]. In her study conducted along the Egyptian Mediterranean coast, Zakaria [91] documented the presence of two siphonophore species, including *Sulculeolaria angusta* and *Abyla trigona* as well as one Hydromedusa species, *Olindias singularis*. These findings represent novel records for the Mediterranean Sea, indicating a migration of these Indian Ocean species from the Red Sea through the Suez Canal.

The Indo-Pacific Chaetognatha, specifically the species *S. neglecta* is highly distributed in the Red Sea and it has been extensively documented by Abouelnaga et al. [4]; this species expanded from the Suez Canal to Port Said. In 2018, an intriguing discovery was made by Heneash et al. [43] in the plankton of Alexandria. It involved the identification of a single, fully developed specimen, which added a significant dimension to the existing body of knowledge in this field. In a groundbreaking study, Abdelsalam and Zakaria [3] made a significant discovery by identifying the presence of *Cranocephalus scleroticus*, an epipelagic amphipod species in the eastern Mediterranean. This finding marked the first documented occurrence of this species in this region. This phenomenon has been documented in the western Mediterranean, Indian Ocean and the Red Sea, as noted by Zakaria [91]. The existing body of literature suggests that, except for the jellyfish species *Rhopilema nomadica*, there needs to be more clear evidence regarding the detrimental effects of Lessepsian migratory zooplankton species on the Egyptian waters of the Mediterranean Sea.

According to Öztürk [66], it has been observed that stressed environments in the Mediterranean are characterized by pollution or physical degradation, exhibit a higher susceptibility to invasion, compared to pristine sites. The theory is supported by the observation that mariculture introductions primarily occur in lagoonal or estuarine habitats and in polluted harbours, where vessel-transported alien species are commonly found [76]. The investigation conducted by Zenetos et al. [96] revealed a notable disparity in the abundance of macrofouling organisms between polluted and non-polluted marinas. Contrary viewpoints; however, have been put forth. In the study conducted by Boudouresque et al. [16], it was found that there exists no discernible correlation between the ecological diversity of the host, the ecosystem number of introductions and the level of imbalance exerted on the ecosystem under evaluation. The present study focuses on assessing the influence of the macrophytes newly introduced on the shallow sub-tidal macro-phytic expansion along the coastline of the Mediterranean in the French region.

To conclude, the issue pertaining to the migration phenomenon from the Red Sea region to the Mediterranean presents a multifaceted and intricate challenge. A combination of biotic and abiotic factors influences zooplankton's distribution and migration patterns. Both climate variability and anthropogenic activities significantly influence the structure of zooplankton communities on the south-eastern Mediterranean coast. The fruitful inauguration of tropical species (indigenous and non-indigenous) with warm water aptitude is closely linked to elevated water temperatures [47]. On the contrary, ballast water is widely recognized as the primary catalyst for introducing non-indigenous marine species. The ballast water tank has the potential to serve as an incubation environment for certain species throughout the cruise. The potential implications of this fact on the introduction of non-indigenous species into the target harbour or adjacent coasts during the emptiness of the ballast tank warrant further investigation [77].

The ongoing immigration process of zooplankton organisms through the Suez Canal is remarkable, and potentially gaining momentum due to the enhanced conditions within the canal. The potential introduction of strange species through the Suez Canal has the potential to exert a positive influence on the marine ecosystem of the Mediterranean Sea [15]. This phenomenon can enhance biodiversity, thereby contributing to the overall stability and improving the health of the well-diversified ecosystem. However, based on the existing scholarly literature, except for the jellyfish species *R. nomadica*, the potential adverse effects of Lessepsian migratory species of zooplankton on the Mediterranean Sea in Egypt remain inconclusive [58].

A crucial requirement lies in establishing a continuous monitoring program to document the most recent occurrences of Erythrean zooplankton species in the waters of Egypt. This program would also closely monitor the distribution and abundance patterns of previously identified strange species in the Egyptian waters of the Mediterranean and the Red Seas. The ultimate objective of such an endeavour is to comprehensively evaluate the potential impacts exerted by these strange species on the indigenous biodiversity of both marine ecosystems. Implementing a comprehensive monitoring program necessitates the inclusion of investigations into the dietary patterns of commercially exploited fish species and other ecologically significant organisms in the Red Sea and the Mediterranean. These studies aimed to ascertain the impact of introduced species on the intricate dynamics of the food web, specifically examining whether these species are favoured as a diet source or remain untouched by the native species. In order to achieve species-level identification, it is imperative to explore the development of a more sophisticated methodology, such as DNA analysis.

5 Exploring Benthic Invertebrates' Migration

The current census provides a comprehensive inventory of migratory species in the Polychaeta (Nereidae) and Serpulidae families and various Indo-Pacific mollusk species. Additionally, newly established species are identified with high certainty. The influx of Crustacea appears to exhibit a relatively slower pace than other taxa. The western basin of the Mediterranean exhibits a comparatively lesser degree of significance in terms of the population increase observed in polychaete, mollusks and decapods. During the initial census conducted in the early 1970s to assess the existence of exotic organisms in the east Mediterranean region, 45 Red Sea native habitat species were documented. Among these species, 26 belong to the Gastropod class, while 19 are classified as bivalves. This significant finding accounted for approximately 9% of the overall mollusk fauna that was previously identified. Within decapods, it has been ascertained that a notable proportion of the overall fauna, specifically 43 species belonging to 19 families, can be classified as Lessepsian migrants, constituting approximately 20% of the total decapod population. The expansion carried out via ships is a valuable mode of transportation for "low probability migrants," for various organisms specially the juveniles that undergo biphasic lifecycles, wherein pelagic larvae drift as plankton.

In a study conducted by Galil et al. [37], a remarkable discovery was made regarding the presence of a staggering number of metazoan species classified as extra-terrestrial entities along the Mediterranean coast. The taxonomic categorization of the strange organisms reveals that the most commonly documented phyla among them are Chordata (22%), Annelida (7%), Mollusca (43%) and Arthropoda (16%). The list provided lacks representation from several phyla, namely the understudied Nemertea, Porifera, Nematoda, Phoronida, Entoprocta, Echiura, Priapula, Pogonophora, Brachiopoda and Sipuncula. The accuracy of the data is presumed to be the highest for large and highly conspicuous species, as these characteristics facilitate their clear differentiation from the genuine biota. The geographic categorization reveals that the predominant native range of the recorded strange taxa is primarily concentrated in the Indo-Pacific Ocean (48%) preceding the Indian Ocean (24%), the Red Sea (17%) and the pantropical regions (6%).

The classification based on the ways of penetration revealed that most strange species entered through the Suez Canal. In contrast, the contribution of vessels and mariculture to the influx of aliens was relatively minimal. It is imperative to exercise caution when utilizing these data, as the route and means of penetration are seldom discernible through direct confirmation. The determination of species' vectors is primarily derived from examining their biological and ecological characteristics, including their known biology and ecology, their habitats in their native and introduced ranges in addition to their dispersal patterns, if available. For instance, in the case of a fouling species commonly found in ports, it is rational to suggest that shipping activities are the most likely vector. The prevailing assumption posits that the migration of Erythrean aliens occurs via the Suez Canal and the coastal regions of the Levant, primarily driven by "natural" dispersal mechanisms such as adult movements, passive or autochthonous active larvae. This dispersal is believed to be independent of any direct or indirect human intervention. Confirming a species' status as a naturally scattering Erythrean alien is supported by a temporal sequence of directional records from the Suez Canal, the Red Sea and the coasts of the Levant. As a viable mechanism, vessel-transported dispersal has been widely acknowledged in the scientific community. Numerous instances have demonstrated the capability of ships to disperse marine organisms across different regions of the globe. The equitable application of this principle must extend to transportation via the Suez Canal. Tugboats and barges that are consistently utilized within the canal may possess a greater proportion of the transportation responsibilities relative to other types of vessels when traversing the entire length of the canal. Coal barges, exemplifying a notable phenomenon, persist at one extremity of the canal for an extended duration before being transported to the opposing extremity, where they continue to reside for an additional prolonged period. According to Winters et al. [87], the duration of time allocated at both ends of the spectrum facilitates two crucial processes: the deposition of larvae onto the barge's surface and the release of eggs or larvae from fully developed organisms.

Over the past seven decades, the Levant region has witnessed significant transformative shifts in its political, economic and social landscape. The discernible influence of alien species on the rate and modalities of their introduction is evident [6]. Despite that the Suez Canal retaining its status as the primary conduit for these species, the introductions' rate facilitated by vessels has exhibited a greater magnitude. In 1950,

56 alien species were documented, with an overwhelming majority of 93% entering the Mediterranean via the Suez Canal. An additional 7% of these species were potentially transported through canals or vessels. Since then, 240 alien species have been recorded, with 80% classified as Erythrean aliens. Among these recent introductions, 9% were potentially transported through canals or vessels, while 10% and 1% were solely vessel-transported and introduced through mariculture, respectively. The surge in the transportation of extra-terrestrial beings via vessels can be ascribed to the concurrent rise in the volume of shipping across the region.

By the end of the 1980s, a comprehensive analysis of various experiments led to the discovery that the presence of Brachidontes harmed the recruitment, survival and growth of Mytilaster. However, despite these findings, researchers argued that the Erythrean mytilid species is unlikely to surpass the native species in competition, suggesting the possibility of coexistence at both local and regional scales [81]. During the late 1990s, an investigation was conducted to address the dynamics of dominance at specific sites. The findings revealed a remarkable and rapid shift in dominance, particularly in areas where mussel beds were previously absent. The study documented the presence of dense populations on rocky platforms, reaching up to 300 specimens per 100 cm^2. This intriguing observation highlights the need to explore further and understand the underlying factors driving such ecological transformations [84]. In a more recent development, it has been observed that the rocks have been completely covered by the Erythrean *B. Pharaonis*, a term referring to the ancient Egyptian pharaohs. It has been a subject of scholarly interest for many years. According to Diga et al. [25], the presence of *M. minimus* was infrequently observed. Establishing extensive Brachidontes beds has impacted the biota inhabiting the rocky intertidal zone. The negative correlation between algae and the Erythrean mytilid, as observed by Galil [36], suggests that the presence of algae hinders the settlement of post-larvae for this species.

Consequently, a change in the environmental status that decreases the cover of algae could have positively impacted Brachidontes. A scarcity of herbivores characterized the south-eastern Levant's rocky shores until the advent of the Erythrean siganid fish. The potential role of the abundant siganids in stimulating population growth is postulated to be linked to their ability to remove algae from the intertidal platform effectively. Larger and more robust Erythrean mytilid displaced the native mussel, which in turn resulted in altered predation dynamics, leading to a substantial increase in the population of the native whelk, *Stramonita hematoma*, which has been observed to exhibit a strong preference for preying on Brachidontes [36].

The Erythrean limpet, scientifically known as *Cellana rota*, was discovered in the Mediterranean region in 1961. Over time, this species has expanded its distribution, and by 2000, it had successfully colonized the Israeli coast. Interestingly, the Erythrean limpet tends to occupy intertidal sites less exposed to strong wave action [20, 82]. In contrast, the native Mediterranean limpet, *Patella caerulea* **(Linnaeus 1758)**, prefers rocky habitats that are directly exposed to the force of the surf. Recently, a study conducted along the Mediterranean coast of Israel reported an intriguing observation regarding the prevalence of the alien limpet in the upper rocky littoral. This invasive species has been observed to gradually supplant the native limpet, which, until a few years ago, exclusively inhabited the same rocks in the Ashdod locality [36]. Moreover, along the coastal regions of Israel, a notable ecological phenomenon has been observed, wherein the indigenous limpet species has been entirely displaced along the southern coast. In contrast, on the central coast, it has significantly colonized approximately 40–50% of the available habitat [84]. The Erythrean jewel box oyster, scientifically known as *Chama pacifica* exhibits a notable disparity in population size when compared to its indigenous counterpart, *C. gryphoides* species, the indigenous to the region known for its distinctive characteristics. The study of *Gaederopus* and *C. gryphoides* is of great academic interest. According to Tsirintanis et al. [84], the presence of these native species as epibionts on the new immigrant species is rare.

In contrast, a growing body of evidence suggests a correlation between alterations in bio-variation modalities in the Mediterranean region and various direct factors, including climatic variations and the introduction of intrusive organisms. In conjunction with the already established drivers of habitat modification, pollution and excessive exploitation, these factors contribute to the evolving understanding of biodiversity dynamics in this area. By the midpoint of the century, it is anticipated that the change in climate and the increase in the invading species will emerge as the primary catalysts behind the decline in biodiversity, raising the susceptibility to extinction among numerous species. This phenomenon will particularly impact those already vulnerable due to diminished population sizes, constrained or fragmented habitats and restricted climatic distributions.

The Erythrean extra-terrestrial beings exhibit a thermophilic nature, tracing their origins back to the warm and equatorial aquatic environments. The correlation between increasing seawater temperature and the consequential effects on the survival, growth and reproduction of the Erythrean aliens, as well as their subsequent competitive advantage over the indigenous Mediterranean biota, has been substantiated by Spanier and Zviely [80]. The strategic positioning of the Israeli coast, situated "downstream" of the prevailing current originating from the opening of the Suez Canal, renders it a primary destination for the initial settlement of Erythrean propagules. The initial documentation of most Erythrean extra-terrestrial beings observed within the confines of the Mediterranean Sea can be traced back to their initial sightings along the Israeli coastline. Given the persistent and uninterrupted progression of two interconnected phenomena, namely the escalation of sea surface temperature and the influx of extra-terrestrial beings, it becomes paramount to augment scholarly investigation pertaining to these multifaceted concerns.

6 Seaweeds Migration

The Mediterranean (IM) coast has documented more than twenty distinct alien species of seaweed. During the initial decade of the twenty-first century, several noteworthy species were documented, including *Codium arabicum* Kützing, *Galaxaura rugosa* (J. Ellis et Solander) J.V. Lamouroux, *Stypopodium schimperi* (Kützing) and *Codium parvulum* (Bory ex Audouin) P.C. Silva [65]. Pacheco et al. [68] demonstrated a notable prevalence observed along the Mediterranean coastlines. The conspicuous manifestation of their existence became readily apparent through substantial drift events, which resulted in vast quantities of algal biomass deposition along the shoreline. This phenomenon clearly indicated the proliferation of invasive seaweeds in the subtidal regions, as documented by Gabriel et al. [35]. The coastal waters of the Mediterranean Sea have been documented to harbor a notable assemblage of macrophyte alien species, which have become widely prevalent.

- The **Rhodophyceae**, commonly known as red algae:
- *Galaxaura rugosa,*
- *Hypneacornuta,*
- *Hypneaesperi,*
- *Lophocladialallemandii,*
- *Sarconemafiliforme,*
- *Solieriadura.*
- **Phaeophyceae**, commonly known as brown algae:
- *Padina boergesenii*
- *Stypopodiumschimperi*
- The **Chlorophyceae**, commonly known as green algae:
- *Acetabularia calyculus,*
- *Caulerpa Mexicana,*
- *Caulerpa racemosa,*
- *Caulerpa scalpelliformis,*
- *Cladophoropsisjavanica,*
- *Codium taylorii.*

7 Migration of Macrophytes

Macrophytes are a group of aquatic plants that play a significant role in various ecosystems. Prior to the construction of the Suez Canal in 1869, numerous species were documented and believed to be indigenous by certain researchers [74]. Notably, *Asparagopsis taxiformis* has been included in this study due to the rapid and recent alterations in its distribution across the Mediterranean region. These changes strongly suggest introducing a cryptic species closely resembling the native Mediterranean variety or the introduction of an exotic genotype originating from a distant population.

The main core of exotic species consists of 110 species, categorized into 1 Magnoliophyta, 22 Chromobionta, 16 Chlorobionta and 71 Rhodobionta. Given the substantial likelihood of the secondary diffusion of exotic species from the NE Atlantic coast into the Mediterranean Sea, it is imperative to acknowledge the presence of 12 additional exotic species that have hitherto remained unidentified in the Mediterranean ecosystem. According to Casoli et al. [18], species are categorized into distinct groups based on their probability of introduction as follows: very high (indicating an introduction with certainty), high (indicating a likely introduction) and medium (indicating a debatable introduction).

The distinction between presumed non-established and established species in the basin is based on their documented presence in the scientific literature. Presumed non-established species are those with only one record. In contrast, established species are characterized by populations with self- maintenance potential supported by at least two published records from different localities or periods.

Due to many factors or vectors, the Mediterranean Sea has introduced macrophytes. These include the transportation of species through the attachment to offshore structures and ships' hulls, commonly known as fouling (e.g., *Antithamnionella* spp.). Additionally, the deballasting of waters and transporting solid materials by ships have also contributed to the introduction of macrophytes. The opening of the Suez Canal has facilitated the entry of species such as *Stypopodium schimperi*. Furthermore, the importation of aquaculture species from their native regions, followed by transfers between basins, has led to the introduction of exotic flora (e.g., the introduction of *Crassostrea gigas* from Japan in the 1970s resulted in the introduction of accompanying exotic flora). Unintentional escapes from private and public aquaria, as observed with *Caulerpa taxifolia*, and the release of species used as baits for fishing such as *Fucus spiralis*, have also played a role in introducing macrophytes in the Mediterranean Sea. Finally, certain epiphytic species such as *Acrochaetium* spp. have undeniably established themselves on their foreign hosts. Once introduced, the proliferation of an exotic species can occur through various vectors, including but not limited to those previously mentioned.

Additionally, human activities such as fishery and ship traffic can serve as conduits for the spread of these species, as they become entangled with anchorages and fishing engines, exemplified by the case of *Caulerpa* spp. The movement of settled organisms on the hulls of vessels represents the earliest known mechanism for introducing species into the marine environment. Over time, the significance of this vector has experienced a decline, leading one to surmise that the majority of macrophytes that once held promise for introduction through fouling have already been introduced. The role of ballast waters as a vector for introducing macrophytes appears insignificant. However, it is not a secondary dispersal vector for species such as *Caulerpa* spp. The primary avenue of diffusion encompasses the aquaculture of shellfish, which is succeeded by ship traffic and the Suez Canal. The likelihood of various species, such as *Codium fragile*, being introduced through multiple pathways, including fouling, ballast waters and aquaculture, is of considerable interest.

The exponential movement of species introduction into the Mediterranean Sea has been observed since the late nineteenth century, with the Indo-Pacific region emerging as the primary source of donor species. The notable surge observed in introductions during the 1970s can be attributed to fortuitous introductions coupled with extensive importations of oysters from Japan, Asia. The proliferating drift observed in marine invasions may have been further amplified by the increased focus on research endeavours following the *Caulerpa taxifolia* incident. In the forthcoming years, it will be imperative to incorporate additional records to complement the existing ones elucidated within this compendium.

8 Conclusion

The comprehensive analysis of marine biodiversity on the Mediterranean coast reveals significant findings about the distribution and migration of marine species. The Mediterranean hosts over 430 marine fish species, with a substantial proportion originating from the Indo-Pacific region. The ecological richness of the Red Sea, demonstrated by its higher species count and population densities compared to the Mediterranean, underscores its role as a primary source of these migratory species. Despite the influx of Lessepsian migrants, no instances of complete displacement of indigenous species have been recorded, indicating underutilized ecological niches in the eastern Mediterranean. However, the potential for future invasions remains high, especially with projected increases in sea surface temperatures.

Zooplankton surveys in the Suez Canal revealed significant migratory behaviors among copepod species, further illustrating the dynamic biotic exchanges between the Red Sea and the Mediterranean. The documented presence of numerous alien benthic metazoan species along the Mediterranean coastline, predominantly from the Mollusca, Chordata, Arthropoda, and Annelida phyla, highlights the increasing influence of invasive species on local ecosystems. Climatic variations, along with invasive organisms, are expected to become the primary drivers of biodiversity changes in the Mediterranean, exacerbating the vulnerability of already endangered species.

9 Recommendations

1. Establish a comprehensive and continuous monitoring program to document the presence and spread of Erythrina and other non-native species in Egyptian waters. This should include regular surveys and data collection on the distribution and abundance of these species in the Red and Mediterranean Seas.
2. Develop and implement strategies to mitigate the impacts of rising sea surface temperatures. This includes identifying and protecting areas that are less susceptible to temperature increases and promoting the resilience of native species through habitat restoration and conservation efforts.
3. Implement proactive measures to manage and control the spread of invasive species. This could involve the development of early detection and rapid response systems, as well as public awareness campaigns to educate stakeholders about the risks and management of invasive species.
4. Prioritize research on the ecological niches and competitive abilities of Red Sea fish species that have a higher propensity for Mediterranean invasion. Understanding these dynamics will be crucial for predicting and managing future invasions.

5. Focus on conserving the indigenous biodiversity of the Mediterranean by protecting critical habitats and supporting the resilience of native species. This includes creating marine protected areas and enforcing regulations to prevent over-exploitation and habitat degradation.
6. Foster international collaboration and information sharing between countries bordering the Red Sea and the Mediterranean. This will facilitate coordinated efforts in monitoring, research, and management of marine biodiversity and invasive species.
7. Conduct thorough impact assessment studies to evaluate the ecological and socio-economic effects of invasive species on Mediterranean ecosystems. This will help in formulating effective management policies and practices.

References

1. Abboud-Abi Saab M, Ouba A (2021) Seasonal and interannual changes in abundance and community structure of tintinnids in the Levantine Sea in relation to hydrographic conditions from 2002 to 2014. Region Stud Mar Sci 47:101990
2. Abdel-Rahman NS (2005) The immigration progress of planktonic Copepoda across the Suez Canal, Egypt. Egypt J Aquat Biol Fish 9(3):59–82
3. Abdelsalam KM, Zakaria HY (2023) First record of the epipelagic Cranocephalus scleroticus (Streets, 1878) (Amphipoda: Hyperiidea) in the Egyptian Mediterranean waters. Egypt J Aq Res 49(2):145–150
4. Abouelnaga Z, EL-Wazeer A, Amr AA, El-Regal MAA (2022) Community structure and spatio-temporal distribution of Chaetognatha near coral reefs on Hurghada coast, Red Sea, Egypt. Egypt J Aq Biol Fish 26(5)
5. Agiadi K, Giamali C, Girone A, Moissette P, Koskeridou E, Karakitsios V (2020) The Zanclean marine fish fauna and palaeoenvironmental reconstruction of a coastal marine setting in the eastern Mediterranean. Palaeobiodiv Palaeoenviron 100:773–792
6. Albano PG, Steger J, Bošnjak M, Dunne B, Guifarro Z, Turapova E, Hua Q, Kaufman DS, Rilov G, Zuschin M (2021) Native biodiversity collapse in the eastern Mediterranean. Proc R Soc B 288(1942):20202469
7. Avşar D (2023) Interactions between the Lessepsian and the native fishes in the Northeastern Mediterranean coast of Türkiye. Acta Biologica Turcica 36(3):2-1
8. Azzurro E, Smeraldo S, D'Amen M (2022) Spatio-temporal dynamics of exotic fish species in the Mediterranean Sea: over a century of invasion reconstructed. Glob Change Biol 28(21):6268–6279
9. Bariche M, Al-Mabruk S, Ates M, Büyük A, Crocetta F, Dritsas M, Edde D, Fortic A, Gavriil E, Gerovasileiou V, Gökoğlu M (2020) New alien Mediterranean biodiversity records (March 2020). Mediterr Mar Sci 21(1)
10. Barroeta Z, Villate F, Uriarte I, Iriarte A (2020) Differences in the colonization success and impact of non-indigenous and other expanding copepod species on the zooplankton of two contrasting estuaries of the Bay of Biscay. Biol Invasions 22:3239–3267
11. Belmonte G, Potenza D (2001) Biogeography of the family Acartiidae (Calanoida) in the Ponto-Mediterranean Province. Hydrobiologia 453/454:171–176
12. Berdugo VIVIANE (1968) Sur la présence dans la Méditerranée orientale de deux espèces du genre Calanopia (Copepoda, Calanoida). Rapports et Procès-Verbaux des Réunions, Commission Internationale pour I'Exploration Scientifique de la mer Méditerranée 19(3):445–446

13. Berumen ML, Roberts MB, Sinclair-Taylor TH, DiBattista JD, Saenz-Agudelo P, Isari S, He S, Khalil MT, Hardenstine RS, Tietbohl MD, Priest MA (2019) Fishes and connectivity of Red Sea coral reefs. In: Coral reefs of the Red Sea, pp 157–179
14. Bianchi CN, Azzola A, Cocito S, Morri C, Oprandi A, Peirano A, Sgorbini S, Montefalcone M (2022) Biodiversity monitoring in Mediterranean marine protected areas: Scientific and methodological challenges. Diversity 14(1):43
15. Biton E (2020) Possible implications of sea level changes for species migration through the Suez Canal. Sci Rep 10(1):21195
16. Boudouresque CF, Blanfuné A, Pergent G, Pergent-Martini C, Perret-Boudouresque M, Thibaut T (2020) Impacts of marine and lagoon aquaculture on macrophytes in Mediterranean benthic ecosystems. Front Mar Sci 7:218
17. Carotenuto Y, Vitiello V, Gallo A, Libralato G, Trifuoggi M, Toscanesi M, Lofrano G, Esposito F, Buttino I (2020) Assessment of the relative sensitivity of the copepods Acartia tonsa and Acartia clausi exposed to sediment-derived elutriates from the Bagnoli-Coroglio industrial area. Mar Environ Res 155:104878
18. Casoli E, Mancini G, Ventura D, Belluscio A, Ardizzone G (2021) Double trouble: Synergy between habitat loss and the spread of the alien species Caulerpa cylindracea (Sonder) in three Mediterranean habitats. Water 13(10):1342
19. Chervinsky J (1959) A systematic and biological comparison between the lizardfish (Saurida grandisquamis) from the Mediterranean and the Red Sea. Fisher Bull Haifa 19:10–14
20. Christiaens J (1967) Présence de la patelle Cellana rota Gmelin en Méditerranée orientale. Bull Mus Natl Hist Nat 38(6):903
21. Cortesi F, Mitchell LJ, Tettamanti V, Fogg LG, de Busserolles F, Cheney KL, Marshall NJ (2020) Visual system diversity in coral reef fishes. In: Seminars in cell & developmental biology, vol 106. Academic Press, pp 31–42
22. Çinar ME, Bilecenoğlu M, Yokeş MB, Öztürk B, Taşkin E, Bakir K, Doğan A, Açik Ş (2021) Current status (as of end of 2020) of marine alien species in Turkey. Plos One 16(5):e0251086
23. Daskalaki E, Koufalis E, Dimarchopoulou D, Tsikliras AC (2022) Scientific progress made towards bridging the knowledge gap in the biology of Mediterranean marine fishes. PLoS ONE 17(11):e0277383
24. Deflem IS, Calboli FC, Christiansen H, Hellemans B, Raeymaekers JA, Volckaert FA (2022) Contrasting population genetic responses to migration barriers in two native and an invasive freshwater fish. Evol Appl 15(12):2010–2027
25. Diga R, Gilboa M, Moskovich R, Darmon N, Amit T, Belmaker J, Yahel G (2023) Invading bivalves replaced native Mediterranean bivalves, with little effect on the local benthic community. Biol Invasions 25(5):1441–1459
26. Dimitriadis C, Fournari-Konstantinidou I, Sourbès L, Koutsoubas D, Katsanevakis S (2021) Long term interactions of native and invasive species in a marine protected area suggest complex cascading effects challenging conservation outcomes. Diversity 13(2):71
27. D'Amen M, Azzurro E (2020) Lessepsian fish invasion in Mediterranean marine protected areas: a risk assessment under climate change scenarios. ICES J Mar Sci 77(1):388–397
28. D'Amen M, Smeraldo S, Di Franco A, Azzurro E (2022) The spread of Lessepsian fish does not track native temperature conditions. ICES J Mar Sci 79(6):1864–1873
29. Echreshavi S, Esmaeili HR, Al Jufaili SM (2022) Goatfishes of the world: An updated list of taxonomy, distribution and conservation status (Teleostei: Mullidae). Fishtaxa-J Fish Tax (23)
30. El-Sherbiny MM, Al-Harbi MA (2020) New morphological and molecular data on the little-known pontellid Calanopia media Gurney, 1927 (Crustacea, Copepoda, Calanoida) from the Red Sea, with notes on its diel vertical distribution. ZooKeys 922:13
31. Evagelopoulos A, Nikolaou A, Michailidis N, Kampouris TE, Batjakas IE (2020) Progress of the dispersal of the alien goatfish Parupeneus forsskali (Fourmanoir & Guézé, 1976) in the Mediterranean, with preliminary information on its diet composition in Cyprus. BioInvasions Records 9(2):209–222
32. Farrag MM, El-Naggar HA, Abou-Mahmoud MM, Alabssawy AN, Ahmed HO, Abo-Taleb HA, Kostas K (2019) Marine biodiversity patterns off Alexandria area, southeastern Mediterranean Sea, Egypt. Environ Monit Assess 191:1–28

33. Fernandez de Puelles ML, Gazá M, Cabanellas-Reboredo M, O'Brien TD (2023) Decadal trends in the Zooplankton community of the Western Mediterranean. Water 15(24):4267
34. Fyttis G, Zervoudaki S, Sakavara A, Sfenthourakis S (2023) Annual cycle of mesozooplankton at the coastal waters of Cyprus (Eastern Levantine basin). J Plankton Res 45(2):291–311
35. Gabriel D, Ferreira AI, Micael J, Fredericq S (2023) Non-native marine macroalgae of the Azores: an updated inventory. Diversity 15(10):1089
36. Galil BS (2023) A sea, a canal, a disaster: the Suez canal and the transformation of the Mediterranean biota. The Suez canal: past lessons and future challenges. Springer International Publishing, Cham, pp 199–215
37. Galil BS, Mienis HK, Hoffman R, Goren M (2021) Non-indigenous species along the Israeli Mediterranean coast: tally, policy, outlook. Hydrobiologia 848:2011–2029
38. Gentilucci M, Moustafa AA, Abdel-Gawad FK, Mansour SR, Coppola MR, Caserta L, Inglese S, Pambianchi G, Guerriero G (2021) Advances in Egyptian Mediterranean coast climate change monitoring. Water 13(13):1870
39. Golani D (2021) An updated Checklist of the Mediterranean fishes of Israel, with illustrations of recently recorded species and delineation of Lessepsian migrants. Zootaxa 4956(1):1–108
40. Golani D, Fricke R, Appelbaum-Golani B (2020) Zoogeographic patterns of Red Sea fishes–are they correlated to success in colonization of the Mediterranean via the Suez Canal? Mar Biol Res 16(10):774–780
41. Golani D, Ritte U (1993). The association between genetic variability and successful colonization in fishes. In: Proceedings of the meeting of the Fishery Society of the British Isles. Conway, Wales
42. Gubanova A, Altukhov D, Stefanova K, Arashkevich E, Kamburska L, Prusova I, Svetlichny L, Timofte F, Uysal ZAHİT (2014) Species composition of Black Sea marine planktonic copepods. J Mar Syst 135:44–52
43. Heneash AM, Alprol AE, El-Naggar HA, Gharib SM, Hosny S, El-Alfy MA, El-Hamid HTA (2022) Multivariate analysis of plankton variability and water pollution in two highly dynamic sites, southeastern Mediterranean (Egyptian coast). Arab J Geosci 15(4):330
44. Hure M, Batistić M, Kovačević V, Bensi M, Garić R (2020) Copepod Community structure in pre-and post-winter conditions in the Southern Adriatic Sea (NE Mediterranean). J Mar Sci Eng 8(8):567
45. Ibrahim O, El-Geziry TM, Khedr A, El-Din KA (2023) Impacts of recent development processes on the temporal and spatial sea-level variations along the Suez Canal. Region Stud Mar Sci 66:103120
46. Isinibilir M, Aker V, Türkeri EE (2022) Summer distribution and community structure of surface water mesozooplankton from the eastern Mediterranean Sea. Oceanol Hydrobiol Stud 51(4):308–324
47. Kalloniati K, Christou ED, Kournopoulou A, Gittings JA, Theodorou I, Zervoudaki S, Raitsos DE (2023) Long-term warming and human-induced plankton shifts at a coastal Eastern Mediterranean site. Sci Rep 13(1):21068
48. Kimor B, Wood EJF (1975) A plankton study in the Eastern Mediterranean Sea. Mar Biol 29:321–333. https://doi.org/10.1007/BF00388852
49. Koutsidi M, Moukas C, Tzanatos E (2020) Trait-based life strategies, ecological niches, and niche overlap in the nekton of the data-poor Mediterranean Sea. Ecol Evol 10(14):7129–7144
50. Lakkis S (1990) Composition, diversite et successions des copepodes planctoniques des eaux libanaises (Mediterrane e orientale). Oceanol Acta 13:489–501
51. Lakkis S, Zeidane R (2004) Exotic species and lessepsian migration of plankton in Lebanese waters, Levantine Basin, Eastern Mediterranean. Rapp Comm Int Mer Medit 37:384
52. Lakkis S (1976) Consideration on the distribution of pelagic copepods Mediterranean off the coast of Lebanon. Acta Adriat 18:39–52
53. Lepoint G, Hyndes GA (2022) Tropicalization of seagrass macrophytodetritus accumulations and associated food webs. Front Mar Sci 9:943841
54. Linnaeus C (1758) Systema Naturae per regna tria naturae, secundum classes, ordines, genera, species, cum characteribus, differentiis, synonymis, locis. Editio decima, reformata [10th revised edition], vol 1. Laurentius Salvius, Holmiae, 824 p

55. Lázaro-Lobo A, Moles AT, Fried G, Verloove F, Antonio Campos J, Herrera M, Goñi E, Bioret F, Buffa G, Fantinato E, Sentinella A (2021) Phenotypic differentiation among native, expansive and introduced populations influences invasion success. J Biogeogr 48(11):2907–2918
56. Madl P (2001). Essay about the phenomenon of Lessepsian Migration. Mar BiolI, Colloquial Meeting of Marine
57. Makris CV, Tolika K, Baltikas VN, Velikou K, Krestenitis YN (2023) The impact of climate change on the storm surges of the Mediterranean Sea: coastal sea level responses to deep depression atmospheric systems. Ocean Model 181:102149
58. Mansour AF, El-Naggar NA, El-Naggar HA, Zakaria HY, Abo-Senna FM (2020) Temporal and spatial variations of zooplankton distribution in the Eastern Harbor, Alexandria, Egypt. Egypt J Aq Biol Fish 24(4):421–435
59. Mavruk S, Toslak C, Yalım FB, Ütük AE, Aktaş Ö, Yılmaz ŞS, Kara A, Yüksek A (2023) Contribution of integrative taxonomy of ichthyoplankton to knowledge on mesopelagic fish biodiversity in the Northeastern Mediterranean. Mar Biodivers 53(1):7
60. Menéndez-Guerrero PA, Green DM, Davies TJ (2020) Climate change and the future restructuring of Neotropical anuran biodiversity. Ecography 43(2):222–235
61. Mohanchander P, Ashiq Ur Rahman M, Premdass K, Lyla PS, Ajmal Khan S (2020) Distribution, morphology and genetic validation of Saurida pseudotumbil Dutt & Sagar, 1981 (Teleostei: Synodontidae) from Indian waters. J Aq Biol Fish 8:18–21
62. Mutlu E, Miglietta C, Meo ID, Deval MC (2022) Spatiotemporal and bioecological distribution of four commercial Mullid species in an ultraoligotrophic Mediterranean gulf. Turk J Zool 46(6):484–499
63. Mutlu E, Meo ID, Miglietta C, Deval MC (2023) Ecological indicative stressors of native vs. non-native fish in an ultra-oligotrophic region of the Mediterranean sea. Sustainability 15(3):2726
64. Nival P, Lombard F, Cuzin J, Goy J, Stemmann L (2020) Zooplankton II. Macroplankton and long-term series. The Mediterranean sea in the era of global change 2: 30 years of multidisciplinary study of the Ligurian Sea, pp 109–146
65. Orfanidis S, Alvito A, Azzurro E, Badreddine ALI, Souissi JB, Chamorro M, Crocetta F, Dalyan CEM, Fortič ANA, Galanti L, Geyran K (2021) New alien Mediterranean biodiversity records (March 2021). Mediterr Mar Sci 22(1):180–198
66. Öztürk B (2021) Non-indigenous species in the Mediterranean and the Black Sea. General Fisheries Commission for the Mediterranean. Stud Rev (87):I-89
67. O'Toole C, Phillips KP, Bradley C, Coughlan J, Dillane E, Fleming IA, Reed TE, Westley PA, Cross TF, McGinnity P, Prodöhl PA (2021) Population genetics reveal patterns of natural colonisation of an ecologically and commercially important invasive fish. Can J Fish Aquat Sci 78(10):1497–1511
68. Pacheco D, Araújo GS, Cotas J, Gaspar R, Neto JM, Pereira L (2020) Invasive seaweeds in the Iberian Peninsula: a contribution for food supply. Mar Drugs 18(11):560
69. Pastor F, Valiente JA, Khodayar S (2020) A warming Mediterranean: 38 years of increasing sea surface temperature. Rem Sens 12(17):2687
70. Patania A, Mutlu E (2021) Spatiotemporal and ecological distribution of megabenthic crustaceans on the shelf-shelf break of Antalya Gulf, the eastern Mediterranean Sea. Mediterr Mar Sci 22(3):446–465
71. Pilowsky JA, Colwell RK, Rahbek C, Fordham DA (2022) Process-explicit models reveal the structure and dynamics of biodiversity patterns. Sci Adv 8(31):p.eabj2271
72. Pisano A, Marullo S, Artale V, Falcini F, Yang C, Leonelli FE, Santoleri R, Buongiorno Nardelli B (2020) New evidence of Mediterranean climate change and variability from sea surface temperature observations. Rem Sens 12(1):132
73. Protopapa M, Zervoudaki S, Tsangaris C, Velaoras D, Koppelmann R, Psarra S, Möllmann C (2019) Zooplankton distribution, growth and respiration in the Cretan Passage, Eastern Mediterranean. Deep Sea Res Part II 164:156–169
74. Ragkousis M, Zenetos A, Souissi JB, Hoffman R, Ghanem R, Taşkın E, Muresan M, Karpova E, Slynko E, Dağlı E, Fortič A (2023) Unpublished Mediterranean and Black Sea records of marine alien, cryptogenic, and neonative species

75. Van Rijn I, Kiflawi M, Belmaker J (2020) Alien species stabilize local fisheries catch in a highly invaded ecosystem. Can J Fish Aquat Sci 77(4):752–761
76. Sandonnini J, Ruso YDP, Melendreras EC, Barberá C, Hendriks IE, Kersting DK, Casalduero FG (2021) The emergent fouling population after severe eutrophication in the Mar Menor coastal lagoon. Region Stud Mar Sci 44:101720
77. Sayinli B, Dong Y, Park Y, Bhatnagar A, Sillanpää M (2022) Recent progress and challenges facing ballast water treatment–a review. Chemosphere 291:132776
78. Shakman EA (2008) Lessepsian migrant fish species of the coastal waters of Libya: Status, biology, ecology. Doctoral dissertation, Rostock, University, Dissertation
79. Shapiro Goldberg D, Rilov G, Villéger S, Belmaker J (2021) Predation cues lead to reduced foraging of invasive siganus rivulatus in the Mediterranean. Front Mar Sci 8:678848
80. Spanier E, Zviely D (2022) Key environmental impacts along the Mediterranean coast of Israel in the last 100 years. J Mar Sci Eng 11(1):2
81. Steger J, Bošnjak M, Belmaker J, Galil BS, Zuschin M, Albano PG (2022) Non-indigenous molluscs in the Eastern Mediterranean have distinct traits and cannot replace historic ecosystem functioning. Glob Ecol Biogeogr 31(1):89–102
82. Steger J, Dunne B, Zuschin M, Albano PG (2021) Bad neighbors? Niche overlap and asymmetric competition between native and Lessepsian limpets in the Eastern Mediterranean rocky intertidal. Mar Pollut Bull 171:112703
83. Tsadok R, Zemah-Shamir Z, Shemesh E, Martinez S, Ramon D, Kolski I, Tsemel A, Tchernov D (2023) Dietary habits change of Lessepsian migrants' fish from the Red Sea to the Eastern Mediterranean Sea. Aquat Invasions 18(4):521–531
84. Tsirintanis K, Azzurro E, Crocetta F, Dimiza M, Froglia C, Gerovasileiou V, Langeneck J, Mancinelli G, Rosso A, Stern N, Triantaphyllou M (2022) Bioinvasion impacts on biodiversity, ecosystem services, and human health in the Mediterranean Sea. Aquat Invasions 17(3):308–352
85. Tüzün S, Gücü AC (2023) Diet variations of Striped Piggy, Pomadasys stridens (Forsskål, 1775) (Teleostei: Haemulidae) in the northeastern Mediterranean Sea. Region Stud Mar Sci 66:103129
86. Velasquez X, Morov AR, Kurt TT, Meron D, Guy-Haim T (2021) Two-way bioinvasion: tracking the neritic non-native cyclopoid copepods Dioithona oculata and Oithona davisae (Oithonidae) in the Eastern Mediterranean Sea. Mediterr Mar Sci 22(3):586–602
87. Winters G, Beer S, Willette DA, Viana IG, Chiquillo KL, Beca-Carretero P, Villamayor B, Azcárate-García T, Shem-Tov R, Mwabvu B, Migliore L (2020) The tropical seagrass Halophila stipulacea: reviewing what we know from its native and invasive habitats, alongside identifying knowledge gaps. Front Mar Sci 7:300
88. Yalgin F, Türker A (2023) Determination of fish diversity in the northern coasts of Cyprus (eastern Mediterranean) by visual census method. Marine Sci Technol Bull 12(1):111–122
89. Yeruham E, Shpigel M, Abelson A, Rilov G (2020) Ocean warming and tropical invaders erode the performance of a key herbivore. Ecology 101(2):e02925
90. Zaghloul WS, Madkour FF, Mohammad SH (2020) Marine gelatinous zooplankton of the Egyptian waters: a review. Egypt J Aquaculture 10(2):35–45
91. Zakaria HY (2006) The zooplankton community in Egyptian Mediterranean waters: a review. Acta Adriat 47(2):195–206
92. Zakaria HY (2015) Article review: Lessepsian migration of zooplankton through Suez Canal and its impact on ecological system. Egypt J Aq Res 41(2):129–144
93. Zakaria HY, Hassan AKM, El-Naggar HA, Abo-Senna FM (2018) Planktonic protozoan population in the Southeastern Mediterranean off Egypt. Egypt J Aq Res 44(2):101–107
94. Zenetos A, Galanidi M (2020) Mediterranean non indigenous species at the start of the 2020s: recent changes. Marine Biodiv Records 13(1):1–17

95. Zenetos A, Albano PG, Garcia EL, Stern N, Tsiamis K, Galanidi M (2022) Established non-indigenous species increased by 40% in 11 years in the Mediterranean Sea. Mediterr Mar Sci 23(1)
96. Zenetos A, Ovalis P, Giakoumi S, Kontadakis C, Lefkaditou E, Mpazios G, Simboura N, Tsiamis K (2020) Saronikos Gulf: a hotspot area for alien species in the Mediterranean Sea. BioInvasions Record 9(4)

Climate Challenges and Resilience Strategies in Egypt's Agriculture and Aquatic Resources

Impact of Climate Change on Water Resources

Mahmoud A. Abu-Zeid, Khaled M. Abu-Zeid, and Mary K. Halim

Abstract Water, or the so-called "Blue Gold," as an indispensable life-giving natural resource, holds significant value and plays a vital role in supporting various life forms and ensuring survival. Nevertheless, it is crucial to acknowledge that freshwater resources are inherently finite, particularly in arid and semi-arid regions. Consequently, conservation and effective governance of these resources assume paramount importance. Climate change (CC) has a direct and indirect impact on the water cycle, influencing both the quantity and quality of water resources required to satisfy the increasing demands of both human livelihoods and ecosystems. It has the potential to contribute to the occurrence of repetitive flooding and drought events, as well as the elevation of sea levels, which can have significant impacts on coastal aquifers. Additionally, it may lead to heightened water temperatures, which can further exacerbate various types of water pollution. The challenges at hand will have significant consequences on various interrelated sectors, including the water, energy and agriculture sectors, public health, as well as the aquatic ecosystems. The demand for water to address these requirements is additionally influenced by climate change. It is apparent that embracing a comprehensive water-energy-food nexus approach, alongside advocating for the utilization of non-conventional water resources, can effectively facilitate the shift towards sustainability. This observation holds significant relevance for national interests, thereby serving as a potential catalyst for active involvement from governments, the private sector, and civil society. The present chapter aims at emphasizing the influence of the climate change extreme events on water resources by examining the close interconnections between climate patterns, freshwater availability, and the biophysical and socio-economic systems at

M. A. Abu-Zeid
Arab Water Council and Ministry of Water Resources and Irrigation, Cairo, Egypt
e-mail: president@arabwatercouncil.org

M. A. Abu-Zeid · K. M. Abu-Zeid
CEDARE and Arab Water Council, Cairo, Egypt
e-mail: kabuzeid@cedare.int; kabuzeid@arabwatercouncil.org

M. K. Halim (✉)
Arab Water Council, Cairo, Egypt
e-mail: maryhalim@arabwatercouncil.org

© The Author(s), under exclusive license to Springer Nature Switzerland AG 2025
M. T. Khalil et al. (eds.), *Climate Changes Impacts on Aquatic Environment*, Earth and Environmental Sciences Library, https://doi.org/10.1007/978-3-031-74897-4_5

both global and regional levels. Additionally, it aims to present advanced technologies and comprehensive solutions to appropriately mitigate the effects of climate change and adapt to them. Furthermore, the chapter aims to enhance the livelihoods of societies who are especially vulnerable to climate change effects, towards attaining climate-resilient communities with the overarching objective of achieving sustainable development in line with the aspired future, while ensuring inclusivity for all individuals. The topic of climate change and its impact on non-conventional water resources is certainly becoming of great importance in the field of environmental studies. It is crucial to explore strategies for both adaptation and mitigation to promote sustainable development to surmount these challenges.

Keywords Climate change · Non-conventional water resources · Adaptation · Mitigation · Sustainable development

1 Introduction

Water plays a crucial role in sustaining various life forms and ensuring their survival. Freshwater resources are becoming increasingly scarce, particularly in arid and semi-arid regions, thereby necessitating stringent methods for safeguarding and properly managing these resources. The effective management of freshwater resources with special focus on sustainability necessitates a holistic view of the intricate interconnections between climate patterns, freshwater availability, and the interplay of biophysical and socio-economic systems. These interconnections operate at various scales, globally, regionally, as well as locally.

In recent years, there has been a notable rise in global average air temperatures and oceanic temperatures, as extensively referenced by the Intergovernmental Panel on Climate Change (IPCC). The frequently occurring heat waves are believed to be significant evidence of climate change, and it is already yielding serious implications on the water resources, with potentially more severe consequences anticipated in the future. In addition to these consequences, it is important to consider the compounding factors of population growth, land-use changes, and urbanization, all of which contribute to the increasing demands for basic needs of water and energy. Furthermore, the continuously escalating living conditions, the evolving agricultural practices, the expanding industrial activities, and the heightened pollution levels further exacerbate the situation. It is also crucial to acknowledge the impact of changing economic activities in this context. It is highly probable that these factors will have negative implications on the water resources. Additionally, it is worth noting that human activities have the potential to pose significant challenges to the availability of freshwater, both in terms of quantity (excessive or insufficient) and quality. The present chapter provides a concise overview of climate change, with special focus on its drivers and influence on water resources at both global and regional levels. The case of the Arab region is specially highlighted, being recognized as the most water-stressed area globally and particularly exposed to the risk of climate change hazards.

2 Climate Change Hazard: Definition and Causes

The proper functioning of natural ecosystems is typically influenced by the climatic patterns that characterize a given region. These patterns can be effectively determined and analyzed by examining such hydro-meteorological variables as temperature, rainfall, moisture content, and airstream velocity [44]. IPCC defined climate change (CC) as "changes in the climate properties that typically persist for decades or longer, due to natural internal or external drivers, or to persistent human interventions and anthropogenic changes in the atmospheric composition or in land use" (IPCC 2022).

According to the UN Framework Convention on Climate Change [43], CC is "the change of climate conditions attributed directly or indirectly to human interventions that alter the composition of the global atmosphere and that are observed over comparable time periods." The American Meteorological Society [1] defines climate change as "any systematic long-term change in the climate components (such as temperature, pressure, or wind velocity) spanning over several decades or longer. Climate change may be due to natural external drivers—such as fluctuations in solar emissions or slight changes in the Earth's orbital features—as well as natural internal processes of the climate system, or human interference."

The compelling forces of climate change disasters are multi-faceted, resulting from the complex interactions among the various systems of the Earth, including the atmosphere, water bodies and land. These changes can arise either from natural processes or human activities, or both, which, in turn, influence such factors as greenhouse gas (GHG) concentrations, aerosol intensities, land use/land cover areas, and solar emission, among others. Moreover, these factors impact the absorption, scattering, and emission of radiation all over the globe in the upper atmosphere and at the Earth's surface.

According to Singh et al. [34], the observed warming in recent decades can primarily be attributed to the escalation in greenhouse gas emissions caused by anthropogenic interventions. Since the onset of the industrial era, estimated to have begun around the year 1750, it can be observed that human intrusions have had an apparent influence on the Earth's climate, predominantly resulting in a warming trend. The primary greenhouse gases, such as carbon dioxide (CO_2), methane (CH_4), nitrous oxide (N_2O), and the halocarbons, are known to be the consequences of man-made undertakings, with tendency to accumulate in the atmosphere, and concentration in the rise over time, as demonstrated in Fig. 1.

The rise of CO_2 levels can be attributed to several significant factors, including the intensified utilization of fossil fuels in transportation, the warming and cooling of buildings, as well as the production of cement and several other commodities. Various human activities have been observed to contribute to the increase of CH_4

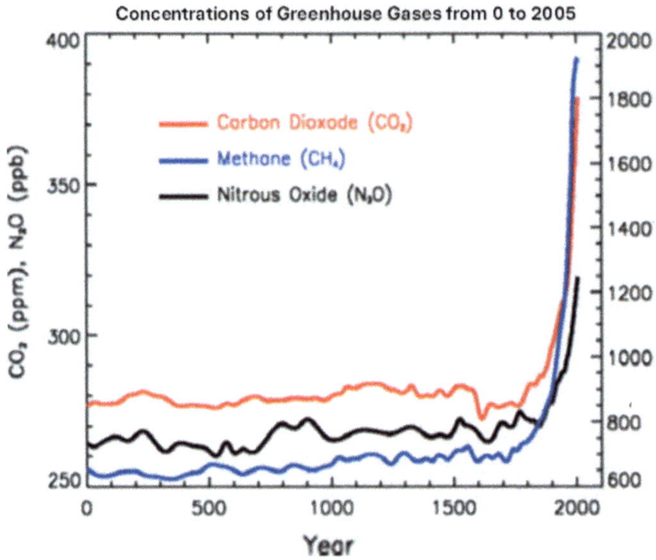

Fig. 1 Atmospheric concentrations of important greenhouse gases over 2000 years [34]. Concentration units are parts per million (ppm) and parts per billion (ppb)

levels, including agricultural procedures, natural gas distribution, and landfills. The rise of N_2O levels is attributed to the utilization of fertilizers and the combustion of fossil fuels. Notably, the utilization of the principal halocarbons, specifically chlorofluorocarbons, in various industrial applications such as refrigeration, has been observed to contribute to the depletion of stratospheric ozone.

The constantly mounting average surface temperature towards the end of the twentieth century, resulting from the emission of greenhouse gases (GHGs) caused by human interference, has already surpassed the critical threshold for various elements of the climate system. The prevailing climate policies place significant emphasis on implementing sustainable measures aimed at achieving long-term reductions in carbon dioxide emissions. It is noteworthy that even in the event of a complete cessation of CO_2 emissions, climate change implications are anticipated to extend for a long duration, spanning approximately 1000 years. Several conferences and fora have been organized worldwide and many institutions were established with the aim of devising strategies to address the negative consequences of climate change and explore innovative solutions for adaptation and mitigation. The UNFCCC, established in 1992, serves as a vital platform for policy development aimed at addressing the emerging climate change challenges. Its primary objective is to stabilize atmospheric greenhouse gases at a level that effectively mitigates the adverse impacts of human activities on the climate system.

The Kyoto Protocol, adopted in 1997, is widely recognized as a fundamental document in the realm of international climate change policy. It represents a crucial milestone as it introduced legally binding restrictions on carbon dioxide and other greenhouse gas emissions for industrialized nations [34].

By the year 2030, it is anticipated that climate change will be clearly manifested through decreased precipitation, significant elevation in average temperatures, and a heightened occurrence of seawater encroachment into coastal aquifers due to rising sea levels and on-going excessive extraction of groundwater. According to the United Nations Development Programme [40], it is anticipated that the phenomenon of urban heat effect, resulting from the process of urbanization, will lead to a projected rise of 3 °C in night-time temperatures.

3 Evidence of Climate Change

The following section examines the dynamic trends in temperature and precipitation indicating climate change phenomena:

(A) **Increases in Temperature**

There is strong evidence indicating that human undertakings have had an apparent influence on the warming of the Earth's atmosphere, biosphere, oceans, and land, where significant and swift variations have taken place on a global scale.

It is worth noting that each of the previous four decades has exhibited a consistent trend of increasing temperatures, exceeding the temperature levels of the preceding decades since the year 1850. According to the IPCC Sixth Assessment Report [24], there has been a marked increase in surface temperature on the global scale during the first two decades of the twenty-first century (2001–2020), amounting to approximately 0.99 (0.84–1.10) °C when compared to the period 1850–1900. The global surface temperature experienced a notable increase of 1.09 (0.95–1.20) °C during the period 2011–2020 in comparison to the reference period of 1850–1900. It is worth mentioning that the land areas witnessed a more substantial rise, with temperatures increasing by 1.59 (1.34–1.83) °C, while the oceanic regions experienced a comparatively lower increase of 0.88 (0.68–1.01) °C. The perceived rise in global surface temperature since the publishing of the 5th IPCC Assessment Report [25] can be primarily attributed to additional warming experienced between 2003 and 2012, with an estimated increase of +0.19 (0.16–0.22) °C. In addition, it is also to be observed that the updated estimate of warming in the IPCC AR6 report [24] was influenced by methodological advancements and the inclusion of new datasets, which in total added approximately 0.1 °C to the overall estimate.

Based on available data, it can be inferred that the probable range of global surface temperature rise by virtue of anthropological interference during the period 1850–1900 to 2010–2019 falls within the range of 0.8–1.3 °C, with a dominant estimate of 1.07 °C. It is plausible that the presence of well-mixed greenhouse gases (GHGs) has contributed to a temperature increase ranging from 1.0 to 2.0 °C. Additionally, various human factors, primarily aerosols, have had a cooling effect on global temperatures ranging from 0.0 to 0.8 °C. Nature-based compellers have caused a slight change in surface temperature worldwide, ranging from − 0.1 °C to + 0.1 °C. Furthermore, core in-house fluctuation has influenced global temperatures within a range of − 0.2 °C to + 0.2 °C. According to the findings of IPCC in the 6th Assessment Report [24], there is a strong likelihood that the increase in well-mixed greenhouse gases (GHGs) has been the primary factor driving tropospheric warming since 1979. Additionally, it is deemed highly probable that the depletion of stratospheric ozone caused by human activities has been the primary driver of cooling in the lower stratosphere from 1979 to the mid-1990s.

In accordance with the IPCC 5th Assessment Report [25], it is anticipated that on the Arab regional level, there will likely be a significant rise in the average annual temperatures in East Africa and the Maghreb states. This increase is projected to exceed 2 °C (°C), with the maximum estimated rise reaching up to 6 °C. These projections are calculated on the basis of the representative concentration pathways (RCP) 2.6 and RCP 8.5 emissions scenarios, respectively, and are expected to occur by the year 2100. According to the findings of the downscaled regional climate modelling conducted for the Arab Region, it has been observed that both models indicate comparable projections of temperature rise ranging from 0 to 2 °C during the period 2011–2041 [41].

(B) **Changes in Precipitation Patterns**

According to the comprehensive analysis conducted by IPCC in the 5th Assessment Report (AR5) published in 2014, there is substantial long-term observational evidence suggesting an apparent link between human activities and alterations in the water cycle since the 1960s. These noticeable signs of human impact can be observed in the atmospheric moisture content, global alterations of precipitation patterns over land, and the more recurrent intensive precipitation phenomena in regions where robust data networks are available. The findings of the IPCC AR5 Report also emphasize the high degree of confidence in the observation that global surface air-specific humidity has experienced a notable increase since the 1970s.

The research conducted by Collins et al. (2013) primarily focused on the examination of various aspects of the water cycle projections, including water vapor, precipitation, surface evaporation, runoff, and snowpack. It is widely acknowledged in academic spheres that there is a high level of confidence in the projection that global precipitation will increase due to global warming. As indicated in the IPCC 5th Assessment Report [25], there may be a potential increase in precipitation exceeding 50% in certain Tropical and Polar Regions approaching the late twenty-first century. On the other hand, there is a likelihood of a decrease in precipitation of 30% or more in significant subtropical areas. In general, there is a noticeable disparity in the average annual precipitation in arid regions compared to humid ones and in dry seasons compared to wet ones. This phenomenon, commonly referred to as the "wet get wetter, dry get drier" pattern, is expected to intensify across a significant portion of the globe, with a high certainty level.

The projected surface evaporation change is expected to exhibit a predominantly positive trend across most oceanic regions, aligning with the general pattern of precipitation change observed over land areas.

In essence, it can be generally observed that there is a correlation between rising temperatures and increased precipitation levels. This phenomenon can be attributed to the fact that warm air has the capacity to retain higher amounts of water vapor. Specifically, a temperature increase of 1 °F can result in a notable rise of approximately 4% in atmospheric water vapor content. Additional factors may also influence precipitation patterns, such as the climatic phenomena known as El Niño and La Niña.

The main concern of heavy precipitation events is frequently highlighted as a prominent focus in reports and assessments examining climate variations, including, for example, those pertaining to the United States. In this arena, the U.S. Global Change Research Program (USGCRP) Indicator Platform, available at http://www.globalchange.gov/browse/indicators, and the reports published by the Environmental Protection Agency (EPA) on climate indicators, accessible at https://www.epa.gov/climate-indicators, are valuable resources for gaining insights into global change and environmental trends.

Regarding the regional perspective, it is observed that precipitation projections exhibit a higher degree of variability compared to temperature projections. It is anticipated that there may be a decrease in precipitation of approximately 40% in the North Africa region towards the termination of the 21st Century. A notable reduction in overall precipitation and the frequency of wet days has been witnessed in North Africa. The incidence of irregular and inadequate rainfall is further aggravated by the presence of extreme temperatures, as referenced by the UNDP [40].

Climate change is certainly a matter of substantial developmental importance for the countries in the Nile Basin region. The average yearly precipitation in the Nile basin region is calculated to be approximately 650 mm. There is considerable variation in rainfall patterns across different countries, characterized by contrasting levels of precipitation. For instance, Egypt experiences relatively low levels of rainfall, while Ethiopia and the countries situated in the Equatorial Lakes Plateau region receive comparatively higher amounts of rainfall. Egypt is known for having a relatively low amount of precipitation compared to other countries. The potential impact of rising temperatures in the Nile Basin region, accompanied by increased evaporation rates and growing water demands, is expected to have implications for the downstream water availability of the Nile. There exists a potential for a notable decrease in Nile streamflow due to climate change, resulting principally from alterations in precipitation patterns. However, it is important to note that studies on this matter have presented conflicting outcomes. The impacts of coastal zones and water resources on agriculture are of significant concern. One prominent consequence is the adverse impact of rising seawater levels on the prime agricultural land in the Nile Delta, which can lead to both inundation and salinization and pose a serious threat to agricultural productivity. Additionally, according to observations highlighted by OECD, any decrease in the availability of Nile water would have detrimental effects on the intensive irrigated agriculture upstream.

4 Climate Change Impacts on the Water Cycle

CC has been observed to have indisputable effects on water resources, quantitatively and qualitatively. CC has demonstrated and is expected to continue to demonstrate influence on the water cycle both directly and indirectly. This influence is manifested in alterations in the precipitation and evaporation cycles, as well as changes in consumption patterns. In turn, evolving consumption patterns and economic development may very likely lead to an increase in demand for water supply.

Throughout history, human societies have consistently encountered challenges of uncertainty and variability in climatic conditions. Water is widely recognized as a crucial resource for sustaining life, fostering sustainable economic development, and facilitating the proper functioning of ecosystems. However, it is an undeniable fact that the availability of water is limited in nature and that extreme climate change events would certainly influence the timing, magnitude, and duration of rainfall and other weather events.

The available evidence strongly suggests that climate variability has experienced a notable increase, hence lowering the confidence in the predictability of water availability due to the shifting and intensification of weather extremes. Consequently, this causes a high uncertainty level regarding the quantity as well as the timing of the water supplies, both on the short- and long-terms. Climate change is commonly considered as a driving factor influencing the supply-side dynamics, which will ultimately shape the availability of water resources.

It is, hence, imperative that the interplay between human demands on water supply (demand-side drivers) and the escalating climate change implications on natural climate patterns should be effectively addressed and managed. The demand-side motivators encompass various socio-economic and demographic pressures, which are influenced by a multitude of factors ranging from technological advancements to institutional and financial circumstances. The management of such 'demand-side drivers' will have significant effects on the climate-related aspects.

4.1 Direct Impacts of Climate Change on the Water Sector

Climate change recurrent extreme phenomena have been detected to have a direct influence on the natural water cycle, causing significant alterations in the quantity and quality of water resources that are crucial for satisfying the increasing demands of both human livelihoods and ecosystems. CC has the potential to contribute to the occurrence of repetitive flooding and drought events, as well as the rise of seawater levels, which can have significant impacts on coastal aquifers that serve as vital water sources for both urban and rural water supply systems. Additionally, the increase in water temperatures and alterations in extreme weather events can potentially intensify various types of water pollution. The changes to the water cycle are anticipated to have significant implications for various interrelated sectors, including water, energy and agriculture sectors, public health, as well as aquatic ecosystems. Climate change has been observed to influence the demand for water to fulfill these needs. The importance of water in fostering sustainable socio-economic development should not be underestimated, yet many countries are currently confronted with a range of water-related challenges, which are further intensified by the consequence of climate change.

The potential CC implications on the water cycle may result in certain regions experiencing decreased precipitation, leading to the transformation of these areas into arid or semi-arid regions and in extreme cases, even desertification. Such potential alterations in water cycles pose a serious risk to the viability of the fragile ecosystems in these areas, thereby jeopardizing the livelihoods of individuals reliant on the invaluable natural resources derived from these ecosystems. Currently, it is evident that a significant portion, exceeding 40% of the Earth's land resources are situated in drylands, encompassing sub-humid, semi-arid, and arid regions. Such zones face imminent challenges posed by the degradation of land and the desertification process. According to the United Nations Convention to Combat Desertification [31], CC has significant direct implications for approximately 250 million individuals while indirectly affecting over a billion people. It is quite expected that the coping mechanisms employed by individuals experiencing recurring episodes of water scarcity may gradually lose their effectiveness or become less suitable in view of the evolving environmental circumstances. The protection of local biodiversity, which plays a crucial role in the long-term viability of ecosystems, may consequently face additional challenges.

It is meanwhile anticipated that various regions will encounter significant rises in the occurrence of disasters, including instances of flooding resulting from the impact of typhoons and hurricanes. Excessive precipitation can potentially surpass the capacity of water channels, leading to the occurrence of flooding events. This phenomenon constitutes a damaging risk to the solidity and cohesion of the water infrastructures as well as the various ecosystems. Evidently, the climate-induced alteration of water cycles will affect the various aspects of the ecosystem, including food production, land utilization, and the survival of plant and animal species.

It is, hence, a must, not an option, to consider climate change when formulating water management strategies, in view of its potential to promote heightened levels of uncertainty and unpredictability in the availability of water resources.

The following section will present the various ways in which climate change directly affects Water Resources, specifically in terms of runoff, floods, droughts, snowmelt and glacier melt, sea-water rise, water quality, groundwater, transboundary waters, agriculture, and ecosystems.

(A) **Runoff**

According to climate projections, as referenced by Singh et al. [34], climate change is expected to pose a remarkable influence on the hydrological system, resulting in potential consequences on river flows and water resources on the regional scale. The occurrence of flooding patterns in space and time can be attributed to the inherent variability in climate. Numerous studies have been conducted to investigate potential patterns in river discharge measurements at various spatial scales. These studies have revealed that certain indicators of flow exhibit noteworthy trends while also establishing statistically significant associations with temperature or precipitation patterns. Furthermore, it is worth noting that human activities have had an undeniable impact on the flow patterns within various catchments worldwide. Extensive research suggests that there is a discernible trend in the alteration of yearly runoff, with certain areas witnessing an increase in runoff, such as high latitudes and certain wide-ranging areas of the United States. Conversely, other regions, including parts of, southern Europe, South America, and West Africa, have experienced a decrease in runoff [28].

The mean runoff change until 2060, as depicted in Fig. 2, is derived from the IPCC Special Report on Emissions Scenario [16], which incorporates data from a comprehensive ensemble of 24 climate model runs. Documented observations regarding changes in runoff patterns in various regions indicated that, in North America's high latitudes, there has been an evident increase in runoff ranging from 10 to 40%. Conversely, in the western USA/northern Mexico, southern Africa, and the Mediterranean, a decrease in runoff ranging from 10 to 30% has been observed. In general, it is anticipated that there will be an expansion of areas experiencing decreased runoff between the late twentieth century and the year 2050.

(B) **Floods**

Floods have been observed to have a considerable impact on the economies of vulnerable regions. This phenomenon is widely recognized as a frequently occurring natural hazard in various parts of the world, with climate change being identified as an aggravating factor [34]. Various factors promote the occurrence of flooding, mainly including heavy rainfall, torrential rain, and snowmelt. The spatial distribution of these factors since 1985 is depicted in Fig. 3. Severe inundations resulting from heavy rainfall—whether of extended or abbreviated duration—have been observed

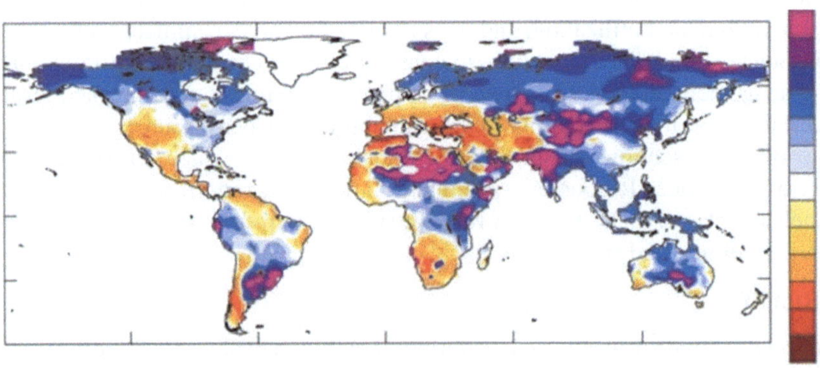

Fig. 2 Annual runoff variation for the period 2041–2060 as compared to 1900–1970, in percentage, according to IPCC SRES A1B Emissions Scenario [28]

in nearly all regions characterized by high humidity, as well as certain semi-arid areas.

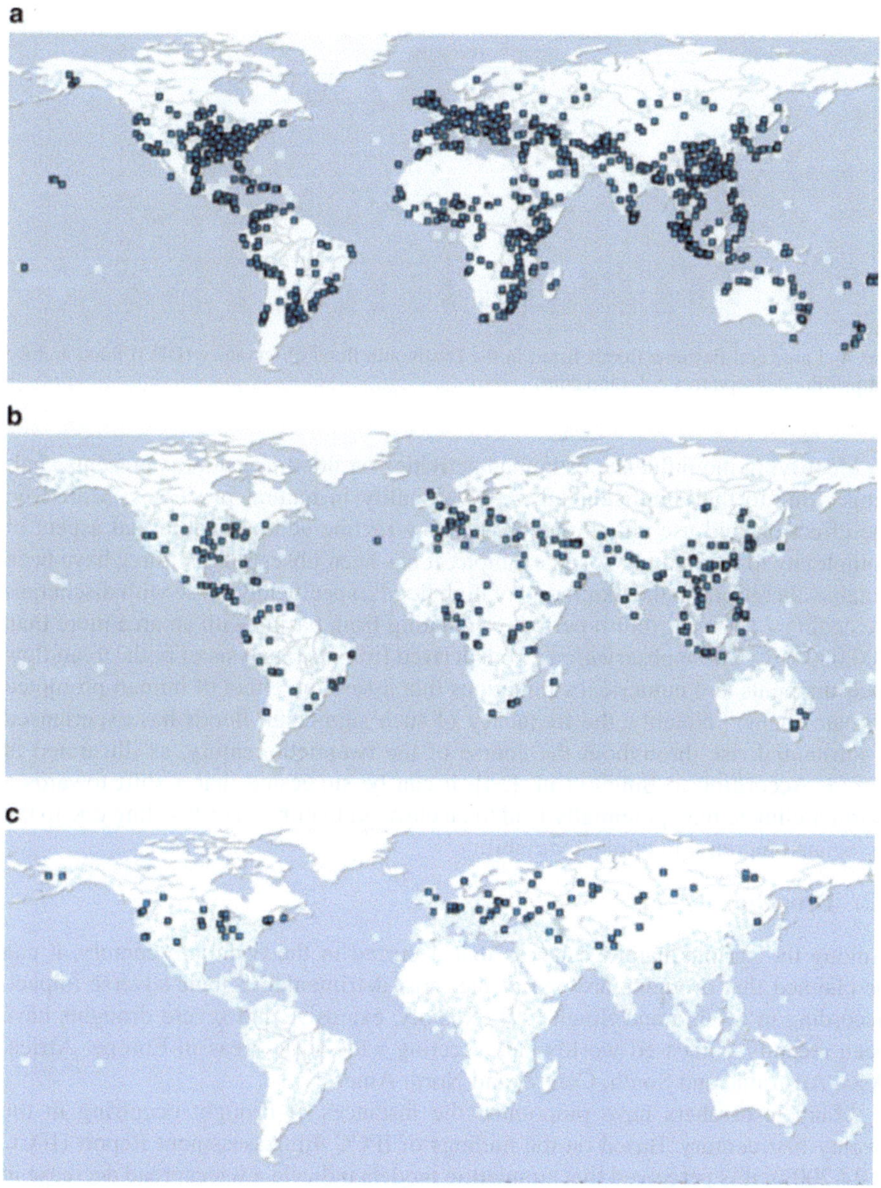

Fig. 3 Spatial distribution of extreme floods from three different sources as referenced by Dartmouth Flood Observatory since 1985: **a** heavy rain **b** brief torrential rain **c** Snowmelt (http://www.dartmouth.edu/~floods/archiveatlas/floodcauselocation.htm) [34]

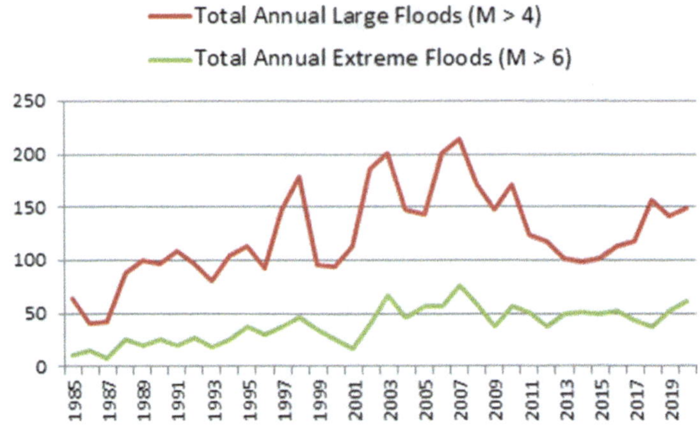

Fig. 4 Large and Extreme floods listed in the Dartmouth flood observatory (DFO) flood archive (https://floodobservatory.colorado.edu/)

Identifying the influence of human activities on flooding patterns presents challenges due to the significant inherent variability in natural processes. Moreover, the effect of land-use alterations on the flow regime adds an additional aspect of complexity to this matter. As an example, it has been observed that there have been notable alterations in the likelihood of high floods, specifically those with discharges exceeding a 100-year return period, originating from basins with an area more than 200,000 km^2. These observations were derived from the analysis of both streamflow measurements and numerical simulations that assess the effect of human-prompted climate change. Notably, the frequency of such significant floods has experienced a substantial rise throughout the course of the twentieth century, as illustrated in Fig. 4. According to Singh et al. [34], it can be suggested that a shift towards a warmer climate may potentially lead to an elevated likelihood of flooding due to the associated increase in climate variability.

(C) **Drought**

Among the various natural hazards that occurred in the twentieth century, it can be claimed that droughts are one of the most detrimental in their adverse impact, according to Mishra and Singh [29]. Notably, extensive and severe droughts have been recently witnessed worldwide, affecting wide-scale areas in Europe, Africa, Asia, Australia, and South, Central and North America.

Many researchers have pinpointed the instances of drought occurring in the twenty-first century. Based on the findings of IPCC 4th Assessment Report (IPCC AR4 2007), it is perceived that simulation models indicate a widespread decrease in moisture levels across most terrestrial regions, a trend that raises concerns regarding the potential occurrence of a global agricultural drought phenomenon towards the end of the century. According to the findings of Singh et al. [34], all model scenarios

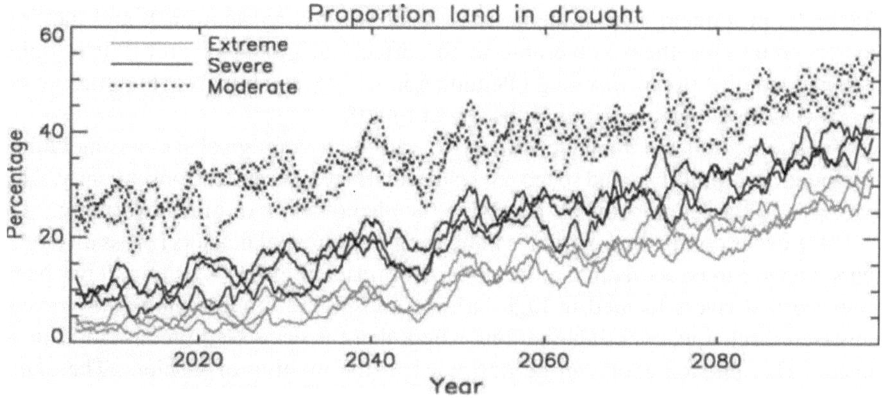

Fig. 5 Proportion of land area in drought for the twenty-first century according to the results from IPCC emissions scenario [34]

indicate a projected decline in soil moisture levels, suggesting that severe soil moisture deficits are expected to expand by double their spatial extent and frequency of occurrence in case of short-term droughts that last for 4–6 months, while long-term droughts lasting over 12 months are anticipated to become three times more prevalent from the mid-twentieth century to the late twenty-first century.

Based on the available data, it is anticipated that there will be a notable rise in the percentage of land area affected by drought in the coming decades. This upward trend is expected to persist throughout the entirety of the twenty-first century, as illustrated in Fig. 5.

Based on the findings presented in the IPCC AR6 Technical Summary [7, 17, 18], it is indicated that there is a projected escalation in drought risks and associated societal harm as global temperatures rise. According to IPCC projections, it is anticipated that a proportion of the population, reaching up to 7%, will potentially be exposed to low total water storage levels, ranging from extreme to exceptional conditions over the course of the twenty-first century. It is also predicted that, by the year 2100, aridity zones may potentially experience an expansion of approximately 25% compared to their spatial extent in 1990.

In recent years, the Arab region, as example, has experienced a notable increase in the occurrence of drought cycles, with frequency and severity that surpassed historical records spanning several centuries within the region. Based on the findings of IPCC, it has been observed that a significant proportion, approximately over 40%, of the Arab region residents encountered adverse climatic events, including droughts, which resulted in various consequences such as food insecurity, erosion of livelihoods, and displacement of a considerable number of people, as highlighted by the UN Habitat report [30].

(D) **Snowmelt and Glacier Melt**

Numerous prominent river systems worldwide are fed by snowpack and melting glaciers, rendering them vulnerable to the effects of global warming. It is quite expected that the global warming phenomenon will exert a remarkable influence on the process of snowmelt and the subsequent runoff.

Glaciers exhibit a notable sensitivity to various hydrological factors, including precipitation, humidity, wind speed, and particularly temperature. Consequently, they serve as a valuable indicator for assessing the phenomenon of global warming.

There exists compelling evidence indicating the retreat of glaciers across all continents, which can be accredited to the apparent impact of global warming. It has been observed that rivers located in high-latitude and high-altitude regions may reveal increased discharge, even in situations where there is decreased precipitation incidences. This phenomenon can be attributed to the melting of glaciers. The alteration in the magnitude and temporal patterns of discharge can potentially lead to notable fluvial geomorphological transformations in river systems, including the widening and deepening of channels, increased meandering and bank erosion, as well as accelerated channel migration [34].

The quantification of societal impacts resulting from retreating glaciers is quite a challenging procedure. The agricultural sector, domestic water supply, and hydroelectric power generation greatly rely on major rivers that receive significant contributions from glacial meltwater. Hence, if the necessary infrastructure is not adequately established, it is plausible that the augmented water resulting from glacial melting could potentially give rise to significant flooding or droughts as the temporal patterns of runoff undergo alterations.

(E) **Sea Level Rise**

The phenomenon of mean sea level rise on the global scale can be attributed to the climate system heating, which has resulted in ice loss on land and thermal expansion due to ocean warming [25]. The phenomenon of thermal expansion was found to account for approximately 50% of the detected sea level rise during the years 1971 to 2018. Additionally, the share of glacier ice loss was estimated to be around 22%, while ice sheets accounted for approximately 20% of the detected sea level rise. Variations in land–water storage were found to contribute approximately 8% to the overall sea level rise during this period. The rate of ice-sheet loss experienced a remarkable four-fold increase between 1992–1999 and 2010–2019. During the period 2006 to 2018, the combined effects of ice-sheet and glacier mass loss emerged as the primary drivers influencing the rise in global mean sea level rise.

It is highly probable that the global mean sea level will experience a sustained increase throughout the twenty-first century because of on-going climate warming. This rise is expected to persist for centuries to millennia, primarily driven by the absorption of heat by the deep ocean and the loss of mass from ice sheets (IPCC AR6 2023).

It is quite anticipated that coastal risks will substantially increase throughout the twenty-first century because of the predicted rise in sea levels. This rise will have major implications on various aspects, including ecosystems, human populations, living conditions, basic infrastructure, food security, cultural and natural traditions,

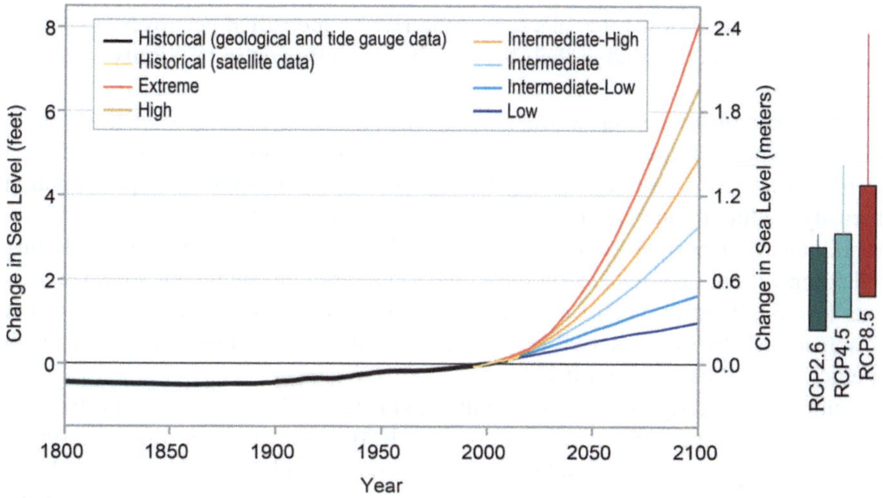

Fig. 6 Historical and projected global average sea level rise. *Source* NCA [30]. https://nca2018.globalchange.gov/downloads. Figure revised in June 2019

and climate mitigation efforts in coastal regions. The challenges associated with urban areas and coastal communities are already being encountered, and they are projected to intensify by 2050 and persist beyond 2100, irrespective of any pause in global warming. According to the Sixth Assessment Report of the Intergovernmental Panel on Climate Change [7, 17, 18], it is projected that by the year 2100, there will be a yearly occurrence of extreme sea level events that have been historically rare, a fact that is expected to further exacerbate the associated risks.

Figure 6 illustrates the historical and projected global average Sea Level Rise from year 1800–2100.

In the United States, certain regions are particularly susceptible to sea-level rise, such as the mid-Atlantic and south-Atlantic states, which are characterized by their low-lying topography and relatively high occurrence of storms. Additionally, the Gulf Coast is also threatened owing to its low-lying topography and the rapid subsidence of its land.

Numerous investigations have been conducted to explore the effects of Sea Level Rise (SLR) on the Nile Delta coastal zones in Egypt. The research conducted by Elshinnawy et al. [12] utilized areal surveying maps to generate a digital elevation model (DEM) for the Nile Delta coastal zones. The findings of this study suggest that a potential rise in sea level by one meter could result in the inundation and subsequent loss of approximately 20–30% of the Nile Delta total area.

(F) **Water Quality**

Climate change models indicate that there is a projected trend of rising temperatures, the impact of which on water quality can be manifested in various manners, including diminished levels of dissolved oxygen, heightened influx of contaminants into water bodies, diminished flow rates in streams and rivers, intensified occurrences of algal blooms, and an augmented probability of saltwater intrusion in proximity to coastal areas.

It has been observed that warmer water has a reduced capacity to retain oxygen, thus indicating that the phenomenon of global warming could potentially result in decreased levels of dissolved oxygen. The potential for heightened precipitation intensity leading to increased runoff and erosion may contribute to an elevated level of pollutant transport. Water quality can be influenced by various factors, including soil composition, geological structures, and topography in catchment areas (such as river basins), the presence of nearby flora, human interventions, rainfall and water flow from nearby land, as well as the interplay of natural, physical, and chemical interactions within the water itself.

Numerous investigations have provided evidence indicating an upward trend in surface water temperature across Europe, North America, and Asia since the 1960s. This increase has been observed to range between 0.2 and 2 °C. The primary driver behind this phenomenon is believed to be atmospheric warming, which can be attributed to the rise in solar radiation. Following the notable drought experienced in 2003, it was observed that the water temperature in the Rhine River exhibited an average rise of approximately 2 °C. Consequently, this led to a decline in the levels of dissolved oxygen (DO) within the river [34].

Climate change was observed to significantly affect various factors, such as air temperature, precipitation intensity, CO_2 levels in the atmosphere, and acid deposition levels. Specifically, considerable increases in dissolved organic carbon (DOC) have been observed in certain regions, including Northern and Central Europe, and North America.

The influence of weather patterns on nutrient loading is not to be under-estimated. The effect of warmer weather on marine bodies can result in elevated nutrient loads in both surface and groundwater. The influence of precipitation patterns, encompassing both seasonal variations and intensity, in conjunction with rising air temperatures, significantly impacts the dynamics and outcomes of pesticide usage.

Numerous scholarly investigations have taken place to examine the possible ramifications of climate risks on water quality in the forthcoming decades. According to global forecasts, it is anticipated that European lakes may experience a rise in water temperature of approximately 2 °C by the year 2070. Nevertheless, it is noteworthy that the extent of this rise may differ according to the specific features of each lake, as well as the season. Consequently, it is expected that shallow lakes, due to their unique attributes, may face the greatest vulnerability to the prospective adverse influences of climate change. Furthermore, it has been anticipated that lakes with short residence times may experience a considerable increase of approximately 92% in their residence time during the summer season by the year 2050. According to George et al. [15], lakes with greater heat storage capacity, such as the deepest ones, tend to exhibit high sensitivity to long-term climate warming. As a result, these lakes are likely to experience elevated winter temperatures. A rise in water temperature can potentially influence the chemical processes occurring in lakes, leading to changes in pH levels and an enhanced generation of alkalinity within the lake ecosystem. An increase in nitrate concentration within rivers may arise because of an augmented occurrence of summertime events. This could potentially trigger a gradual release of nitrates from soils, subsequently leading to their transportation into watercourses during the onset of damp seasons. Other research indicated that there may be a potential increase in nitrate concentration within the aquifer layers of the Seine basin in the years 2050 and 2100. These increases are attributed to high precipitation levels, resulting in enhanced soil leaching. Additionally, it has been observed that a Norwegian river basin may experience a 40–50% surge in nitrate flux between 2070 and 2100. This phenomenon is also linked to amplified precipitation and subsequent soil leaching, as reported by Singh et al. [34].

(G) **Groundwater**

It is widely acknowledged that groundwater has a substantial contribution to the overall global freshwater supply, accounting for more than 89% of the total volume available. It has been observed that a significant number of aquifers are transboundary in nature, with water shared by more than one basin [2].

It is also commonly believed that global warming may affect groundwater resources through potential modifications in precipitation and temperature patterns. Moreover, this situation may be aggravated by the issue of over-exploitation. The process of groundwater recharge can be influenced by various factors, such as alterations in land-use/land-cover, urbanization, deforestation, modifications in agricultural practices, and shifts in soil characteristics. These changes, which can occur gradually over a prolonged duration, have the possibility to impact the infiltration capacity.

According to Singh et al. [34], there is a significant decrease in computed groundwater recharge in various regions, such as north-eastern Brazil, southwest Africa, and along the southern border of the Mediterranean Sea, under different climatic scenarios. This decrease may amount to more than 70%. According to the available data, it has been observed that certain regions, namely the Sahel, the Near East, Northern China, Siberia, and the western USA, are projected to experience a considerable increase in groundwater recharge of over 30% by the 2050s. In response to the growing concerns regarding the prospects of groundwater resources, UNESCO-IHP (International Hydrological Programme) has initiated the Groundwater Resources Assessment under the Pressures of Humanity and Climate Changes (the so-called GRAPHIC) project with the aim of comprehensively investigating the complex relationship between groundwater and the water cycle on the global scale, as well as its vital role in supporting ecosystems and human societies. Moreover, the project seeks to address the potential challenges posed by the joint impacts of the increase in population and extreme climate change incidences [42]. The study covers a global scope, spanning across all continents, and employs a diverse range of contemporary technologies to effectively evaluate and monitor alterations in groundwater resources.

In addition, it is worth noting that coastal groundwater aquifers may be affected by salinization by virtue of potential sea water intrusion resulting from the rise in sea levels attributed to climate change.

(H) **Transboundary Waters**

In the contemporary global context, it is worth noting that a significant number of river basins, over 270 basins, are shared by two or more sovereign states. Similarly, a comparable number of shared groundwater aquifers traverse more than two states. Frequently, these interconnected water bodies lack legally binding agreements as far as the sharing of water resources between them is concerned.

In the absence of established agreements, there is a tendency for unilateral actions that may lead to over-exploitation, wastage, and degradation of the limited transboundary water resources. The increasing competition for transboundary water resources in the twenty-first century is expected to significantly amplify the likelihood of intense social disruptions and conflicts in various regions [2].

The allocation and management of a shared watercourse, given its complex and delicate nature, have prompted numerous instances of concern and have presented opportunities for both conflict and cooperation [34]. Global warming is widely recognized as a potential challenge to international relations concerning transboundary basins in view of its impact on the hydrological cycle, which consequently disrupts the surface and groundwater resources quantitatively and qualitatively. According to the 3rd IPCC's Assessment Report [19], it is indicated that in situations where conflicts arise, the occurrence of climate change events is expected to aggravate rather than alleviate matters due to the uncertainty related to the future availability of resources it entails. A significant consequence of climate change on treaties between competing users, whether they are within a specific zone or involve upstream and tail-end parties, is that assigning privileges in absolute terms may potentially give rise to additional future conflicts, particularly when the total absolute quantity of available water may vary.

There is a diverse range of international, regional, and sub-regional legal conventions and agreements pertaining to water-related matters currently in existence. The primary international legal agreement concerning international water resources management is the "UN Convention on the Law of Non-Navigational Uses of International Watercourses" that was adopted by the UN General Assembly in 1997 and came into effect in 2014 following the ratification of 35 countries. The Convention was initiated with the aim of establishing a comprehensive framework that guarantees the effective utilization, conservation, management, and protection of international watercourses. Additionally, it seeks to enhance the optimal and sustainable development of these watercourses, with a special focus on satisfying the demands of both current and future generations. Nevertheless, it is worth mentioning that there are still several countries that have not yet fully embraced the Convention, particularly those that share major river basins. For several years, the Helsinki Rules have also been recognized as a valuable outline for guiding Transboundary River basin management, emphasizing the holistic approach of considering the entire drainage basin.

It is noteworthy to acknowledge that the 1997 UN Convention represents the sole treaty that governs the shared freshwater resources management on a global scale. It can be regarded as a Framework Convention, as it offers a comprehensive set of principles and regulations that can be adapted to accommodate the unique characteristics of specific international watercourses, including those found in the Middle East region [2].

As far as Groundwater is concerned, transboundary aquifers represent a valuable and often overlooked resource that presents an opportunity for fostering international cooperation. A comprehensive analysis has revealed the presence of 59 transboundary aquifers in the Americas, 38 in Africa, 12 in Asia, and 63 in south-eastern Europe.

It is widely acknowledged that the water quality found in aquifers is frequently of high calibre, rendering it suitable for direct human consumption. Nevertheless, it is worth noting that aquifers can be considered as delicate and vulnerable systems. In the event of depletion or pollution of such aquifers, the recovery process will probably take a prolonged time spanning several centuries. Considering a growing reliance on groundwater reservoirs, it is noteworthy that transboundary aquifers have historically received limited consideration within the realm of international law. Whereas the existing regulatory framework for transboundary surface waters is robust, the same level of development is yet to be achieved for transboundary aquifers.

In recent years, agreements pertaining to transboundary aquifers have notably emerged. The riparian countries of the Nubian Sandstone Aquifer system, namely Egypt, Sudan, Libya, and Chad, have successfully established a collaborative joint Authority. The Authority is tasked with a range of important responsibilities, including the collection and maintenance of data, the execution of studies, the formulation of plans and programs for water resources development and utilization, the implementation of common groundwater policies, the provision of technical personnel training, and the examination of the environmental implications associated with water resources development [2].

In response to the mounting issue of water stress in the domain of shared river basins and groundwater aquifers, a number of over 30 governments and organizations have made the decision to collaborate to enhance cross-border water cooperation. Numerous on-going international initiatives are dedicated to achieving a mutually agreed and enforceable treaty for transboundary groundwater aquifers. The primary objective is to establish a framework that promotes collaborative interactions among riparian nations that share the same aquifer, ensuring that "no harm" is inflicted upon any of the involved parties.

At the regional level, it is worth noting that the Arab region, for instance, exhibits a significant reliance on shared water resources. Many Arab countries depend on water supplies that are shared with neighbouring Arab states or countries beyond the region. A significant proportion, specifically over one-third, of the freshwater resources in the region are derived from external sources. Additionally, it is noteworthy that among the 22 Arab countries, 14 countries share a surface-water body [11]. Examples of transboundary waters in the Arab region include the Tigris-Euphrates waterway, which involves Turkey, Syria, Iraq, and Iran as riparian countries, as well as the River Nile, with the participation of 11 African riparian countries, two of which are situated within the Arab Region.

The interdependence on these resources has given rise to various hydro-diplomatic initiatives and multilateral treaty endeavors, exemplified by the 1959 Nile Agreement between Egypt and Sudan.

A remarkable instance of collaboration within the Nile Basin can also be observed through the establishment of the Nile Basin Initiative (NBI) in 1999. This initiative serves as a distinct platform for the nations within the Nile region to engage in a cooperative endeavour, with the aim of achieving concrete advantages within the Basin and fostering a strong basis of trust and confidence [2]. Nevertheless, it is worth noting that the agreement in question has encountered several challenges stemming from the unilateral actions taken by certain Nile Basin countries. These actions involved signing the agreement prior to achieving a consensus on certain crucial articles, thereby resulting in an agreement that is incomplete and lacks inclusivity. Consequently, the agreement has fallen short of attaining its intended objectives.

In year 2011, Ethiopia established the Grand Ethiopian Renaissance Dam (GERD) on the Blue Nile, a decision made independently without prior consultation with Egypt and Sudan, the downstream countries. In the year 2015, the nations of Egypt, Sudan, and Ethiopia came together to sign the "Declaration of Principles on the Grand Ethiopian Renaissance Dam" with the aim of finding a resolution to the ongoing dispute surrounding the dam. The agreement pertains to Ethiopia's on-going erection of the Grand Ethiopian Renaissance Dam on the Blue Nile, a project that has generated significant controversy. A key provision of the agreement is the need to establish a consensus on the regulations governing the initial filling and subsequent operation of the dam. The urgent need for a comprehensive and mutually agreed-upon binding agreement on the filling and operating rules, as well as a mechanism for coordination in dam management among the three countries, is crucial for achieving peace and development in the basin. However, it is important to note that despite Ethiopia's on-going fourth year of dam filling, an agreement has not yet been reached with the two downstream countries. Considering the potential adverse consequences of the Grand Ethiopian Renaissance Dam (GERD) on water availability downstream of the Blue Nile in Sudan and Egypt, it is worth exploring the potential role of climate change as a mitigating factor. It is hypothesized that climate change could potentially result in increased runoff into the Blue Nile, thereby positively contributing to its average river flows [5].

In the context of shared river basins, it is imperative to establish agreements that foster mutually beneficial outcomes and ensure the absence of negative impacts throughout the basin. It is widely acknowledged that the development of an international river necessitates collaborative efforts among the riparian countries. The examination of climate change effects on transboundary waters is of considerable significance, particularly for downstream nations like Egypt. It is imperative to conduct comprehensive studies on climate change implications both upstream and beyond the borders of these downstream countries.

(I) **Agriculture**

The agricultural sector has been acknowledged as a substantial supplier to greenhouse gas emissions. This is primarily attributed to various agronomic practices such as land renovation, including ploughing, cultivation, and deforestation practices. Additionally, the use of organic and inorganic manures can lead to the volatilization of greenhouse gases. Methane emissions from ruminant livestock and paddy rice cultivation also contribute to the overall greenhouse gas emissions associated with agriculture. Moreover, the agricultural sector is considered a chief man-made source of methane, which is known for its substantial global warming potential.

Roughly speaking, 70% of the global freshwater supply is allocated for agricultural purposes, and around 30 developing nations currently encounter water scarcity challenges. According to Fischer et al. [14], it is projected that by the year 2050, the number of water-scarce countries will rise to approximately 55, most of them being located in developing countries. The issue of water shortage, coupled with the deterioration of cultivable land, emerges as a principal impediment to the augmentation of agricultural productivity. The susceptibility of the agricultural sector to climate fluctuations primarily stems from alterations in precipitation and temperature patterns. Accordingly, the potential consequences on the agricultural domain have raised concerns regarding the extent of global food sustenance in the future. Many nations heavily rely on agriculture as a vital component of their economies, hence the negative consequences of climate change extreme events on the agricultural arena could be strongly connected with poverty and could have a discernible impact on numerous developing countries. In Africa, it has been estimated that a considerable proportion of the population, approximately 60–70%, relies on employment for earning their living on the agricultural sector which contributes an average of approximately 34% to the gross domestic product (GDP) per country. Notably, as far as the West African Sahel region is concerned, agriculture and stock farming engage more than 80% of the population residing in rural areas according to Singh et al. [34]. Various investigations have revealed that the agricultural sector's susceptibility is reliant upon certain factors such as the native biological settings, humidity, crop cultivation schedule, available indigenous knowledge and evidence-based information, besides awareness of projected climate variations. Moreover, the high unpredictability of climate impacts poses an added challenge that agriculturalists and stakeholders must surmount.

Anthropogenic-driven climate change is believed to have substantial influence on agricultural systems and consequently agricultural productivity, which can be attributed to various factors such as alterations in precipitation patterns, temperature fluctuations, the fertilizing effect of carbon dioxide (CO_2), variations in climate conditions, and changes in surface water runoff. Also, the interplay between temperature and soil humidity influences the span of the cultivation and harvesting period, crop development and the water needs. In regions with arid and semi-arid conditions, high temperatures may restrain the crop cycle, hence diminishing overall crop productivity.

(J) **Ecosystems**

Global climate change has resulted in modifications in the natural and biotic schemes on various scales. This can be attributed to the abrupt augmentation in the energy equilibrium of the globe, consequently affecting the ecosystems, which are the cornerstones that support human society. This phenomenon has the potential to induce abrupt and irreversible consequences that fundamentally alter the ecological dynamics and ecosystem structure, thereby potentially yielding significant implications on human society. The global ecosystem is influenced by various factors that have the potential to significantly impact its operationalism. Such factors include, but are not restricted to, the historical fluctuation and extreme levels of CO_2 and climate, both of which have played a crucial role in shaping the ecosystem over time. Additionally, human activities, such as agricultural practices, nitrogen accumulation, and contamination, among others, have also contributed to changes in the ecosystem. Furthermore, natural disturbances, like wildfires, have an important role in shaping the ecosystem. Even restrained changes in management operations within specific cultivated areas, such as the intensification of agricultural practices, can have notable effects on the ecosystem. The impact of operational diversity, habitat loss, and fragmentation on ecological dynamics, particularly as related to biodiversity, has been widely acknowledged in the scientific community [13].

Deserts, being one of the most expansive native biosystems, are anticipated to encounter frequently recurrent incidences of sporadic climate events, potentially leading to an escalation in inter-annual variability in the coming years. The probability for desertification vulnerability is expected to increase because of the escalating occurrence of severe droughts on a global scale. For instance, in the Americas, there are projections indicating significant expansion of temperate deserts under climate scenarios where CO_2 levels are doubled. Furthermore, it is quite expected that climate change will also affect the desert ecosystems biodiversity.

Climate change extreme events can also have direct impacts on inland aquatic ecosystems through increases in temperature and CO_2 concentrations. Additionally, according to Meehl et al. [27], it can also indirectly affect these ecosystems by causing changes in hydrology due to alterations in regional or global precipitation patterns. Over and above, higher temperatures can have adverse effects on various organisms, including microorganisms, benthic invertebrates, and numerous fish species. It is highly probable that significant alterations will take place in the species types, growth seasons, and the establishment of planktonic assemblies, as well as their complex food mesh connections.

4.2 *Indirect Impacts of Climate Change on the Water Sector*

The water scarcity mounting challenge, including drought, desertification, and related challenges, is currently impacting a significant portion, about one-third, of the global inhabitants. As anticipated, these challenges will continue to intensify, leading to further implications on consumption patterns, migration trends, and various socio-economic aspects of people's livelihoods in various regions worldwide.

(A) **Migration**

The passive effects of climate change include various supply-side effects, such as increased risks of water scarcity, floods, glacial melting, and sea level rise, as previously outlined, are known to contribute to the potential acceleration of human migration.

Rural–urban migration and migration prompted by political conflict and environmental crises are additional demographic factors that are increasingly influencing water resources and allocations. According to the UN World Water Development Report 3, titled "Water in a Changing World" [46], it is estimated that there exists a range of 24 million to nearly 700 million people are environmentally displaced individuals, who are likely displaced due to water-related factors.

Such phenomenon of human migration could have significant implications on the prospective development initiatives aimed at mitigating future challenges related to water availability. The intricate nature of understanding the relationship between migration and environmental factors, particularly as related to water resources, stems from the fact that individuals depend on the natural environment for their sustenance, whether directly or indirectly. Furthermore, it is worth noting that the interplay between development policies, and political and economic stability can substantially affect both migration movements and water resources availability. Considering the intricate nature of these circumstances, it becomes a real challenge to accurately measure the extent of potential migration that may arise due to environmental factors [46].

At the Arab regional level, the challenge of water scarcity and poverty compels individuals to migrate towards densely populated urban areas in pursuit of employment opportunities. This influx of people places additional strain on the already overburdened infrastructure, thereby exacerbating existing costs and pressures. The correlation between climate crises and social unrest stemming from climate-induced migration has been widely recognized and extensively studied. The civil war in Syria has been associated with the occurrence of a five-year drought in the country starting in 2007, along with various other contributing factors. The occurrence of such a severe drought resulted in an unprecedented level of poverty, thereby leading to the migration of individuals towards the outskirts of Syria's major urban centers. It is noteworthy that these cities were already grappling with the challenges posed by population expansion, meanwhile, the increase in the number of refugees and the subsequent strain on the inadequate infrastructure added more pressure on the underlying grievances, hence playing a pivotal role in the uprising of 2011.

The phenomenon of state failure, uncontrolled migration, and ungoverned spaces has been observed to have a direct correlation with the facilitation of armed groups and terrorists. These actors exploit the vulnerabilities of poor individuals, thereby increasing their own numbers. The intersection of various factors, such as inadequate governance, high population density, and escalating costs, can contribute to the deterioration of infrastructure. This, in turn, can lead to challenging circumstances for local communities, especially during the summer season when the combination of intense heat and insufficient rainfall can result in crop failures and limited availability of water and electricity resources. This has become an evident driver of widespread protests and disturbances across the region.

(B) **Changing Consumption Patterns**

The significant influence of climate change on water resource availability is quite evident, affecting mainly the supply side. Human demands also play a role in exacerbating the pressures on the water supply as they interact with climate change. Meanwhile, it can be observed that the primary factors contributing to increased water demand are associated with population expansion during the early phases of a nation's development. As societies progress and individuals experience economic growth, there is a natural inclination towards increased consumption, including the utilization of water resources.

As nations progress in their development, there is a noticeable increase in the demand for non-food commodities and services, which often possess significant ecological and water footprints. In contrast to developed nations, where there is a growing emphasis on promoting water footprint reduction among consumers and corporations, it is worth noting that significant quantities of water are utilized in the production and processing of non-food stuff and facilities. This so-called virtual water content contributes to the existing challenges related to water resource availability and quality. The perception of 'virtual water' was hence introduced to indicate the indirect utilization of water that exits a country through exports and enters another country through imports as an inherent component of goods that require water for production [46].

The management of water resources encounters challenges due to the limited availability of indigenous knowledge and data necessary for effective decision-making and the formulation of sustainable long-term plans. Many countries have limited knowledge regarding the comprehensive understanding of water usage, including its various purposes, as well as the quantity and quality of available water resources. There is limited awareness regarding the extent to which water withdrawal can potentially lead to adverse environmental impacts, as well as the substantial financial investments being made in water management and infrastructure. The extreme climate change events definitely add further complexities to these existing uncertainties.

(C) **Socio-economic Impacts**

Evidently, the climate change phenomenon can have a tremendous effect on the nations' security and societal cohesion by exacerbating socio-economic ruptures and undermining trust in public institutions. The problem can be pertinently described as a series of interconnected challenges that converge to generate a cascade of issues at the local, national, and geopolitical scales. The situation commences with state institutions that have experienced a decline in their effectiveness, ultimately leading to areas without effective governance. These ungoverned spaces become fertile ground for the proliferation of extremist armed groups and criminal organizations. Consequently, this situation triggers the displacement of populations within the affected region and prompts a significant influx of refugees, impacting not only the countries in the immediate vicinity but also extending beyond their borders [33].

5 Climate Change Adaptation/Mitigation Solutions in the Water Sector

The global community is currently facing unprecedented temperatures and severe weather patterns, which necessitate immediate attention and action. Topics related to ecological and CC impacts, such as clean and renewable energy, sustainable development, environmental safeguarding, CO_2 radiation and contamination control, as well as food and water security, are on top of the agendas of numerous countries. The development and implementation of policies, plans, directive guidelines, and innovative technologies aimed at addressing environmental challenges, adaptation and mitigation measures, and promoting sustainable development are of utmost importance for the long-term well-being and survival of humanity. Certain subjects that were previously considered as strategies to safeguard future generations have now become immediate concerns. This shift in priority is attributed to the rapid urbanization and population expansion, which has occurred without taking into consideration sustainable measures. Consequently, this has resulted in a swift disruption of the delicate balance of our planet. In essence, the available time to address these issues is much shorter than once previously estimated.

Statistical data demonstrate that the majority of natural disasters, approximately over 70%, can be attributed to the incidence of extreme climate conditions and patterns, and water-related events. These factors pose significant challenges to achieving sustainable development, particularly as far as poverty alleviation is concerned. One potential approach to address these concerns involves the integration of disaster mitigation and risk management strategies into comprehensive development planning. Toward this end, it is imperative to establish an enhanced knowledge base. Additionally, it is crucial to foster the understanding and engagement of policy-makers, civil society, and the public in acknowledging the interdependence of sustainable development, poverty alleviation, and ecosystem conservation. It is noteworthy that the mitigation of natural hazards and their consequences is an integral component of achieving these goals.

Furthermore, it is imperative to formulate and apply effective adaptation policies and plans. To effectively mitigate greenhouse gas emissions, it is necessary to adopt a twofold approach: reducing the reliance on fossil fuels and concurrently increasing the utilization of alternative clean energy sources such as solar energy, wind, hydro, and biomass. This can be further complemented by implementing energy conservation strategies. It is imperative to prioritize the reduction of deforestation and the implementation of reforestation initiatives to effectively enhance carbon dioxide sinks. Further investigation is warranted to enhance comprehension of climate processes and mitigate uncertainties in climate projections. The utilization of climate data, analyses, and information is crucial in the planning processes, as emphasized by Jain [26].

In this regard, it is to be noted that any approach aimed at understanding and managing risks should be comprehensive in the sense that it should seek an appropriate balance between conservation and use of natural resources on one hand and meeting socio-economic aspirations on the other. In this context, there is also a need to determine the extent of resources available and their sensitivity to risks before embarking on any development goals. These resources would be in the form of human capability, technological tools, and financial means [3].

- **Mitigation Measures**

The variability in rainfall patterns, which may result from climate change implications, along with the increased evaporation rates in reservoirs that store water, are emerging climatic risks that require both immediate and long-term mitigation measures [2].

Advancing climate mitigation efforts towards achieving sustainable development necessitates not only hastening the rate of progress but also effectively tackling the fundamental factors that contribute to vulnerability and emissions. Focusing on these drivers fosters the involvement of diverse communities, sectors, stakeholders, regions, and cultures in just, equitable and inclusive processes that aim to enhance the health and well-being of individuals and the whole planet. Examining climate change through a justice lens entails prioritizing certain aspects, namely: (i) safeguarding vulnerable communities against the repercussions of climate change, (ii) mitigating the consequences of low-carbon transitions, and (iii) establishing a fair and equitable global decarbonization framework [20].

The temporal aspects of implementing mitigation measures and their efficacy will bear considerable implications for overarching long-term sustainable development outcomes. Ambitious mitigation efforts can be regarded as a crucial factor in facilitating the achievement of the global Sustainable Development Goals (SDGs). The adoption of coordinated cross-sectoral approaches to climate mitigation can effectively address synergies and mitigate potential trade-offs. This approach is valuable in managing the interplay between different sectors and ensuring the alignment of sustainable development objectives. This task necessitates the implementation of comprehensive planning strategies that incorporate policy frameworks capable of addressing multiple objectives and impacts. The presence of robust inter-dependencies and cross-sectoral linkages presents a range of possibilities for achieving synergistic outcomes while also necessitating careful consideration of the trade-offs associated with various mitigation options and technologies. The successful implementation of climate change mitigation policies requires the adoption of coordinated sectoral approaches, which should prioritize the integration and coordination of interactions between different sectors and ensure active participation of local communities in the development of new products, as well as in the production and consumption practices.

Over the course of several decades, efforts were exerted to mitigate the effects of climate change by comprehending its fluctuations across decadal, annual, and seasonal timeframes, with the aim of fostering the development of climate forecasting techniques, risk assessment strategies related to natural disasters, and diversification of crops and livelihoods. Various forms of adaptations have been widely implemented on the global scale. The following examples pertain specifically to sectors associated with water.

- **Drought**: The potential for mitigating the impacts of drought can be explored through the application of conventional rainwater harvesting techniques and water-conservation procedures. Additionally, the establishment of shelter belts and windbreaks can contribute to enhancing the resilience of rangelands. In the context of Sudan (Africa), the establishment of revolving credit funds could be considered to support drought management efforts. In regions such as Mexico and Argentina, introducing drought-resistant vegetation, amendment of cultivation dates, as well as diversification of crop varieties can be explored to enhance agricultural resilience. Furthermore, the compilation of products as economic investments and the establishment of native financial channels may prove beneficial in managing drought-related challenges. In the aftermath of drought events, it is important to consider the implementation of employment programs within national government initiatives. This can provide opportunities for affected communities and contribute to their recovery. Additionally, aiding small subsistence farmers in increasing crop production can be a valuable measure to enhance their resilience in countries like Botswana.
- **Sea-level rise**: Examples from Egypt include the installation of robust infrastructure in regions susceptible to coastal erosion, coupled with the establishment of a comprehensive local CC scheme that effectively incorporates climate-related considerations into Egypt's overarching policies. In the Philippines, several key initiatives have been undertaken to face the threats caused by natural hazards, particularly cyclones. These initiatives include risk monitoring and evaluation, upgrading skills for the appropriate design of shoreline defense systems, building of cyclone-resistant lodgings, and revisiting construction standards. Implementation of the Flood Protection Act and Shoreline Protection Strategy can be considered as proactive measures that enable the integration of emerging climate trends. These measures also involve the construction of a storm surge barrier, which takes into consideration the potential impact of a 50-cm rise in sea levels, as observed in the Netherlands [34].
- **Adaptation Measures**

Though mitigation of anthropogenic climate change is of utmost importance, yet it is imperative that all nations adapt to climate change, particularly developing countries, being more often susceptible to its implications and are likely to experience the most severe and immediate consequences. And even if kind of stabilization of greenhouse gas concentrations perceived in the forthcoming decades, it is inevitable that certain CC consequences will continue to exist, such as the escalating water stress in numerous regions, the intensification of extreme climate episodes, and the possibility of significant population displacement.

Climate change undoubtedly presents a novel challenge to the development and execution of adaptation policies. This is due to the various dimensions involved in adapting to climate change including diverse domains, mainly water resources, agriculture, and industry. Adaptation efforts must also consider the different spatial scales, ranging from local to regional levels. Moreover, the actions required for adaptation should encompass physical, technological, investment, regulatory, and market-based approaches. It is also necessary that adaptation strategies be tailored to different climatic zones, such as dryland areas, floodplains, mountains, and arctic regions.

The successful implementation of proactive adaptation necessitates the prevalence of enabling policy conditions across various levels. At the national level, it is imperative to expand and enhance water governance by integrating with non-water sectors. Besides, there should be concerted efforts to promote access to technology, science, and information in order to facilitate informed planning. Moreover, it is crucial to carefully evaluate development initiatives to identify potential maladaptations related to water. On the regional level, it is imperative to prioritize the emphasis on collaborative water management for shared surface and groundwater. Numerous models are available that facilitate the equitable sharing of water resources while also promoting rational management practices. As for the international and global scale considerations, augmenting financial resources to support investments in water-related projects is a compelling argument, particularly emphasizing the reinforcement of infrastructure [34].

Climate change adaptation initiatives encompass a range of strategies aimed at enhancing the resilience and adaptive capacities of individuals who have been displaced due to climate-related water challenges. These adaptation initiatives involve the utilization of environmentally friendly reconstruction methods and passive building strategies, enhancing the resilience of communities through integrated natural resource management practices, and expanding the green open spaces which serve as protective measures against dust storms, desertification, and sand encroachment in urban areas. Furthermore, the strengthening of both governmental and community capacities is prioritized with the aim of effectively managing flash floods by implementing infrastructure that is resilient to such extreme flooding events.

From a regional standpoint, it is important to acknowledge the wide range of water challenges associated with climatic conditions, such as water scarcity and droughts, particularly in the Arab region. Considering this, it is crucial for Arab cities to consider innovative approaches while incorporating climate change adaptation measures into their initial urban design and progressive processes. By so doing, these cities can enhance their resilience and minimize the vulnerabilities faced by both their inhabitants and infrastructure. This aligns with the objectives of the Global Sustainable Development Goals, the Paris Agreement, and the New Urban Agenda. Climate change adaptation solutions in the Arab region have the potential to leverage various climate finance opportunities. It is advisable to prioritize investments in people-centered mobility and resilient infrastructure while also ensuring the protection of coastal urban areas and the promotion of sustainable and climate-resilient livelihoods [30].

Given the current and anticipated water scarcity, the utilization of **non-conventional water resources (NCWR)** has emerged as an indispensable strategic measure for the Arab region.

The analysis of water conditions in the Arab region reveals that Non-Conventional Water Resources (NCWR) constitute approximately 8% of the total water resources available on the regional scale. One of the notable components of Non-Conventional

Water Resources (NCWR) is **Treated Wastewater (TWW)**, which is commonly referred to as Grey Water and which has been recognized as a significant yet under-utilized resource, often described as the "untapped opportunity" or "The Renewable Water Resource of the Future." It is worth mentioning that the volume of produced wastewater, which may also include industrial wastewater, reaches approximately 23.45 billion cubic meters per year. However, out of the total amount, only 6.34 BCM/year, which accounts for approximately 27.4%, undergoes primary, secondary, tertiary, or advanced degrees of treatment within the Arab countries.

Another significant non-conventional water resource that merits attention is **agricultural drainage water**, which has a total potential of 33.90 BCM. This resource is frequently recycled in various Arab countries and can, therefore, be considered as a valuable component in the overall water balance.

One of the most expensive forms of Non-Conventional Water Resources is **Desalinated Water**, which is also commonly referred to as Silver Water. Seawater desalination currently represents a modest 7% of the overall non-conventional water resources (NCWR) in the Arab region, equivalent to a total volume of 4.16 billion cubic meters (BCM). Nevertheless, it is increasingly recognized as a crucial water resource in many Arab countries, particularly in the Gulf countries [4].

These sources have the potential to contribute to addressing the gap between supply and demand to enhance agricultural production. And though the use of non-conventional water seems to be simple, yet it is multi-faceted, as it has multi-disciplinary inter-linkages with different sectors, such as: environment, health, industry, energy, agriculture, domestic, etc., sometimes with conflicting objectives, different agendas and overlapping responsibilities.

Evidently, non-conventional water stands at the forefront for meeting the future demands of adaptation to climate change. However, its development and management need adequate knowledge and capacities. For the Way Forward, the proposed actions could take place by providing the enabling environment for NCWR development and operation and identifying NCWR-related portfolio of projects which could be further supported for soliciting financing through local, regional, and international funding institutions.

The successful implementation of measures to address climate change will require a strong and unwavering dedication from leaders and relevant stakeholders, including Governmental authorities, NGOs, and civil communities on the global scale. It is imperative that public policy regarding key water services and functions place high priority on enhancing competencies and institutions, as well as guaranteeing the required infrastructure investment to achieve long-term water security.

It is a must not an option that the world should take prompt and collective action to effectively address the pressing issues of climate change. Only by so doing, we can secure economic, environmental, and social stability, while also preventing a potential worldwide water scarcity.

6 Assessment of Climate Change Adaptation/Mitigation Costs in the Water Sector

Quantifying the precise economic impact of climate change on water resources poses a considerable challenge. However, a large number of scholarly research sheds light on the substantial costs associated with such impacts.

- In compliance with the **2016 World Bank** report [35], an assessment was conducted to evaluate climate change implications on water resources and the economy by large. The research findings suggest that by the year 2050, there is a projected decline in freshwater quantity due to climate change, which could potentially yield a 6% reduction in the Gross Domestic Product (GDP) of certain regions.
- The **2014 Global Commission on the Economy and Climate** report [36] dealing with "Better Growth, Better Climate" provides an evaluation of the economic consequences associated with climate change. It highlights the considerable risks that climate change causes to water resources, particularly in regions that are more susceptible to its impacts. The report emphasizes the importance of implementing proactive adaptation measures to mitigate costs and address these vulnerabilities.
- The **2018 IPCC** [21] Special Report on Global Warming of 1.5 °C investigates the effects of global warming and emphasizes the water resources' susceptibility to climate change. It underscores that increased water scarcity and fluctuations in rainfall patterns, in addition to the more frequent natural climatic hazards can result in significant economic ramifications.
- The **2020 UNDP** [39] Human Development Report explores the complex interplay between climate change, water, and human advancement. It highlights the economic effects of CC on water resources, encompassing detrimental effects on infrastructure, diminished agricultural output, and escalated healthcare expenditures.

The COP27 (UN Climate Change Conference), held in Sharm El-Sheikh, Egypt, in November 2022, has ended with a significant resolution to create a novel fund aimed at addressing "loss and damage." By virtue of this fund, countries responsible for substantial carbon emissions are committed to compensate nations that are vulnerable and experiencing adverse climate impacts. This resolution holds great significance as it follows a prolonged period of nearly three decades of legal appeals, thereby establishing a notable precedent in the realm of climate justice. The outcome serves as a compelling impetus to advance towards a sustainably-secure future.

7 Recommendations and the Way Forward

Given the prevailing climate change and variability, it is evident that the hydrological cycle and interconnected domains such as water, forest, and land are being significantly impacted. Consequently, it is has become a must not an option to adopt an integrated approach that focuses on effectively managing space, land, and water resources. This approach is regarded the sole channel to facilitate mitigation, adaptation, and disaster preparedness, thereby safeguarding essential livelihood aspects such as food and energy security, socio-economic advancement, ecological conservation, etc.

The following recommendations are of utmost importance in alleviating the adverse influence of climate change on water resources:

General Recommendations

- Supporting establishment of a "Damage and Losses Fund" and financing infrastructure projects to overcome risks of droughts, floods, and rainfall in the most vulnerable regions [6].
- Promoting dialogue on how to restore the Earth's hydrological balance through climate change adaptation and mitigation measures.
- Climate and the environment as fundamental bases for achieving the SDGs. Therefore, we must be noting the necessity of anchoring approaches to climate action according to the principle of "leaving no one behind."
- Working towards progress across four key dimensions: mitigation, adaptation, finance, and loss and damage, with a special focus on moving from words to action.
- The need for scaling up climate action and ambition, especially for implementing commitments and following-up on promised financial and technical support.
- The international community should take into consideration the environmental, climatic, developmental, and humanitarian impacts of the political decisions taken and that political decisions do not lead to a decline in climate, environmental and development action [10].

Recommendations Concerning Climate Change and Water Resources

- Strengthening cooperation and integration between countries and placing "Water" at the heart of climate action with the aim of promoting adaptation and mitigation measures to face CC adverse effects on Water Resources.
- Enhancement of Global Climate Models (GCM) to improve CC projections and advancement of hydrological and hydrogeological mathematical modeling.
- Ensuring technology transfer to improve rainfall forecasts, predictions and early warning systems.
- Climate-induced droughts and hotter temperatures require new Integrated Water Resources Management strategies and Implementation plans for water supply.

- Importance of implementing nature-based solutions and green technology that contribute to climate change mitigation and resilience, to fill the gap for water access and increase resilience.
- The International community should promote the development and commitment to treaties on the appropriate management of transboundary waters taking into account projections of climate change impacts.
- It is necessary to promote the use of new non-conventional water resources that has become an indispensable strategic option to achieve water security and adapt to climate-related hazards towards sustainable development in countries suffering from water scarcity.
- Importance of water desalination projects and the safe reuse of treated wastewater as an urgent necessity to meet the growing demand for water. This should be part of the green circular economy that the world is trying to achieve nowadays to reduce emissions and enhance resilience to climate change.
- Good governance is an essential factor in the implementation of NCWR projects, meanwhile adopting a nexus approach between the water-energy-food sectors and their relation to the environment.
- Partnership, integration, and common understanding of the role of all stakeholders (especially cooperation between Governments and private sector) are necessary to create promising opportunities for investment in NCWR projects.
- Water resources projects are usually expensive and require the firm commitment of financing institutions to provide necessary funds for projects that help overcome water scarcity problems.
- Innovation and technology, such as artificial intelligence and nanotechnology, are crucial factors in advancing the agenda of using NCWR in an economic and environment-friendly manner.
- There is urgent need to create a favourable investment environment to attract sponsors to the vital water-related sector, considering the financial, economic and environmental measures, while investing in infrastructure to enhance water supply and easy access to clean water and improve sanitation services.
- Education and awareness are among the key factors to increase understanding of the importance of using NCWR and public acceptance of the idea of safe water reuse.
- Enhancing women's capacity development and leadership in climate action and emphasizing the importance of their role and participation.
- Developing an interactive map using satellite images, RS techniques and GIS, to determine the nature of water resources, and the available water quantities and expected water uses, while linking the obtained information to increasing population rates and planning for future demands.

8 Conclusions

Numerous empirical findings, including the rise in mean air and oceanic temperatures on the global scale, as well as the melting of snowflake and ice, validate the perception that the Earth's climate is undergoing a warming trend which has manifested noticeable effects on the global, regional, and local levels, particularly within various water resource sectors. Based on comprehensive analyses of existing research within this domain, the following conclusions can be derived:

- Evidence-based investigation reveals notable alterations in the large-scale hydrologic cycles, considering both spatial and temporal dimensions. These observations include the rise in precipitation levels in elevated areas of the north hemisphere, since 1970 and onward. Additionally, there is an increased occurrence of intense precipitation events, modifications in runoff patterns, diminished snow cover, and changes in the glacial runoff magnitude and time.
- Findings from global climate models indicate that an increase in rainfall intensity in high latitudes and a decrease in lower mid-latitude expanses is anticipated throughout the twenty-first century. This shift in precipitation evidences is expected to contribute to high risks of both floods and droughts in various regions, owing to the variability in precipitation intensity. By the middle of the twenty-first century, it is quite expected that water quantity and annual waterway flow will probably increase in high latitudes. Conversely, numerous arid and semi-arid regions are expected to experience a water resources declining curve.
- Food security, among other aspects, may face potential vulnerability due to anticipated water resources alterations quantitatively and qualitatively. This vulnerability is particularly noted in regions characterized by dry and semi-dry environments, as well as in Asian and African mega deltas.
- The prospective negative effect of climate change on water quality is a matter of concern. It is anticipated that various factors such as elevated water temperatures, extreme precipitation patterns, repetitive occurrences of floods and droughts, as well as pollution, may contribute to a decline in water quality. This decline can be attributed to imbalances in multiple elements, including deposits, nutritive components, dissolved organic carbon, pathogens, insecticides, salts, and warm-air contaminants.
- The water resources quantity, accessibility and quality are anticipated to exert significant effects on both ecosystems and human well-being. These impacts are anticipated to be aggravated by the rise in sea levels, which will consequently lead to the expansion of saline groundwater aquifers and estuaries. Accordingly, there is a projected decline in the availability of fresh water for both coastal communities and ecosystems.
- For efficiently managing water resources, it is advisable to employ a range of strategies that take into account the availability and demand for water at various levels, including local, regional, and continental scales. These strategies should be tailored to meet the diverse needs associated with water usage. Some recommended approaches include the implementation of water conservation measures,

enhancing water use efficiency through recycling, promoting the utilization of non-conventional water resources, establishing water markets and engaging in virtual water trade, as well as improving storage infrastructure to serve as crucial resources during periods of drought. Furthermore, it is essential to enhance decision-making processes by applying robust models that account climate change implications on the water cycle. This necessitates comprehensive awareness of the doubts that may worsen the influence of extreme climate fluctuations.

Evidently, the climate-induced effects on water resources in countries already grappling with water scarcity are of utmost importance for achieving sustainable development. The recurring occurrence of droughts and the escalating water demands to satisfy the needs for sustainable development are further compounded by climate change and rising temperatures. Consequently, it is imperative to explore innovative strategies for adapting to these evolving circumstances.

For a long time, there has been a tendency among governments and stakeholders to approach water and climate change as separate and isolated domains. However, it is essential for policy-makers and top managers to realize that efforts to mitigate emissions and implement adaptation initiatives are inherently linked to effective water management. Similarly, addressing issues such as repairing leaky pipes, rehabilitating mangroves, and enhancing access to sanitation and other water services contribute to the development of climate resilience. It is imperative that these two agendas converge to foster a future that is resilient to both water-related challenges and climate change impacts [45].

Coordinated actions are needed by governments, as well as regional/international organizations and various stakeholders if water security, and consequently food and energy security, is to be achieved. The Water Action Agenda, which is the principal output of the [38] Water Conference, has compiled more than 700 obligations targeting the march towards a water-secure future. Within the framework of the 2018–2028 Water Action Decade, the international community promises to promote the water agenda by enhancing on-going schemes and action plans and stimulating water action to realise the 2030 Sustainable Development Agenda, in particular SDG 6 related to "Water and Sanitation for All." The UN Plan outlines an ambitious target to advance progress across sectors during the Water Action Decade. Accordingly, the UN and partners have initiated the SDG 6 Global Acceleration Framework, as part of the Water Action Decade to achieve the SDGs by 2030, in order to join forces among the global community entities and deliver fast results at all appropriate scales and at the country level. Efficiently tackling the global climate-related water challenges is fundamental to steer the path towards a future of global collaboration and effective integrated multi-lateral coordination [38].

No doubt, water possesses the capacity to significantly influence the lives of a countless number of individuals. We should hence capture this potential to guide us towards the attainment of PEACE. There is every reason to be optimistic that future generations will inhabit a world characterized by harmonious water relations, provided that all nations collectively strive towards this noble objective.

References

1. AMS (2021) Glossary of meteorology. American Meteorological Society (AMS), Boston, MA, USA. http://glossary.ametsoc.org
2. Abu-Zeid M (2014) Transboundary waters: from conflict to cooperation (Keynote Paper—Arabic & English). Arab Water Counc Sci J (Al-Maa) 5(2)
3. Abu-Zeid M (2009) Climate change and its impact on water resources, with special focus on the Arab Region and Egypt. Keynote Paper, Arab Water Forum, Cairo, Egypt
4. Abu-Zeid M, El-Atfy H (2017) Use of non-conventional water resources towards sustainable development in the Arab Region. Arab Water Counc Sci J (Al-Maa) 8(2)
5. AbuZeid K (2021) Potential transboundary impacts of the Grand Ethiopian renaissance dam under climate change and variability. In: Diop S et al (eds) Chapter 16 in book: climate change and water resources in Africa: perspectives and solutions towards an imminent water crisis. Springer Nature Switzerland AG 2021. ISBN 978-3-030-61224-5 (https://doi.org/10.1007/978-3-030-61225-2_16)
6. COP 27 (2022) COP27 outcome: reflections on the progress made, opportunities missed. From Africa Renewal. By: Fazal Issa. December 2022 (https://www.un.org/africarenewal/news/cop27)
7. Climate Change 2022: Mitigation of climate change. Working Group III contribution to the sixth assessment report of the intergovernmental panel on climate change
8. Collins M, Knutti R (2013) Long-term climate change: projections, commitments and irreversibility. In: Stocker T et al. (ed) Book: Climate change 2013—The physical science basis (pp 1029-1136, Chapter: 12). Cambridge University Press
9. Dartmouth Flood Observatory (DFO) (https://floodobservatory.colorado.edu/)
10. EDF (2022) Environment and development forum: the road to Sharm El-Sheikh climate change COP27, September 2022, Cairo, Egypt
11. ESCWA (2022) Impact of climate change on shared water resources in the Euphrates basin. ESCWA Publication: E/ESCWA/CL1.CCS/2021/RICCAR/Technical Report 11, September 2022
12. Elshinnawy IA, Foad IE, Salama IM, Issa UH (2017) Impacts of sea level rise on coastal flooding of Nile Delta, Egypt (https://www.researchgate.net/publication/334031298)
13. Fahrig L (2003) Effects of habitat fragmentation on biodiversity. Annu Rev Ecol Evol Syst 34:487–515
14. Fischer G, Shah M, van Velthuizen M, Nachtergaele FO (2001) Global agro-ecological assessment for agriculture in the 21st century. International Institute for Applied Systems Analysis, Luxemburg, Austria
15. George G, Hurley M, Hewitt D (2007) The impact of climate change on the physical characteristics of the larger lakes in the English Lake District. Freshw Biol 52:1647–1666
16. IPCC SRES (2002) IPCC Special Report on Emissions Scenario (A1B)
17. IPCC (AR6) (2022) Annex II: glossary. In: Möller V, van Diemen R, Matthews JBR, Méndez C, Semenov S, Fuglestvedt JS, Reisinger A (eds) Climate change 2022: impacts, adaptation and vulnerability. Contribution of working group II to the intergovernmental panel on climate change sixth assessment report AR6. Cambridge University Press, UK, pp 2897–2930. https://doi.org/10.1017/9781009325844.029
18. IPCC AR6 Cross-chapter paper 3 (CCP3): deserts, semiarid areas and desertification. In: Pörtner H-O, Roberts DC, Tignor M et al (eds) Climate change 2022: impacts, adaptation and vulnerability. Contribution of working group II to the sixth assessment report of the intergovernmental panel on climate change. Cambridge University Press, Cambridge, UK and New York, NY, USA, pp 2195–2231. https://doi.org/10.1017/9781009325844.020
19. IPCC (2001) Climate change 2001: Synthesis report. In: Watson RT, the Core Writing Team (eds) A contribution of working groups I, II, and III to the 3rd assessment report of the intergovernmental panel on climate change. Cambridge University Press, Cambridge, UK, and New York, NY, USA, p 398

20. IPCC AR6 Technical Summary (2022) Climate change 2022: mitigation of climate change. Working group III contribution to the sixth assessment report of the intergovernmental panel on climate change. ISBN 978-92-9169-160-9
21. IPCC (2018) IPCC special report on global warming of 1.5 °C (https://www.ipcc.ch/sr15/)
22. IPCC AR4 (2007): Climate Change 2007: Synthesis Report. Contribution of Working Groups I, II and III to the Fourth Assessment Report of the Intergovernmental Panel on Climate Change [Core Writing Team, Pachauri, R.K and Reisinger, A. (eds.)]. IPCC, Geneva, Switzerland, 104 pp.
23. IPCC AR6 (2023): Climate Change 2023: Synthesis Report. Contribution of Working Groups I, II and III to the Sixth Assessment Report of the Intergovernmental Panel on Climate Change [Core Writing Team, H. Lee and J. Romero (eds.)]. IPCC, Geneva, Switzerland, pp.
24. IPCC (AR6) (2021) Climate change 2021: the physical science basis. Summary for policymakers. Working group I contribution to the intergovernmental panel on climate change sixth assessment report. Switzerland, ISBN 978-92-9169-158-6
25. IPCC (AR5) (2014) Climate change 2014: Synthesis report. In: Core Writing Team, Pachauri RK, Meyer LA (eds) Contribution of working groups I, II and III to the fifth assessment report of the intergovernmental panel on climate change. IPCC, Geneva, Switzerland, p 151
26. Jain PC (2003) Greenhouse effect and climate change: scientific basis and overview. Renew Energy 3(4–5):403–420 (June-July 1993)
27. Meehl GA et al (2007) Global climate projections. In: Solomon S, Qin D, Manning M, Chen Z, Marquis M, Averyt KB, Tignor M, Miller HL (eds) Climate change 2007: the physical science basis. Contribution of working group I to the 4th assessment report of the IPCC. Cambridge University Press, Cambridge, UK, pp 747–845
28. Milly PCD, Dunne KA, Vecchia AV (2005) Global pattern of trends in streamflow and water availability in a changing climate. Nature 438:347–350
29. Mishra AK, Singh VP (2010) A review of drought concepts. J Hyrol 391:201–216
30. NCA (2018) Fourth national climate assessment Report. Chapter 2: our changing climate. U.S. Global Change Program, Washington, DRC 20006, USA (https://nca2018.globalchange.gov)
31. NCCD (2008) 2008 World Day to combat desertification. United Nations convention to combat desertification. 17 January 2018
32. Obasi GOP (2003) Managing risks—water and climate. Keynote address by Secretary-General, WMO, presented at the Pan-African implementation and partnership conference on water. Addis Ababa, Ethiopia, December 8, 2003
33. Ranj Alaaldin (2022) Climate change may devastate the Middle East. Here's how governments should tackle it. Planet Policy, March 14, 2022
34. Singh VP, Mishra AK, Chowdhary H, Khedun CP (2014) Climate change and its impact on water resources. In: Wang LK, Yang CT From: handbook of environmental engineering, volume 15: modern water resources engineering. © Springer Science + Business Media, New York. https://doi.org/10.1007/978-1-62703-595-8_11 (https://www.researchgate.net/publication/314210788)
35. The World Bank (2016) High and dry: climate change, water, and the economy. DC, USA
36. The Global Commission on the Economy and Climate (2014) Better growth, better climate. New Climate Economy Report, c/o World Resources Institute, Washington, DC 20002, USA
37. UN Habitat (2021) Climate change in the Arab Region: challenges and opportunities. Roundtable 4 concept note. World Cities Day: adapting cities for climate resilience. Luxor, Egypt
38. UN (2023) Water Action Agenda operations concept note (https://sdgs.un.org/sites/default/files/2022-11/.pdf)
39. UNDP (2020) Human development report 2020: the next frontier: human development and the anthropocene. New York
40. UNDP (United Nations Development Programme) (2018) Climate change adaptation in the Arab States: best practices and lessons learned (www.adaptation-undp.org)
41. UNEP/ROWA (2015) Climate change in the Arab region, United Nations Environment programme, issues brief for the Arab Sustainable Development Report, Regional Office for West Asia

42. UNESCO-IHP (2008) Groundwater resources assessment under the pressures of humanity and climate changes. United Nations Educational Scientific and Cultural Organization, Paris. (IHP/2008/GW/GRAPHIC)
43. UNFCCC (UN Framework Convention on Climate Change) (2009) Fact sheet: the need for mitigation. UNFCCC, Bonn, Germany
44. WAGRA (The Water and Geotechnical Research Association, Afghanistan) (2020). https://watgeora.org/climate-change
45. WRI (World Resources Institute) (2023) UN 2023 water conference. New York, March 2023. https://www.wri.org/insights/un-water-conference-2023
46. WWDR-3 (UNESCO, 2009) World Water Assessment Programme, 2009. The United Nations World Water Development Report 3: water in a changing world. UNESCO Publishing, Paris, France and Earthscan, London. www.unesco.org/water/wwap

Climate Change Impacts on Egyptian Fisheries and Aquaculture

Sahar Fahmy Mehanna

Abstract The rapid growth of the global population and the rising demand for seafood are occurring alongside a concerning decline in food resources, particularly fisheries. The Earth's oceans harbour a diverse array of over 30,000 fish species, many of which face potential threats from pollution, overfishing, illegal, unreported, and unregulated (IUU) fishing practices, invasive species, and atmospheric changes. With approximately 200 million individuals worldwide relying on fishing for sustenance, adopting sustainable fishing practices is imperative to prevent the depletion of fish populations. Given the significant global reliance on fisheries, it is crucial to consider the impacts of various challenges, particularly climate change, on these resources. Identifying and implementing practical adaptations to develop sustainable strategies resilient to climate change is essential. Climatic variation affects wildlife and biodiversity across terrestrial and aquatic ecosystems, exacerbating pre-existing stressors such as invasive species, diseases, and habitat loss. The potential decline in the maximum catch of various fish stocks in certain seas by up to 30% by the 2050s can be attributed to ocean warming, acidification, sea-level rise, and deoxygenation. Furthermore, atmospheric variations could lead to a projected decline of 10–40% in species suitable for marine aquaculture in tropical and subtropical regions by the 2050s. Understanding the impact of climate change on crucial commercial fish species and taking proactive measures to address these effects is crucial for promoting sustainable fishing practices. Fish stocks and marine habitats are vulnerable to the adverse effects of physical and biogeochemical changes in the oceans, directly linked to the increasing levels of greenhouse gases. These alterations significantly impact the United Nations' Sustainable Development Goals. This chapter aims to provide marine stakeholders with the necessary information to assess the influence of climatic variation on Egyptian fisheries and formulate appropriate adaptation strategies.

Keywords Egypt fishery resources · Global warming · Acidification · Deoxygenation · Monitoring · Mitigation · Governance

S. F. Mehanna (✉)
National Institute of Oceanography and Fisheries, NIOF, Cairo, Egypt
e-mail: sahar_mehanna@yahoo.com

© The Author(s), under exclusive license to Springer Nature Switzerland AG 2025

M. T. Khalil et al. (eds.), *Climate Changes Impacts on Aquatic Environment*, Earth and Environmental Sciences Library, https://doi.org/10.1007/978-3-031-74897-4_6

1 Introduction

Aquaculture and fisheries are essential for ensuring food security, enhancing food supply, and supporting livelihoods both locally and globally. Approximately 500 million individuals globally rely on fisheries and aquaculture for their livelihoods, and fisheries products contribute about 15% of animal protein consumption for a population of three billion. Edible aquatic creatures, including various fish species, possess significant nutritional value, making them a prominent commodity in the global food trade for both developing and developed nations. According to the Food and Agriculture Organization [13], global fish production was estimated at approximately 179 million tons, with aquaculture contributing 82.1 million tons (46% of the total production).

However, the primary concern is the sector's capacity for sustainable and rapid growth to meet the anticipated future demand, further compounded by the rapid expansion of the global population and the influences of climatic variation. Alongside well-documented challenges such as overexploitation, habitat degradation, pollution, eutrophication, and invasive species, climate change has emerged as a significant concern for global food production, posing substantial risks to both the quantity and quality of agricultural output [18, 32, 5]. Furthermore, the anticipated consequences of climate change pose an escalating threat to food security, particularly regarding the availability of dietary protein [24]. Oyinlola et al. [33] postulated that climate fluctuations could result in a decline of up to 30% in the maximum catch potential of various fish stocks in certain seas by the 2050s. Additionally, these changes may lead to the loss of 10–40% of species deemed suitable for marine aquaculture in tropical and subtropical regions.

Climate change is characterized by long-term alterations in weather patterns over short (ten years) or extremely long (million(s) year(s)) periods [21, 39]. Human activities' role in climate change is widely acknowledged, particularly concerning the utilization of fossil fuels like gas, coal, and oil for energy generation [4, 10, 12, 17, 23, 34]. Additionally, forest deterioration and human-induced denudation [36, 25] significantly contribute to greenhouse gas (GHG) emissions. The rise in the concentration of GHGs such as nitrous oxides (N_2O), carbon dioxide (CO_2), fluorinated gases, and methane (CH_4) in the air is attributed to anthropogenic activities. Climatic fluctuation impacts have been documented across numerous significant economic sectors and services globally [13, 22, 38, 40].

Climate change is anticipated to significantly impact fisheries and aquaculture due to various factors, including acidification, alterations in sea temperatures and circulation patterns, heightened occurrence and intensity of hazardous events, rising sea levels, and consequent ecological transformations. The impacts of climate change can be categorized into direct and indirect effects, encompassing changes in marine productivity, shifts in species distribution and seasonal patterns, modifications to habitats and food webs, as well as consequences for fishery and aquaculture costs, productivity, and the livelihoods and safety of fishing communities [8, 3]. Specifically, the rise in water temperature and subsequent alterations in habitats and food

Table 1 Summary for both physical and biological impacts of climate change on fisheries

Physical	Biological
Temperature	Species distribution
Stratification	Primary productivity
Coastal upwelling	Stock productivity
Sea levels	Species substitution
Acidification	
ENSO	
Currents	

availability prompt fish migration toward cooler, more productive waters. Consequently, numerous regions worldwide are anticipated to experience a decline in fishing prospects, while other areas will witness the emergence of new fishing opportunities (Table 1).

This chapter discusses the impacts of climate change on Egypt's fisheries resources and the adaptation strategies to mitigate these negative impacts. Moreover, the findings will help managers, policymakers, and researchers suggest and implement adaptation plans to address climate change's negative impacts on fisheries resources.

2 Egyptian Fisheries

In 2020, Egypt's fisheries and aquaculture sectors contributed approximately two million metric tons of fish, primarily for human consumption. Over the past three decades, fish production in Egypt has grown significantly, reaching 2.1 million tons in 2020 from approximately 346,000 tons in 1990, a remarkable growth rate of 460%. Compared to the modest 31% growth in natural resource utilization between 1990 and 2020, the aquaculture sector experienced a remarkable surge of 2502% in production during this period. Coastal areas in Egypt significantly contribute to the overall production of wild fisheries. However, pollution poses a substantial challenge, negatively impacting fish stocks' productivity and quality [27]. Marine resources face significant threats of irreversible habitat loss, ecological functions, and biodiversity loss due to pollution, overfishing, climatic alterations, harmful fishing methods, competing demands from human activities, various industrial uses, and unsustainable coastal area development. The issue of illegal, unreported, and unregulated (IUU) fishing remains a significant obstacle to sustainable fisheries [27]. Additionally, inadequate governance, management, and practices pose further challenges. The government has identified several key opportunities to address the challenge of providing highly nutritious food to Egypt's growing population. These opportunities include promoting sustainable and responsible fisheries administration, diminishing overfishing, implementing innovative and environmentally friendly methods in aquaculture, and preserving the health of the marine ecosystem. By focusing on these areas, the government aims to ensure nutritious food availability while safeguarding the long-term sustainability of Egypt's aquatic resources.

In Egypt, fish production is derived from three primary sources: inland and marine fisheries and aquaculture. Marine fisheries encompass the Red Sea and the Mediterranean, while inland fisheries include the River Nile, lakes, irrigation and drainage canals, and lagoons. Analyzing Egypt's fish production over the past three decades (1990–2020) reveals that most of the catch comes from inland waters, specifically lakes and the Nile River. These inland waters accounted for approximately 55% of the total landing in the 1990s but significantly declined to only 14% in 2020 (Fig. 1). The share of total fish production from Egypt's marine fisheries sector experienced a significant decline from approximately 24% in the 1990s to a mere 5% in 2020 [28, 29, 27]. In contrast, aquaculture initially contributed about 21% to the overall fish landing in Egypt during the 1990s but has since grown significantly, emerging as the country's predominant source of fish production. As of 2020, aquaculture accounted for approximately 80% of Egypt's total fish production [28, 29, 27, 16].

Despite the significant increase in fish production in Egypt, reaching approximately 2.1 million tons in 2020, with 20% from fishing operations and 80% from aquaculture, the growing burden of population growth and increasing demand for fish consumption per capita necessitates a re-evaluation of priorities. It is crucial to exploit available fisheries' resources rationally, effectively, and sustainably. Like most nations worldwide, Egypt recognizes the imperative of prioritizing, managing, and conserving fisheries resources. These renewable and productive sources of sustenance possess the potential to contribute significantly to national development and income, provided their sustainability is maintained. However, Egypt's fisheries resources are under significant pressure due to the various aforementioned challenges. In addressing these challenges, climate change emerges as a significant driver of transformations within the fisheries sector, impacting both the environment and local communities. The diverse implications of climate change necessitate a comprehensive understanding and proactive measures to safeguard the long-term viability and sustainability of Egypt's fisheries resources.

3 Fisheries of Egyptian Marine Water Bodies

Egypt's marine water bodies include a coastal stretch of approximately 2400 km and a continental platform spanning about 87,200 km^2. The inland fisheries sector covers around 10,160 km of shoreline, divided into segments such as 2140 km for coastal lakes, 1188 km for inland lakes, 5238 km for Nasser Lake, and 1532 km for the Nile River. In 2018, fish production from these key resources reached 373,300 tons, valued at about 10.7 million Egyptian pounds. The fishing industry significantly contributes to the national economy, accounting for 9.3% of the agricultural GDP and 5.1% of the total GDP. Over the past decade, marine fish landings in Egypt's

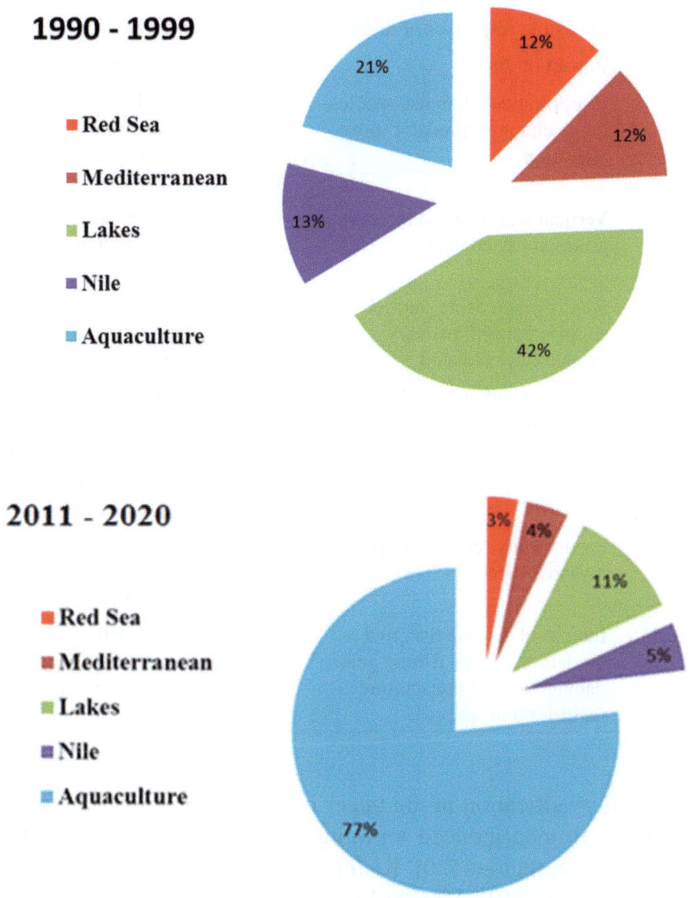

Fig. 1 Variant fisheries resources contributing to fish production in Egypt

economic zone have shown variability. According to GAFRD [16], the catch declined to 104,600 tons in 2018 from 127,800 tons in 2009. In the same year, Egypt faced a significant gap between fish production and consumption, importing approximately 350,000 tons of marine products at a total cost of around 400 million US dollars [16] to address this shortfall [27].

4 Climate Change Impacts on Fisheries

According to the Intergovernmental Panel on Climate Change [20], the ocean absorbs about 93% of the excess heat from human-induced greenhouse gas emissions, primarily affecting the surface water (0 to 700 m deep). This warming contributes to

Table 2 Impacts and possible responses of different climate drivers on fisheries

Climate factor	Impact on fish	Management response
Temperature	Physiological changes, species range changes, predator–prey alteration	Establishing MPAs, sound scientific research, observation and monitoring advanced systems, shifting to passive fishing gears
Salinity	Vertical stratification increasing, productivity changes	Continuous observation from surveys, more studies on fish behavior and physiology
Sea circulation	Run-off increasing, nutrient supply reduced, primary productivity reduced	Observations, ecosystem monitoring systems, improved and direct science surveys on ecosystem monitoring
Sea level rise	Breeding and nursery habitat loss, mariculture reduction and damage	Monitoring and observation systems, coastal area protection, integrated tracking of coastal water systems
Acidification	Coral bleaching, increased mortality	Sound science, ecosystem monitoring, and observation
Climate variability	Productivity reduction, increased invasive species	Improved catch recording and observation systems, life history and spatial range monitoring
Dangerous/bad weather	Increased disease risk, more predators, loss of fishing gears, damage/loss of aquaculture facilities and stocks	Improved ecosystem monitoring and observations, sound science, innovative technology on materials and fishing gears

increased thermal stratification in the upper ocean, influencing carbon cycling and nutrient processes. Human-induced warming has also been observed at depths up to 2000 m in some ocean regions [20]. Rising temperatures have been linked to more frequent marine diseases [19]. Maynard et al. [26] suggested that disease outbreaks due to rising temperatures might be as significant a factor in coral bleaching as temperature increases. These diseases can severely impact human health, aquaculture, and fishing industries, causing substantial financial losses [37]. Table 2 summarizes the different impacts of climate factors on fisheries and aquaculture.

5 Impacts on Species Distribution, Fisheries Productivity, and Abundance

Climate change is expected to affect ecosystem productivity, species distribution, and fisheries abundance. It can alter predator–prey dynamics, although the extent of these changes remains uncertain, necessitating further research on climatic influences on phenology and food web dynamics. Climate change impacts on fisheries are mixed; some regions face negative consequences while others might see benefits. Global warming affects the distribution and abundance of fisheries through temperature fluctuations and primary production changes. Rising ocean temperatures can alter aquatic habitats, prompting species migrations to cooler areas, affecting predator–prey relationships, and reducing exploitable biomass due to decreased primary production.

Habitat Loss

The habitat of fisheries species is crucial for their distribution, abundance, and yield. Climate change is anticipated to significantly impact fish populations and their habitats. Rising global temperatures affect fish stocks' abundance, migratory patterns, and mortality rates, influencing the feasibility of cultivating specific fish species in certain regions. Coral bleaching, driven by global warming, threatens fish populations and fisheries by degrading essential habitats. Species distribution shifts in response to climate changes have been documented across all major oceanic regions [35]. Ling et al. noted the significant impact of sea urchin poleward shifts due to global warming, transforming reefs into "urchin barrens" unsuitable for many temperate fish species.

Diseases

Climate change is expected to alter the distribution of diseases in marine ecosystems. Environmental parameters, particularly water temperature, influence disease prevalence and transmission among fish species. Eisenlord et al. [11] reported a significant decline in sea star populations due to a wasting disease exacerbated by ocean warming. Maynard et al. [26] linked increased seawater temperatures to the proliferation of lobster shell disease in New England. Burge et al. [7] analyzed the global dissemination of marine diseases and pathogens due to climate change.

Change in Behavior

Ocean acidification affects fish sensory capabilities and behavior. Elevated CO_2 levels impair olfaction, vision, and hearing in marine species, as shown by Munday et al. [30, 9] and Ferrari et al. [15]. Acidification significantly impacts juvenile fish's ability to differentiate water sources and select predator-free habitats. These sensory and behavioral changes increase predation risk and decrease survival rates, as reported by Munday et al. [31] and Ferrari et al. [14].

Economic Effects of Climate Change

Climate change's impact on fish populations has significant social and economic ramifications for stakeholders, including workers, coastal communities, and consumers. The economic consequences vary, with some regions facing negative effects and others benefiting. Key impacts include changes in catch value, production costs, employment, distributional effects, community economies, and long-term profitability. Mitigation and adaptation strategies are essential for addressing these challenges.

Mitigation

Mitigation efforts aim to reduce or reverse the anthropogenic factors contributing to climate change [1]. Strategies include reducing greenhouse gas emissions through sustainable practices, adopting clean energy, promoting electric vehicles, implementing energy-efficient systems, and tree planting. These measures improve air quality, reduce healthcare costs, and enhance energy efficiency. Effective mitigation relies on collective efforts from individuals, governments, businesses, and stakeholders.

Adaptation

Adaptation involves adjusting to climate change's impacts to ensure long-term sustainability. Strategies must be tailored to the specific environmental conditions of affected areas, considering population dynamics, community characteristics, and existing industries. Adaptation measures include developing climate-resilient built environments, protecting vulnerable habitats, managing water resources, reinforcing infrastructure, and enhancing disaster risk management.

Resiliency

Resilience refers to the ability to recover from adverse events, such as climatic alterations. Achieving resilience involves individuals, communities, businesses, and sectors collaborating to adapt effectively to climate impacts [1]. Measuring resilience is challenging due to diverse potential outcomes but should be seen as an indication of the field's diversity [2, 6].

6 Conclusion

Fisheries and aquaculture play a crucial role in food security and livelihoods in developing nations. Climate change poses significant threats to marine ecosystems and fisheries, necessitating active engagement and well-designed policies for adaptation and mitigation. Enhanced scientific research, stakeholder collaboration, and effective governance are essential for addressing climate-related risks and ensuring the sustainability of fisheries.

Recommendations

To address climate change's impacts on fisheries and aquaculture, the following recommendations are proposed:

- Establish effective communication channels with stakeholders to convey information about climate change impacts.
- Enhance best practices and research on fish behavior based on sound science.
- Encourage nature-based innovative solutions.
- Protect ecosystems, particularly nursery and spawning areas.
- Focus on herbivore aquaculture and sustainable seafood demand.
- Improve ecosystem observation systems.

– Preserve vulnerable species components.
– Implement integrated water system tracking.
– Shift to sustainable fishing gear.
– Adopt flexible policy and management strategies.
– Promote climate change education and awareness.

References

1. ACT (2018) Mitigation, adaptation, and resilience: climate terminology explained. Retrieved from: https://www.hidropolitikakademi.org/tr/news/22267/mitigation-adaptation-and-resilience-climate-terminology-explained
2. Aldunce P, Beilin R, Howden SM Handmer J (2015) Resilience for disaster risk management in a changing climate: practitioners' frames and practices. Global Environ Change 30. https://doi.org/10.1016/j.gloenvcha.2014.10.010
3. Badjeck MC et al (2010) Impacts of climate variability and change on fishery-based livelihoods. Marine Policy 34(3):375–383. https://doi.org/10.1016/j.marpol.2009.08.007
4. Barange M, Bahri T, Beveridge MCM, Cochrane AL, Funge-Smith S, Paulain F (2018) Impacts of climate change on fisheries and aquaculture, synthesis of current knowledge, adaptation and mitigation options. FAO, Rome
5. Beach RH, Viator CL (2008) The economics of aquaculture insurance: an overview of the U.S. pilot insurance program for cultivated clams. Aquac Econ Manage 12:25–38. https://doi.org/10.1080/13657300801959613
6. Borquez R, Aldunce P, Adler C (2017) Resilience to climate change: from theory to practice through co-production of knowledge in Chile. Sustain Sci 12:163–176. https://doi.org/10.1007/s11625-016-0400-6
7. Burge CA, Mark Eakin C, Friedman CS, Froelich B, Hershberger PK, Hofmann EE, Petes LE, Prager KC, Weil E, Willis BL, Ford SE, Harvell CD (2014) Climate change influences on marine infectious diseases: implications for management and society. Ann Rev Mar Sci 6:249–277. https://doi.org/10.1146/annurev-marine-010213-135029
8. Daw T, Adger WN, Brown K, Badjeck MC (2009) Climate change and capture fisheries: potential impacts, adaptation, and mitigation. In: Cochrane K, De Young C, Soto D, Bahri T (eds) Climate change implications for fisheries and aquaculture: overview of current scientific knowledge. FAO Fisheries and Aquaculture Technical Paper. No. 530. FAO, Rome, pp 107–150
9. Dixson DL, Munday PL, Jones GP (2010) Ocean acidfication disrupts the innate ability of fishto detect predator olfactory cues. Ecology Lett 3:68–75. https://doi.org/10.1111/j.1461-0248.2009.01400
10. Doubleday ZA, Clarke SM, Li X, Pecl GT, Ward TM, Battaglene S et al (2013) Assessing the risk of climate change to aquaculture: a case study from southeast Australia. Aquacult Environ Interact 3:163–175. https://doi.org/10.3354/aei00058
11. Eisenlord ME, Groner ML, Yoshioka RM, Elliott J, Maynard J, Fradkin S, Turner M, Pyne K, Rivlin N, van Hooidonk R, Harvell CD (2016) Ochre star mortality during the 2014 wasting disease epizootic: role of population size structure and temperature. Philos Trans R Soc Lond B Biol Sci 371(1689): 20150212. https://doi.org/10.1098/rstb.2015.0212
12. Environmental Protection Agency (2016) Sources of greenhouse gas emissions. Retrieved from: https://www.epa.gov/ghgemissions/sources-greenhouse-gasemissions
13. FAO (2020) The state of world fisheries and aquaculture 2020. In: Sustainability in action. FAO, Rome
14. Ferrari MCO, Dixson DL, Munday PL, McCormick MI, Meekan MG, Sih A, Chivers DP (2011) Intrageneric variation in antipredator responses of coral reef fishes affected by ocean

acidification: implications for climate change projections on marine communities. Glob Chang Biol 17:2980–2986
15. Ferrari MC, Manassa RP, Dixson DL et al (2012) Effects of ocean acidification on learning in coral reef fishes. PloS one 7
16. GAFRD (1990–2020) Annual fishery statistical books from 1990 to 2020. Agriculture and land Reclamation Ministry, Egypt
17. Gao Y, Yu G, Yang T, Jia Y, He N, Zhuang J (2016) New insight into global blue carbon estimation under human activity in land-sea interaction area: a case study of China. Earth Sci Rev 159:36–46. https://doi.org/10.1016/j.earscirev.2016.05.003
18. Hamdan R, Othman A, Kari F (2015) Climate change effects on aquaculture production performance in Malaysia: an environmental performance analysis. Int J Bus Soc 16:364–385. https://doi.org/10.33736/ijbs.573.2015
19. Harvell C et al (1999) Emerging marine diseases--climate links and anthropogenic factors. Science 285(5433):1505–1510. https://doi.org/10.1126/science.285.5433.1505
20. IPCC (2013) Summary for policymakers, the physical science basis. Contribution of working group I to the fifth assessment report of the Intergovernmental Panel on Climate Change. Cambridge University Press, Cambridge; New York, NY
21. IPCC (2014) Climate change 2014: synthesis report. Contribution of working groups I, II, and III to the fifth assessment report on the Intergovernmental Panel on Climate Change. Core writing team, R. K. Pachauri and L.A. Meyer. Intergovernmental Panel on Climate Change, Geneva, 151 pp. Available online at: http://www.ipcc.ch/pdf/assessmentreport/ar5/syr/SYR_AR5_FINAL_full_wcover.pdf
22. IPCC (2018) Global warming of 1.5 °C. In: Masson-Delmotte V, Zhai P, Pörtner H-O, Roberts D, Skea J, Shukla PR, Pirani A, Moufouma-Okia W, Péan C, Pidcock R, Connors S, Matthews JBR, Chen Y, Zhou X, Gomis MI, Lonnoy E, Maycock T, Tignor M, Waterfield T (eds) An IPCC special report on the impacts of global warming of 1.5 °C above pre-industrial levels and related global greenhouse gas emission pathways, in the context of strengthening the global response to the threat of climate change, sustainable development, and efforts to eradicate poverty
23. IPCC (2019) Special report on climate change, desertification, land degradation, sustainable land management, food security, and greenhouse gas fluxes in terrestrial ecosystems, summary for policymakers approved draft. IPCC, Geneva
24. Kandu P (2017) Papua New Guinea. Impacts of climate variations on local fisheries and aquaculture resources in PNG. In: Ramos EJ (ed) Ecological risk assessment of impacts of climate change on fisheries and aquaculture resources. APEC Ocean and Fisheries Working Group), Peru, pp 45–49
25. Khaine, I, Woo, SY (2015) An overview of interrelationship between climate change and forests. For Sci Technol 11:11–18. https://doi.org/10.1080/21580103.2014.932718
26. Maynard J, van Hooidonk R, Eakin CM, Puotinen M, Garren M, Williams GJ, Heron SF, Lamb J, Weil E, Willis B, Hervell CD (2015) Projections of climate conditions that increase coral disease susceptibility and pathogen abundance and virulence. Nat Climate Change 5:688–694. https://doi.org/10.1038/nclimate2625
27. Mehanna SF (2021) Egyptian marine fisheries and its sustainability. In: Galanakis CM (eds) Sustainable fish production and processing. Academic Press, Elsevier, pp 111–140, 325 p
28. Mehanna SF (2020a) Challenges faced the small-scale fisheries and its sustainable development. ICAR—Central Marine Fisheries Research Institute, Research Centre Mangalore, 7–10 January 2020
29. Mehanna SF (2020b) An overview of the aquaculture sector in Egypt: current trend and the development strategies. Tropentag 2020, 9–11 September, Germany
30. Munday PL, Dixson DL, Donelson JM, Jones GP, Pratchett MS, Devitsina GV et al (2009) Ocean acidification impairs the olfactory discrimination and homing ability of marine fish. Proc Natl Acad Sci USA 106:1848–1852. https://doi.org/10.1073/pnas.0809996106
31. Munday PL, Dixson DL, Mccormick MI, Meekan M, Ferrari MCO, Chivers DP (2010) Replenishment of fish populations is threatened by ocean acidification. Proc Nat Acad Sci Unit States Am 107:12930–12934

32. Myers SS, Smith MR, Guth S, Golden CD, Vaitla B, Mueller ND et al (2017) Climate change and global food systems: potential impacts on food security and undernutrition. Annu Rev Public Health 38:259–277. https://doi.org/10.1146/annurev-publhealth-031816-044356
33. Oyinlola MA, Reygondeau G, Wabnitz CCC, Cheung WWL (2020) Projecting global mariculture diversity under climate change. Glob Change Biol 26:2134–2148
34. Palmer T, Stevens B (2019) The scientific challenge of understanding and estimating climate change. Proc Natl Acad Sci USA 116:24390–24395. https://doi.org/10.1073/pnas.1906691116
35. Poloczanska ES, Brown CJ, Sydeman WJ, Kiessling W, Schoeman DS, Moore PJ, Brander K, Bruno JF, Buckley LB, Burrows MT, Duarte CM, Halpern BS, Holding J, Kappel CV, O'Connor MI, Pandolfi JM, Parmesan C, Schwing F, Thompson SA, Richardson AJ (2013) Global imprint of climate change on marine life. Nat Clim Change 3:919–925
36. Riphah SU (2015) Global warming: causes, effects, and solutions. Durreesamin J. 1:1–7
37. Rose JB, Epstein PR, Lipp EK, Sherman BH, Bernard SM, Patz JA (2001) Climate variability and change in the United States: potential impacts on water and foodborne diseases caused by microbiologic agents. Environ Health Perspect 109(suppl 2):211–221. https://doi.org/10.1289/ehp.01109s2211
38. Troell M, Eide A, Isaksen J, Hermansen Ø, Crépin AS (2017) Seafood from a changing Arctic. Ambio 46:S368–S386. https://doi.org/10.1007/s13280-017-0954-2
39. Yazdi SK, Shakouri D (2010) The effects of climate change on aquaculture. Int J Environ Sci Dev 1:378–382. https://doi.org/10.7763/IJESD.2010.V1.73
40. Zolnikov TR (ed) (2019) Global adaptation and resilience to climate change. Palgrave Studies in Climate Resilient Societies (Bern). https://doi.org/10.1007/978-3-030-01213-7

Impact of Climate Change on Egyptian Agriculture, Challenges, and Opportunities

Ayman F. Abou-Hadid

Abstract The current chapter delves into the intricate relationship between agriculture and climate change, highlighting the multifaceted impacts of environmental factors on agricultural activities worldwide. It emphasizes the critical role of adaptation strategies in ensuring food security and agricultural sustainability in the face of climate variability. Focusing on Egyptian agriculture as a case study, the chapter explores the vulnerability of agricultural systems to climate-related risks such as drought, temperature variations, and rising sea levels. It introduces the concept of Climate Smart Agriculture (CSA) as an integrated approach to managing agricultural activities efficiently, focusing on increasing productivity, enhancing resilience, and reducing emissions. Through a combination of research findings and innovative practices, the chapter underscores the importance of sustainable water resource management, biological improvement of crops, and technological innovation in mitigating the adverse effects of climate change on agriculture. The chapter provides valuable insights into the challenges and opportunities for adapting agriculture to a changing climate landscape, with implications for global food security and rural livelihoods.

Keywords Adaptation · Food security · Resilience · Climate Smart Agriculture (CSA) · Water resources · Temperature variations · Precipitation · Sustainability

1 Introduction

Agriculture, one of the major economic activities globally, serves as the primary source of food for humans and provides a significant portion of animal feed. Additionally, it supplies raw materials for numerous industries, encompassing plant production, animal husbandry, fisheries and aquaculture, and forest management.

The success of agricultural endeavours hinges greatly on environmental conditions and balanced climatic variations. Precipitation is the primary water source for agriculture, either directly meeting water needs in rainfed agriculture or indirectly

A. F. Abou-Hadid (✉)
Faculty of Agriculture, Ain Shams University, Cairo, Egypt
e-mail: ayman_abouhadeed@agr.asu.edu.eg

© The Author(s), under exclusive license to Springer Nature Switzerland AG 2025
M. T. Khalil et al. (eds.), *Climate Changes Impacts on Aquatic Environment*, Earth and Environmental Sciences Library, https://doi.org/10.1007/978-3-031-74897-4_7

through water streams and river basins. Moreover, precipitation plays a vital role in recharging underground aquifers in various regions. Adequate rainfall is imperative for productive agriculture; insufficient rain can lead to drought, negatively impacting agricultural output. Conversely, excessive rainfall may trigger flooding and soil erosion, both of which can have devastating effects on agricultural productivity.

Temperature plays a crucial role in crop growth. Increasing temperatures and higher carbon dioxide concentrations can enhance crop yields. However, surpassing the optimal temperature range for crops can inhibit plant growth and escalate water evapotranspiration, increasing water requirements. Elevated temperatures affect plant production and intensify heat stress on animals, leading to reduced growth and activity levels. Temperature variations can disrupt plant growth cycles, altering the availability of commodities in the market and potentially reducing crop productivity. Climatic variations also affect the health of plants and animals, rendering them more susceptible to infections and causing economic damage. Consequently, the variability in climate significantly impacts agricultural income, thereby affecting farmers, farmworkers, and local traders, ultimately destabilizing rural communities.

Considering these interconnections between climate change and agriculture, this chapter aims to offer a comprehensive understanding of their dynamics. By identifying challenges, proposing solutions, and emphasizing the importance of adaptation strategies, the chapter aims to facilitate sustainable agricultural development in the face of climate change.

2 Climate Smart Agriculture

Agricultural activities are rapidly spreading across the planet due to the exponential increase in population. New lands are being cultivated in territories that were previously untouched. However, despite advancements in agricultural sciences and techniques, specialists often need help finding quick and accurate solutions to diverse problems. Compounding this challenge is the accelerated pace of climate change, which complicates decision-making using conventional methods. Recognizing these issues, many scientists consider climate-smart agriculture to be the model for the future of agriculture.

Climate-smart agriculture is an integrated approach to managing agricultural activities, aiming to address interconnected issues in food production efficiently and effectively. It seeks to achieve increased productivity, enhanced resilience, and reduced emissions in a timely manner. Doing so can increase sustainable food production and improve livelihoods, particularly for the rural poor. Additionally, it can mitigate vulnerability to both biotic and abiotic threats to agricultural production systems and rural communities. Moreover, it contributes to lower greenhouse gas emissions and improves the overall carbon footprint of agriculture.

3 Impact of Climate Change on Agriculture

Everyone is increasingly feeling the effects of climate change and its impacts on various human activities. Farmers and rural inhabitants are acutely aware of how climate change affects agriculture. Successful farming and crop production rely on healthy, fertile soil, stable weather conditions, and a consistent water supply throughout the growing season. The impacts of climate change on agriculture manifest in several ways, including:

(a) Climate change can trigger extreme weather events such as floods, severe droughts, strong winds, and sudden temperature fluctuations. Plants and animals exposed to such events undergo severe stress. For instance, hot winds can disrupt the pollination of fruit trees, leading to the loss of flowers and fruits at early stages.
(b) Changing temperature profiles can alter the growth cycles of various crops, affecting normal planting dates and the duration of the growing season. This may necessitate reconsidering crop rotation practices, especially in intensive agricultural systems.
(c) Precipitation patterns will change, affecting both the timing and quantity of rainfall. In arid regions, the productivity of rain-fed agriculture is expected to decrease.
(d) Rising sea levels pose a serious threat to river deltas and low-lying areas. Some lands may become submerged underwater, while others may face salinization due to the intrusion of saline water into delta soils. River deltas are often densely populated agricultural regions known for their fertility.
(e) The impact of rising sea levels on deltas may lead to the emigration of farmers from affected regions, posing significant social challenges.

Addressing these impacts requires proactive measures to adapt agricultural practices to changing environmental conditions and mitigate the effects of climate change on food production and rural livelihoods.

4 Effects of Climate Change on Agriculture

The impacts of climate change on agriculture will lead to several severe effects:

(a) Food security will be at risk due to changes in cultivation dates for major crops and increased temperatures, which will elevate water consumption. Many areas already have water shortages, leading to plant water stress and reduced yields. This reduction in crop productivity will significantly lower farm incomes and diminish farmers' living standards. Moreover, the need to import more commodities from regional and international markets will rise, exacerbating pressure on already strained supply chains. Consequently, food security will be jeopardized worldwide.

(b) Land health and soil stability will be adversely affected by climate change. Drought events will negatively impact both natural flora and rainfed agricultural lands. Extreme flooding may occur, resulting in the loss of natural vegetation, land degradation, and heightened vulnerability to future climatic shocks.
(c) Increased conflicts over water in rainfed areas and overgrazing will diminish the stability of domestic animal populations.
(d) Climate change will disrupt local communities by destroying farms, reducing farm incomes, and increasing poverty. In such circumstances, migration may become the only viable option for farmers who are compelled to seek livelihoods elsewhere.

5 The Future of Egyptian Agriculture Considering Climate Change and Regional Conditions

5.1 Current Situation

Agriculture plays a vital role in the Egyptian economy, absorbing approximately 55% of the labour force. It also consumes nearly 80% of the country's water resources and contributes around 14% of the total national income. Given Egypt's location in a hyper-arid region, its agriculture is highly sensitive to climate change, particularly reliant on the Nile River, making it vulnerable to the impacts of climate variability.

It is crucial that the national strategy for climate change adaptation prioritizes the quality and efficiency of agricultural inputs. Currently, the cultivated land area in Egypt spans approximately 8.44 million feddans (1 feddan = 4200 square meters, 1 fedddan = 0.42 ha, 1 feddan = 1.034 acres), with 80% located in the Delta and Nile Valley (old lands) and the remainder situated in the outskirts of the valley and Delta (new lands). The productivity and suitability of agricultural land vary significantly depending on factors such as salinity and groundwater levels.

Projections suggest that the cultivated area is expected to expand to 11.5 million feddans by 2030. Egypt's plant production is diverse, driven by multiple seasons (winter, summer, nili) and a wide range of agricultural products, including field crops, vegetables, orchards, fodder, oil crops, sugar crops, and others.

Despite having a land area of only 8.44 million feddans, Egypt manages to cultivate crops across 17 million feddans, a figure anticipated to increase to between 20 and 22 million feddans by 2030. This growth is attributed to the high productivity of current crops and agricultural varieties, which have been enhanced by adopting modern technologies and advancing breeding programs.

5.2 Coastal Areas

Coastal areas along the Mediterranean Sea are vulnerable to the threats posed by rising sea levels. This includes both natural protection areas, such as the Nile Delta and Alexandria coastal zone, which feature beaches, sand dunes, longitudinal limestone formations, and industrial zones protected by marine walls and barriers. These areas are particularly at risk and require future adaptation measures to bolster their resilience against rising water levels. It is crucial to fortify these regions to prevent the inundation or salinization of the Delta lands.

Egypt's water resources are both limited and relatively stable. However, there has been a noted decrease in the efficiency of water usage in agriculture. This decline is attributed to a 30% decrease in water transport efficiency and a 50% reduction in the effectiveness of field irrigation. Such inefficiencies significantly constrain the country's ability to expand its agricultural sector in the short term and hamper its capacity to address potential increases in evaporation rates due to rising temperatures.

5.3 Animal and Fish Production

Buffaloes, cattle, and sheep are integral components of livestock production in Egypt, providing both red meat and milk. Fish and poultry, on the other hand, are the primary sources of white meat. The livestock sector contributes approximately 42.9% to the agricultural output, underscoring its critical role in ensuring food security and supporting economic activities.

The Agricultural Development Strategy, extending until 2030, aims to increase dairy production to 9.5 million tons, red meat to one million tons, poultry to 1.4 million tons, and fish to 1.4 million tons annually. Achieving these targets, among other objectives, necessitates safeguarding this livestock wealth from diseases and ensuring sustainable farming practices.

Egypt's annual fish production stands at 1.1 million tons, with fish farming accounting for approximately 72.76% of the total fish production in the country.

6 The Impact of Climate Change, Risks, Disasters, and Crises in the Agricultural Sector

Salinization of land in the Delta, coupled with flooding of agricultural areas north of the Delta due to decreased rainfall on the North Coast, poses significant challenges. These challenges are exacerbated by the decline in rain-fed agriculture, dwindling aquifer water levels, and the looming threat of desertification. Climate change is expected to reduce crop productivity further, alter agricultural landscapes, and facilitate the spread of fungal plant diseases. Agricultural lands in the Delta are particularly vulnerable, especially those adjacent to the Mediterranean coast.

Given these anticipated conditions, urgent action is necessary to implement programs that enable adaptation to the expected impacts of these changes on Egyptian agriculture. Various predictions exist regarding the rates of temperature change and rising water levels in the Delta region. Below, we will examine the anticipated impacts of temperature changes of up to two degrees Celsius and sea level rise of up to one meter above the current level.

7 Results of Sensitivity Studies to Climate Change

These results are based on field experiments aimed at collecting data for different models, which undergo a calibration process to ensure accurate predictions under Egyptian conditions. Simulation studies have been conducted across various agricultural climatic zones, spanning periods from 25 to 40 years. These studies reveal significant impacts of climate change on crop productivity and water consumption.

For instance, simulations indicate that a two-degree Celsius rise in temperature will lead to a 9% decrease in wheat crop productivity and a 6.2% increase in water consumption compared to current conditions. This could result in an 18% shortage in water if temperatures rose by four degrees Celsius. Similarly, maize yield is projected to decline by 19% by mid-century, with a 3.5 °C temperature increase and an 8% rise in water consumption. Rice yield may decrease by 11%, with a 16% increase in water consumption. Being highly sensitive to temperature changes, Tomatoes could see a 14% decrease in productivity with a two-degree Celsius rise and a 51% decrease with a 3.5-degree Celsius rise.

Furthermore, climate change is expected to have varied impacts across different crops. Sugar cane productivity may decrease by 24.5%, accompanied by a 2.3% increase in water consumption and a 25.6% decrease in yield per water unit. Conversely, cotton productivity may increase by 17% with a two-degree Celsius temperature rise, with water consumption increasing by 4.1–5.2%. Under conditions of high-temperature increase (four degrees Celsius), cotton productivity could rise by 31%, with water consumption increasing by about 10%.

By the middle of this century, water consumption for most major crops is projected to increase due to climate change-induced warming. Water consumption changes for winter crops may range from -2% for barley to + 2.5% for wheat. Summer sunflower crops may see a 6% increase, maize an 8% increase, cotton a 10% increase, soybeans a 15% increase, rice a 16% increase, and sugarcane a 2.3% increase.

8 The Risks of Climate Change and Regional Conditions on Egyptian Food Security

Egyptian agriculture is confronted with numerous threats stemming from climate change, directly impacting food security. One such threat is the rising level of the Mediterranean Sea, which will elevate the salinity and groundwater levels in agricultural lands. This rise in salinity, coupled with increased salinity in northern freshwater lakes, will result in the loss of fertile agricultural areas and a reduction in plant and animal production. Additionally, changes in fish populations, which serve as a primary source of protein in Egypt, will occur, further affecting food availability, particularly for the poor.

The consequences of these changes extend beyond agriculture, leading to displacement of populations due to flooding, reduced fertility, or lack of alternative employment opportunities. Egypt heavily relies on food imports, with rates reaching 50% for wheat and 90% for oils. Consequently, food security may be vulnerable to economic crises, given the anticipation of high import bills. Moreover, without adequate investment in agro-technological development to adapt to climate change, there is a risk of facing technological crises.

Furthermore, there are ideas that merit careful consideration and specialized study, such as reducing rice cultivation and replacing sugar cane with beets, considering the water-intensive nature of these crops. Additionally, the shift towards growing short-staple cotton to meet local factory demands could pose challenges in maintaining and improving the quality of Egyptian cotton.

Considering these challenges, there is a need to focus on agricultural development in Africa, with particular attention to enhancing cooperation with countries like Ethiopia. Strengthening partnerships in various fields will address mutual challenges and foster sustainable agricultural practices.

9 Adaptation Possibilities

9.1 Future Trends of Cultivation

According to a study conducted by Khater et al. [6], an agricultural survey utilizing satellite imagery was conducted to assess land cover in the Nile Delta. The data obtained revealed that the total area of the Delta was 2.9 million Feddan. However, discrepancies were observed between the survey results and official estimations for specific crops. For instance, the cultivated area of wheat, as per the survey, was approximately 2.5 million feddan, which was 13% less than the official estimate. Similar disparities were observed for barley, with the survey estimating 148 thousand feddan compared to the official report of 181 thousand feddan, and for cotton, where the survey estimated 250 thousand feddan compared to the reported 284 thousand feddan.

These discrepancies resulted in an overestimation of the water budget. With the looming threats of climate change potentially reducing available water and an increasing population demanding more agricultural products, it was concluded that a redesign of crop patterns is necessary. The cultivation area should be based on satellite imagery to facilitate better utilization of agricultural lands and water resources.

9.2 *Improvement of Sugarcane*

Sugarcane is a significant crop in Upper Egypt, yet it poses a challenge due to its high water requirements. However, an experiment conducted by Gaber et al. [4] tested various new breeds of sugarcane that exhibited increased growth and sugar content even under water stress conditions. This suggests that these new breeds require less water to produce the same amount of sugar, offering a potential solution to maintain sugar production amidst lower water availability resulting from climate change.

9.3 *Removing Metal Contaminants from Wastewater.*

One strategy to adapt to climate change and cope with reduced water availability is by utilizing recycled water. However, a significant challenge associated with recycled water is the concentration of hazardous metals it may contain. Abou-Hadid et al. [2] investigated the production of efficient carbon fibre from various solid waste residuals to adsorb hazardous metals from wastewater samples. Effective removal of hazardous elements from wastewater necessitates using reliable technology and suitable functional materials.

The study found that carbon fibre derived from agricultural solid waste was a promising and cost-effective adsorbent for wastewater treatment applications. Specifically, two types of carbon fibre were synthesized from different agricultural wastes: rice husk and sugarcane bagasse. These carbon fibres were demonstrated to be effective in removing contaminants from wastewater, highlighting their potential for widespread use in wastewater treatment processes.

9.4 *Water Catchment Potentials on the Northwest Coast of Egypt*

Egypt is a hyper-arid region with the highest levels of water scarcity globally. The country's northwest coast is particularly vulnerable to a significant reduction in water resources due to climate change. To address this challenge, the first step towards adaptation involves assessing the potential for rainwater catchment in the region.

In a study conducted by Khater et al. [6], the rainwater catchment potentialities in the northwest coast of Egypt were investigated using remote sensing and geographic information systems. The findings revealed that the vegetation cover in the study area needs to be increased to sustain long-term agriculture, even to support the local population. However, field surveys suggested the feasibility of cultivating certain winter crops that require minimal water, such as wheat and barley.

Additionally, it is crucial to preserve fig plants in this area, which rely on scattered rains and fog water droplets on their broad leaves for sustenance. Constructing small dams and water reservoirs can help harvest water for human and animal consumption. Furthermore, adopting new agricultural technologies, such as greenhouses and soilless culture, is recommended to produce high-value crops with limited water resources in the region.

9.5 Grey Water Use and Its Footprint in Agriculture

Water footprint analysis typically offers comprehensive insights into water resources management. Its significance becomes even more pronounced when water resources are limited. Abd-Elsalam et al. [1] conducted an experiment to assess the water footprint of potato plants cultivated using grey water during winter seasons. The study examined various nitrogen levels in potatoes and found that higher nitrogen levels led to increased vegetative growth and yield. Consequently, the water footprint of potatoes also increased with elevated nitrogen levels. It is essential to recognize that the water footprint is a multidimensional indicator, encompassing both water consumption and the type of pollution involved.

9.6 Climate Change and Potato

Planting dates can significantly impact crop performance by subjecting plants to varying weather conditions, particularly during sensitive growth stages. In a study conducted by Meligy et al. [7], potatoes were cultivated on three different dates, with water added at three levels for each planting date. The results indicated that delaying the planting date reduced potato yield, primarily due to increased temperatures during the tuber maturity stage. Consequently, it was concluded that if global temperatures continue to rise, the production of potatoes is expected to decrease if cultivation dates remain unchanged.

9.7 Remote Sensing Estimation of Evapotranspiration

Evapotranspiration plays a pivotal role in water utilization in agriculture, with major crops, including wheat, among the highest agricultural water consumers. Sustainable management practices in crop production are essential for optimizing water use efficiency.

In a study conducted by Gamal et al. [5], actual daily evapotranspiration (ET) data collected through a remote sensing model were compared and validated with Energy Balance (EB) flux tower field measurements. The findings revealed that remote sensing offers a reasonable and cost-effective method for estimating evapotranspiration. This advancement holds promise for enhancing agriculture's water management practices, enabling adaptation to potential climate change scenarios.

9.8 Biological Improvement of Abiotic Stress

The impact of climate change is expected to manifest in global warming, increased sea water levels leading to higher salinity and extreme weather conditions such as droughts. Afifi et al. [3] have contributed significantly by providing insights into adapting to these three climate change stressors. The study involved the collection of ninety-eight isolates of Trichoderma from the rhizosphere and seeds across sixteen governorates in Egypt. Certain isolates exhibited high performance under both in vitro and ex vivo pot experiments, particularly against heat, salinity, and drought stresses.

The experiments yielded compelling evidence that these isolates could aid in mitigating salinity, heat, and drought stresses. Such observations hold the potential for enhancing phytosanitary services for growers and agricultural researchers, particularly in arid regions, thus promoting sustainable utilization in anticipation of climate change impacts.

10 Conclusion

In conclusion, the intricate relationship between climate change and agriculture presents multifaceted challenges that require proactive and innovative solutions. As elucidated throughout this chapter, agriculture, being a cornerstone of economies worldwide, is profoundly influenced by climatic variations, which impact crop yields, livestock health, and water availability. The consequences of climate change on agriculture extend beyond economic realms, posing threats to food security, rural livelihoods, and environmental sustainability.

The concept of climate-smart agriculture emerges as a promising approach to navigate the complexities of agricultural production amidst changing climatic conditions. By integrating adaptive strategies, enhancing resilience, and mitigating emissions, climate-smart agriculture not only enhances productivity but also fosters sustainability and improves livelihoods, particularly in vulnerable rural communities.

The case of Egyptian agriculture serves as a poignant illustration of the intricate interplay between climate change and regional conditions. With Egypt's heavy reliance on the Nile River and its susceptibility to rising sea levels, salinization, and water scarcity, the agricultural sector faces imminent threats. However, the chapter outlines various adaptation possibilities, ranging from redesigning crop patterns based on satellite imagery to harnessing innovative technologies for wastewater treatment and rainwater harvesting.

Furthermore, advancements in biotechnology, such as the biological improvement of crops to withstand abiotic stresses, offer promising avenues for enhancing agricultural resilience in the face of climate change. Nevertheless, effective adaptation requires a comprehensive approach encompassing policy interventions, technological innovations, and stakeholder collaborative efforts.

In essence, addressing the impacts of climate change on agriculture necessitates a holistic and coordinated approach that integrates scientific knowledge, technological innovation, and policy coherence. By embracing adaptive strategies and fostering sustainable practices, agricultural systems can mitigate the adverse effects of climate change, ensure food security, and safeguard the livelihoods of millions dependent on agriculture worldwide.

11 Recommendations

- Adopt climate-smart agriculture.
- Improve water use efficiency.
- Optimize crop patterns.
- Develop drought-resistant crops.
- Promote sustainable livestock and fish farming.
- Enhance coastal protection.
- Utilize recycled water.
- Invest in rainwater harvesting.
- Adopt green technologies.
- Enhance soil health.

References

1. Abd-Elsalam MM, Farag AA, El-Shinawy MZ, Abou-Hadid AF (2022) Effect of different nitrogen rates on gray water and water footprint to potato. Arab Univ J Agric Sci 30(2):1–9. https://doi.org/10.21608/ajs.2022.110065.1445
2. Abou-Hadid AF, El-Behairy UA, Elmalih MM, Amdeha E, El Naggar AMA, Taha MH, Hussein AEM (2022). Production of efficient carbon fiber from different solid waste residuals for adsorption of hazardous metals from wastewater samples. Biomass Conv Biorefinery. https://doi.org/10.1007/s13399-022-03097-6
3. Afifi HH, Hassan NA, Abou-Hadid AF, Madkor MA (2021) The ability of selected *Trichoderma* spp. to improve wheat (*Triticum asetivum* L.) tolerance under heat, salinity, and drought stresses through seed treatments. Plant Cell Biotechnol Mol Biol 22(47–48):61–74. https://www.ikprress.org/index.php/PCBMB/article/view/6906
4. Gaber AA, Abou-Hadid AF, El-Gabry YA, Ebid MHM (2021) Morphological and physiological study for sugarcane early selection to drought tolerance. Plant Arch 21(1):1935–1944. https://doi.org/10.51470/PLANTARCHIVES.2021.v21.no1.269
5. Gamal R, El-Shirbeny M, Abou-Hadid A, Swelam A, El-Gindy A-G, Arafa Y, Nangia V (2022) Identification and quantification of actual evapotranspiration using integrated satellite data for sustainable water management in dry areas. Agronomy 12(9):2143. https://doi.org/10.3390/agronomy12092143
6. Khater AA, Abou-Hadid AF, El-Behairy UA, Aboelghar MA, Ali AM (2019) Studying rainwater catchment potentialities in the northwest coast of Egypt using remote sensing and geographic information system. Arab Univ J Agric Sci 27(3):1955–1966. https://www.ajs.journals.ekb.eg/article_76135.html
7. Meligy MM, Abou-Hadid AF, El-Shinawy MZ, El-Behairy UA (2020). Impact of climate change on water requirements and the productivity on potato crop. Egypt J Horticult 47(1):57–68. https://doi.org/10.21608/ejoh.2020.27403.1130

Breeding Plants Resilient to Climate Change

Naglaa A. Abdallah

Abstract Climate change is increasingly impacting biodiversity, agricultural production, and food security, leading to climate-driven extinctions. In plants, it affects species distribution, extinction rates, reproduction timings, and growing season lengths. Climate change has also disrupted marine, terrestrial, and freshwater ecosystems worldwide, causing the loss of local species, increased diseases, and mass animal mortality. Anticipated future climate changes include rising temperatures, more severe droughts, rising sea levels, potential decreases in rainfall, regional flooding, and reduced water availability. These factors could severely threaten agricultural production and food security, including production, access, and prices. Insect attacks will occur more frequently as a result of rising temperatures exacerbating the effects of drought and decreasing soil moisture. Using advanced breeding techniques, crop varieties that are climate-resilient must be developed in order to both adapt to and mitigate the effects of climate change. By creating environmentally friendly plant varieties with high yields, reduced pesticide requirements, and pest resistance, plant breeding can increase food production per unit area. Novel breeding programs can significantly impact crop improvement by targeting precise genome changes. Genomic-assisted breeding assists in annotating information obtained from pan-genomes, helping capture lost genes that can optimize breeding programs. New breeding techniques using CRISPR/Cas genome editing are promising candidates for promoting sustainability and environmental protection. Through their application, beneficial climate-resilient crops that target both biotic and abiotic stresses have been developed, greatly enhancing crop performance. de nova Building resistance against biotic and abiotic stress has many uses for CRISPR/Cas systems, such as base editing, prime editing, and epigenome editing. Combining genome editing with speed breeding can result in crops that are climate-adapted, which is essential for maintaining global food security.

N. A. Abdallah (✉)
Department of Genetics Faculty of Agriculture, Cairo University, Giza, Egypt
e-mail: Naglaa.abdallah@agr.cu.edu.eg

National Biotechnology Network of Expertise (NBNE), Cairo, Egypt

© The Author(s), under exclusive license to Springer Nature Switzerland AG 2025
M. T. Khalil et al. (eds.), *Climate Changes Impacts on Aquatic Environment*, Earth and Environmental Sciences Library, https://doi.org/10.1007/978-3-031-74897-4_8

Keywords Genomic-assisted breeding · CRISPR/Cas · Base editing · Prime editing · Epigenome editing phenotyping · Speed breeding · Artificial intelligent

1 Introduction

Climate change impacts agriculture through both direct effects, such as physiological, phenotypic, and morphological impacts on plant growth, alterations in landscapes, and heat waves, as well as indirect effects like changes in soil fertility, water quality, increased pests/diseases, heat/drought/flood events, rising sea levels, and pollution. Variability in climate conditions like droughts, heat, and flooding primarily affects agricultural productivity and food security. Crop production worldwide is expected to be seriously threatened by extreme climate disruptions, which are predicted to produce unstable crop yields [61]. Drought stress coupled with higher temperatures considerably reduces the yield and photosynthesis rates of vegetable crops. Wheat productivity is expected to decrease by 6.0%, rice productivity by 3.2%, maize productivity by 7.4%, and soybean productivity by 3.1% for every degree Celsius increase in the world's average temperature [9, 70, 82, 116]. Climate-resilient crops will require innovative technologies as land becomes more scarce, and the world's population continues to rise, predicted to reach 9.7 billion by 2050 [4]. Farmers must modify their management strategies and grow more climate-resilient crops with enhanced resistance to biotic and abiotic stresses in difficult environments in order to adapt to climate variability [88].

Crop domestication through plant breeding has been used to select desirable traits from wild relatives since 10,000 years ago. In order to produce highly productive, climate-resilient plant varieties that can feed the world's growing population, plant breeding is crucial to agriculture. Developing climate-resilient crops necessitates access to genomics, phenomics, and genetic diversity among various germplasms, which can be employed in smart breeding programs, genome editing, and artificial intelligence tools [24]. Furthermore, genomic-assisted breeding aids in examining crop pan-genomes and leveraging and restoring vital lost genes to optimize breeding programs and introduce desired traits. Speed breeding enables swift gene identification and ultimately offers an excellent blueprint for crop enhancement. Through the use of cutting-edge plant breeding techniques, which includes genome editing, many crops have been successfully modified to become resistant to both biotic and abiotic stress. Cutting-edge technology in contemporary plant breeding, combined with effective agronomic practices like microbiome applications, can be utilized to produce climate-resilient superior genotypes that address food security challenges. It is necessary to implement multidisciplinary breeding platforms, including big data analytics tools and high-throughput phenotyping methods, to create climate-adapted crops that support worldwide food security.

2 Plant Breeding as a Solution

Scientists can improve crop productivity and adjust crops to changing environmental conditions through plant breeding. Breeding techniques have advanced many important crops, such as sugarcane, soybeans, rice, wheat, and maize. In response to rising food demands, the Green Revolution of the 1960s significantly increased the yield potential of the most economically significant crops, such as rice and wheat [24]. Hybridization and traditional breeding methods were used to select elite crop varieties.

While conventional breeding strategies have successfully improved crops by incorporating traits from wild relatives, they face limitations due to their lengthy process and issues like a genetic drag from limited recombination, erosion of genetic variation, hybridization bottlenecks, and time-consuming phenotyping experiments for selection. The Green Revolution improved agriculture tremendously, but it also reduced the genetic diversity of crops, which resulted in the loss of elite genes (Fig. 1).

Since climate change demands faster breeding cycles, new breeding technologies are needed. The creation of commercial varieties using fundamental breeding processes is an ongoing, long-term endeavor that involves continuously crossing germplasm and selecting individuals with desirable traits.

Targeted genes/QTLs can be transferred to plant genomes more quickly and easily by using marker-assisted selection (MAS) in breeding programs. Single nucleotide polymorphism (SNP), restriction fragment length polymorphism (RFLP), random amplified polymorphic DNA (RAPD), simple sequence repeat (SSR), competitive allele-specific PCR (KASP), and cleaved amplified polymorphic sequence (CAPS) are among the molecular crop breeding techniques that have been identified.

Speed breeding protocols have been established to accelerate crop generation time for various crop improvements [105], using artificial lighting. In speed breeding, plants are exposed to extended photoperiods with optimal light intensity under controlled temperatures, which enhances photosynthesis activity, leading to reduced generation time and early seed development [23]. Additionally, speed breeding has been successfully used to produce four generations of crops per season rather than the usual one or two, including canola, wheat, chickpea, barley, and others [105].

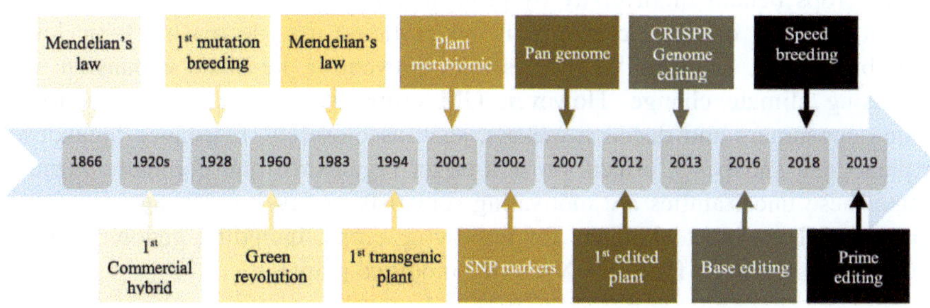

Fig. 1 Milestones of key achieved by conventional and modern plant breeding

Furthermore, speed breeding can help improve crops by identifying potential genes to be used in genomic-assisted breeding approaches, genotyping by sequencing, genomic selection, and creative breeding methods [75].

3 Smart Breeding Strategies for Mitigating Climate Distractions

Genetic crosses and mutation screening are examples of traditional breeding techniques that require a lot of labor and time. Through DNA modification of seed and plant cells, stress-tolerant crop varieties with desired traits must be developed in order to address the many direct and indirect challenges that climate change presents to agriculture. Biotech crops are essential to achieving the following goals: reducing food insecurity and undernutrition in low-income countries, combating climate change-related food production declines, feeding 9.7 billion people by 2050, and helping to achieve the SDG2 goal of ending hunger by 2030.

Genetic engineering

Modern breeding techniques, such as genetically modified (GM) crops and genome editing, can significantly enhance breeding efficiency and expedite crop improvement. GM crops have made substantial progress in crop improvement over the past three decades. The target gene must be cloned and altered; the host plant must be transformed using biolistic or Agrobacterium-mediated transformation; the DNA from the organism exhibiting the desired trait must be extracted, and transgenic plants expressing the desired trait must be screened in order to create genetically modified crops. Before being commercialized, developed plants must receive regulatory approval, which can take up to 15 years. Long-lasting transgenic tomatoes were the first approved crop to be commercialized in 1994. Only eight commercial traits—affected growth/yield, abiotic stress tolerance, insect resistance, disease resistance, herbicide tolerance, nematode resistance, pollination control system, and modified product quality—have been commercialized out of a total of 46 GM traits developed in 32 crops [39].

GM crops benefit biodiversity by protecting farmland biodiversity, preserving varietal diversity in many crops, reducing pesticide use, decreasing toxic levels in herbicide use, lowering CO_2 emissions, preventing farmland expansion, and addressing climate change. However, GM crops have raised several concerns among consumers and decision-makers, such as biosafety, resistance breakdown in pathogens and pests, effects on non-target organisms, and commercialization costs. These uncertainties are motivating scientists to develop cutting-edge (next-generation) breeding techniques for improving crops, including genome editing, which adds little to no foreign DNA to the modified plants.

Genome editing

The ability to modify gene expression through next-generation breeding via genome editing has revolutionized crop enhancement. A recent technique for accurately altering DNA sequences to improve desired traits in crops is the clustered regularly interspaced short palindromic repeat (CRISPR)-CRISPR-associated protein (CRISPR-Cas) system [2]. This system is straightforward, precise, and economical. When it comes to improving nutrient content and mitigating biotic and abiotic stresses, this method is preferred over alternative genome editing techniques. Moreover, when plant cells are exposed to the CRISPR/Cas system, a double-strand break occurs at the target site close to the PAM sequence. This break is subsequently fixed by the cellular machinery through the processes of homologous recombination (HR) or non-homologous end joining (NHEJ) [2].

Principal crops have been effectively edited by CRISPR/Cas systems to become resistant to both biotic and abiotic stress. They have been utilized to eliminate genes linked to crop susceptibility to disease, including the OsERF922 gene, ALB1 and RSY1 genes [29] for blast resistance, and USTA and UvSLT2 genes to stop smut disease in rice. Powdery mildew spread in wheat can be inhibited by knocking out the TaMLO and TaEDR1 genes [99, 110]. According to Tashkandi et al. [93], TYLCV accumulation was decreased by utilizing the CRISPR-Cas system to mutate the SlPelo gene in tomato plants and the Su eIF4G gene in rice, thereby showing virus resistance. Drought advancement has also been achieved by introducing the AGROS8 gene through CRISPR-Cas9.

Initially, modified plants were created using the CRISPR/Cas9 and CRISPR/Cpf1 (Cas12a) systems, which allowed for the knock-in or knock-out of desired sequences from DNA templates (HR) or knock-out (indel mutation). For the purpose of enhancing editing and gene expression more precisely, new generation CRISPR-Cas systems have been developed, including prime editing, base editing, epigenome editing, and CRISPR mobility through grafting.

Base editing

Elite traits can vary due to mutations resulting in a single base change [32]. Through modifications to the CRISPR-Cas system, scientists were able to precisely point mutation in plants by changing one base of DNA to another without the need for a repair template. Base editing is a new technique that replaces a single base by converting cytosine (C) to uracil, which starts cytosine base editing (CBE) and causes C.G to T.A transitions. This is done by combining CRISPR/nCas9 (Cas9 nickase) with a cytidine deaminase. By combining tRNA adenosine deaminase (TadA) with nCas9, adenine base editing (ABE) has been developed to convert an A-T base pair to a G-C base. Economically important crops like wheat, and maize [119], cotton [71], and rice [36], have all seen the application of CBE. Additionally, ABE has been used in wheat and rice [28, 101].

Prime editing

Small indels and base substitutions for transition and transversion have been made possible by prime editing, which has been shown to be a flexible and accurate method of genome editing [1]. Moreover, it permits the introduction at the target site of all 12 known bases. In order to insert new genetic information into a particular DNA location, the reverse transcriptase (RT) engineered to work with nCas was combined to create the prime editing system. The reverse transcriptase template and primer-binding site are fused with the gRNA sequence to create the prime editing gRNA. The most economically significant crops, such as wheat and rice, have been edited using prime editing [12, 35, 51, 52, 55, 107].

3.1 Epigenome Editing

Fusing dead Cas9 (dCas9) with epigenetic effector domains allows for the precise targeting of promoter and enhancer regions, which in turn modifies gene activation or repression. This allows for the introduction of epigenetic changes (methylases/demethylases) to target genes. Using endogenous DNA for cytosine methylation with MQ1 or DNMT3A and cytosine demethylation with Tet1 can be used in epi-editing. Additionally, the system can be used to modify the accessibility of the transcriptional machinery and change the structure of the chromatin by methylating histones at arginine and lysine residues. This can change the expression of a gene. By using this technique, crop improvement programs can be accelerated by controlling the expression of critical genes linked to biotic and abiotic stressors [87].

3.2 CRISPR Mobility Through Grafting

Grafting involves attaching non-genetically modified shoots (the upper part of the plant) to an edited rootstock. A recent method has been developed to edit plants using transcript mobility, preventing the introduction of foreign DNA during the editing process. It involves fusing tRNA-like sequence (TLS) motifs to Cas9 and gRNA in the constructed vector, which is then used to obtain edited plants. These plants can be employed to serve as the target plant's rootstock when grafting. Transcripts of Cas9-TLS and gRNA-TLS have the ability to travel from root to shoot, which can lead to tissue editing in recipient-grafted shoot tissues [108]. The CRISPR mobility technology can be applied to major crops like maize, wheat, and rice for mass production, without removing transgenes in the regenerated plants.

- ***Non-GM Genome Editing Approaches***

DNA-free editing is likely to be more acceptable to consumers and decision-makers. This can be achieved using nanoparticle transformation, such as polyethyleneimine (PEI)-coated Fe3O4 magnetic nanoparticles [100], virus particles like Sonchus yellow net rhabdovirus (SYNV) for transforming the CRISPR-Cas system [62], graft-mobile gene editing [108], or Agrobacterium-mediated plant transformation, followed by transgene elimination in the segregated plants. Carbon nanotubes (CNTs) carrying plasmid DNA have recently been demonstrated to be useful for plant transformation. Nanotubes can deliver CRISPR-Cas vectors as a non-integrative, transient gene editing system by diffusing through plant cell walls. Low concentrations of carbon nanotubes are non-toxic to biological systems and can provide an easy and efficient mechanism for transporting CRISPR vectors for plant gene editing, applicable to any genotype. In rice, carbon nanotubes fused to CRISPR-Cas vectors were used to edit the phytoene desaturase (PDS) gene [20].

4 Application of Biotech Crops for Climate Resilient Agriculture

Abiotic tolerance genes have been incorporated into transgenic crops for multiple economically significant crops, including wheat, maize, and rice (Table 1). Stress-related structural genes (which are in charge of osmolyte biosynthesis, such as proline, glycine/betaine, and stress-induced LEA proteins) and regulatory genes (like dehydration-responsive element-binding factors and NAC transcription factor genes) have been used to engineer plants that carry genes for managing water stress. Genetically modified agriculture (GM) has produced salt-tolerant crops; some are presently undergoing final field trials prior to commercialization. Many stress-related genes related to salt tolerance have been found and used to create plants that are tolerant of salt. These genes include salt overly sensitive (SOS), GmCLC1 and GsCLC-c2, DREB1B and DREB1F, and OsMYB6 [56, 67, 86, 92, 106]. Heat stress-induced plant recovery has been linked to transgenic plants that express heat shock proteins (HSPs). In stressful situations, HSPs bind and stabilize denatured proteins to stop them from aggregating.

Insect-resistant GM crops, such as those using *Bacillus thuringiensis* (Bt) genes, have higher crop yields and reduced pesticide usage compared to non-GM adopters. Insect-resistant biotech crops require fewer pesticide applications and decreased pesticide use. For many important crops, disease-resistant varieties have been created to boost yields while lowering the usage of toxic chemical pesticides.

Growing biotic-resistant and abiotic-tolerant crops through genome editing has been made possible in large part by the CRISPR-Cas system. There have been reports of enhanced agronomic traits and stress tolerance to biotic and abiotic stresses (Table 2). Therefore, it was found that improving drought tolerance in tomatoes required knocking out the SlLBD40 gene [57]. Moreover, maize required substituting a stronger ARGOS8 gene promoter [85]. Furthermore, mutated TaSal1 wheat lines showed enhanced drought tolerance and closed stomata [2]. Drought-tolerant rice was created by utilizing the CRISPR/Cas9 system to knock down the OsERA1 gene and

Table 1 A list of typical genetically modified (GM) crops that are resistant to biotic stressors and abiotic stresses

Species	Trait targeted	Transferred gene(s)	Benefit as a result of stress	References
Abiotic stress				
Barely	Salt tolerance	*AtAVP1*	Greater shoot biomass and grain yield	Schilling et al. [80]
Rice	Salt tolerance	*SAMDC*	Accelerated growth of seedlings	Roy and Wu [76]
Rice	Salt tolerance	*P5CS*	Able to produce flowers and seeds	Karthikeyan et al. [46]
Rice	Heat tolerance	*OsRab7*	Higher yield	El-Esawi and Alayafi [21]
Rice	Drought	*AtDREB1A*	Sufficient in both vegetative and reproductive phases	Ravikumar et al. [74]
Wheat	Salt	*betA*	Increased germination rates, more tillers, and greater grain yields	He at al. [30]
Wheat	Drought	*HaHB4*	Increased numbers of fertile florets per plant, tillers per spike, and spikelets per spike	González et al. [25]
Wheat	Heat	*TaHsfC2a*	Enhanced thermotolerance	Hu et al. [34]
Maize	Salt and drought	*ZmbZIP4*	Increased synthesis of ABA and root development	Ma et al. [63]
Maize	Drought	*ARGOS8*	Enhanced the amount of grain produced per acre by five bushels	Shi et al. [85]
Maize	Heat and drought	*OsMYB55*	Reduced leaf damage and increased plant biomass	Casaretto et al. [13]
Cotton	Salt	*AhCMO*	Increased yield of seeds	Wang et al. [100]; Zhang et al. [111]
Cotton	Salt and drought	*AtNHX1, AtAVP1*	Increased fiber yield in dryland and low-irrigation environments	Shen et al. [84]
Tomato	Salt	*PgNHX1, AVP1*	Better survival rate	Bhaskaran and Savithramma [10]

(continued)

Table 1 (continued)

Species	Trait targeted	Transferred gene(s)	Benefit as a result of stress	References
Tomato	Heat	*APX*	Enhanced tolerance to heat stress	Bhaskaran and Savithramma [10]; Zhang et al. [114]
Biotic stress				
Maize	Insect resistance	cry1Ab + cry3Bb1	Target European corn borer, corn rootworm	Dowd et al. [19]; Li et al. [53]; Sanchis [77]
Maize	Funagl resistance	chalcone isomerase 3-like (CI3)	Target Fusarium and pathogenic fungi	Dowd et al. [19]
Rice	Bacterial resistance	Xa23	Target blight disease	Ji et al. [44]; Wang et al. [103]
Rice	Virus resistance	RNA interference (siRNAs)	Target the spherical and bacilli viruses of rice tungro	Le et al. [50]; Sharma et al. [83]
Potato	Insect	cry1Ac	Target Leptinotarsa decemlineata	Amiri and Bakhsh [5]; Davidson et al. [17]
Potato		alfAFP	Target Veticillim	Gao et al. [22]
Potato	Virus	RNA polymerase	Target Potato virus X	Bai et al. [7]; Liu et al. [58]

enhance primary root development [68]. OsRR22 mutant rice produced by CRISPR/Cas9 showed improved salt tolerance in seedlings [113]. Additionally, through over-expressing the GmNAC06 gene in soybeans using CRISPR/Cas9-based gene editing technology, glycine betaine and proline accumulation were able to improve salinity tolerance while preserving ionic homeostasis [51].

5 Pan-Genomes for Crop Improvement

The term "pangenome" refers to the entire gene pool found in different individuals within a species. It involves variable genes (shared by some group members but absent in others) found in the dispensable genome and core genes found in the core genome of every individual [94]. The creation of crop varieties for the next generation will be greatly impacted by a full grasp of genes and the regulatory mechanisms that govern key crop traits. A pan-genome workflow is shown in Fig. 2.

The recovery of genes lost in wild-type genomes during the process of crop domestication is aided by crop pan-genome studies. A systematic approach to gathering information on genotypic and phenotypic differences is provided by the crop pan-genome, which includes landraces, cultivated varieties, and wild relatives of crops.

Table 2 List of representative biotic- and abiotic-tolerant crops developed by genome editing

Species	Trait targeted	Gene(s) edited	Benefit in response to stress	References
Abiotic stress				
Rice	Drought	*OsERA1*	Increase root growth	Ogata et al. [71]
Rice	Salt		improves salt stress resistance in rice	Alam et al. [3]
Rice	Herbicide tolerance	*OSALS*		Wang et al. [106]
Rice	Drought tolerance	OsEBP89		Zhang et al. [117]
Wheat	Drought tolerance	*TaSal1*	Stomata closure response and ABA	Abdallah et al. [2]
Wheat	Drought tolerance	TaDREB2 and TaERF3		Kim et al. [52]
Tomato	Drought tolerance	*SlGID1*		Illouz-Eliaz et al. [45]
Tomato	Salt tolerance	*SlHyPRP1*		Tran et al. [100]
Potato	Drought tolerance	StFLORE		Ramírez Gonzales et al. [77]
Soybean	Drought tolerance	*GmHdz4*		Zhong et al. [109]
Soybean	Salt tolerance	*GmAITR*		Wang et al. [106]
Biotic stress				
Rice	Bacterial	*OsSWEET14*	Bacterial leaf blight	Arulganesh et al. [7]
Rice	Fungal	*Bsr-d1, Pi21* and *ERF922*	Rice blast	Zhou et al. [43]
Rice	Virus resistance	*eIF4G*	Rice tungro spherical virus	Kumam et al. [51]
Wheat	Fungal resistance	*TaMLO-A1*	Powdery mildew	Wang et al. [107]
Maize	Virus resistance	*ZmGDIα*	Rice black-streaked dwarf virus	Liu et al. [59]
Tomato	Bacterial resistance	*SLDMR6-1*	Bacterial speck	Thomazella et al. [96]
Tomato	Fungal resistance	*SlPMR4*	Powdery mildew	Santillan Martinez et al. [78]
Tomato	Virus resistance	*TOM1*	Tomato brown rugose fruit virus	Ishikawa et al. [41]; Tashkandi et al. [93]

This allows for the identification of genes that are missing from reference genomes [16]. This strategy is also a great genomic-based way to comprehend how genetic diversity contributes to crop improvement. Knowing accessory genomes can help find elite cultivars with stress-responsive genes for both biotic and abiotic stresses [8]. Furthermore, pan-genomes have identified multiple presence/absence variations of genes that respond to biotic stress in different species [15]. In addition, a number

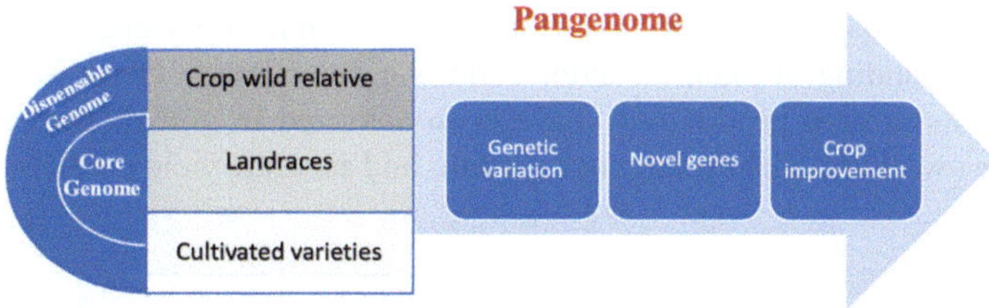

Fig. 2 Pan-genome assembly workflow for agricultural enhancement

of hotspots linked to environmental stressors have been found by SNP studies [18]. The pangenomes of eighteen elite lines of wheat revealed a large number of genes and SNPs linked to crucial agronomic characteristics [104]. Moreover, in breeding programs for significant crops, yield-related genes have been strictly selected during breeding, and alleles for improved products have been identified [14, 37, 95].

Several challenges exist in pangenome studies, such as accurate annotation, assembly, and economic feasibility. Short genomic reads from next-generation sequencing (NGS) can hinder repetitive region assembly; however, longer reads using single-molecule sequencing can result in high-quality genome assembly but with lower accuracy. For pangenome studies, access to a thoroughly annotated reference genome is required. Although scarce, functional datasets linked to pangenomes are essential for establishing a linkage map between trait diversity and pangenomes. Furthermore, interpreting pangenome data can be highly challenging due to the size and complexity of some genomes, like hexaploid wheat [16, 38].

Pan-genome mapping has been used to study complex stress-related gene sets, like biotic stress tolerance, that may be used to improve crops. Pan-genome analyses of crops such as rice, soybean, chickpea, Brassica, and Brassica oleracea have revealed a large number of genes related to abiotic and biotic stress [8, 79, 89, 98, 115].

6 Plant Phenotypic

Breeders have been able to consistently increase crop yields in a positive way owing to the vast amounts of data generated by phenomics and genomics research [11]. Determining the interaction between plants and their surroundings is largely dependent on plant phenotyping. Combining various omics approaches with climate and environmental information, known as plant phenotyping, can be used to improve plant breeding programs. This integrated information is utilized from the ground up to develop elite crop varieties and create next-generation crops. Plant phenotyping involves acquiring, organizing, and evaluating datasets to design intelligent models that predict plant growth under varying environmental conditions [33].

Artificial intelligence systems have been developed using phenotypic data and applied in agriculture for automation or digitalization purposes by creating intelligent predictive models. These systems are intended to improve plant health, including characteristics linked to abiotic and biotic stresses and crop yield, and provide a deeper understanding of plant behavior under various climatic circumstances [42]. Improvements in crop productivity have been achieved in greenhouses and fields through the use of artificial intelligence systems and accurate yield prediction models [31, 45].

7 Nanotechnology for Precision Delivery of Fertilizers and Pesticides

Nanotechnology provides precise delivery, especially in harsh environmental conditions like high heat, drought, acidity, and light. Many studies on the use of nanotechnology for sustainable agriculture have been carried out during the previous 20 years [81]. In agriculture, nanoparticles are essential since they boost crop yield, suppress infections, and get rid of unwanted weeds and insects. Nanotechnology has the ability to improve the efficacy and safety of pesticides, aside from its primary application in precision agriculture [72]. Through lowering the volume and concentration of synthetic pesticides used for pest control, the use of nanopesticide formulations could minimize plant damage, environmental pollution, pest resistance, and economic loss [91]. Solid nanoparticles, soluble in water, have been successfully employed to control a wide range of insects while leaving minimal environmental residues [26]. Active ingredients, such as pesticides or fertilizers, are encapsulated into appropriate nanocarriers. Polycaprolactone is cost-effective and naturally degradable in the environment, making it a popular choice for nanofertilizer and nanopesticide particles.

8 Conclusion

Climate change is severely impacting global food security, making it crucial to breed crop plants that can mitigate environmental stresses, resist diseases and pests, and have enhanced yield potential. Genome-assisted breeding has replaced phenotype-based breeding in the evolution of plant breeding. Innovative pan-genome techniques enable the detection of genetic variations and recovery of lost genes, particularly in wild relative crops. Assembled pan-genome data integrate genome information into the phenome, accelerating trait-specific breeding.

A new era of smart breeding has been brought about by the development of biotech crops, speed breeding, and artificial intelligence applications. Environmentally resilient crops that can tolerate a range of biotic and abiotic stresses while maintaining high yields could be developed with the help of biotech plants, such as transgenic and genome-edited plants. However, complicated laws and drawn-out procedures restrict the use of commercialized genetically modified food crops.

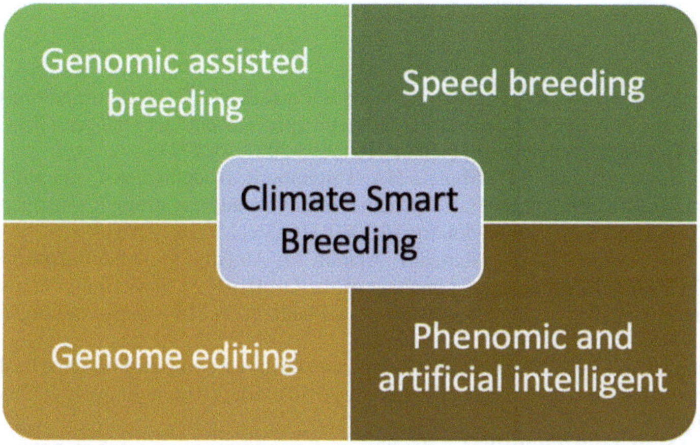

Fig. 3 Climate resilience in agriculture using the intelligent breeding approach

Genome editing has opened the door for plant scientists to accurately manipulate genomes without introducing foreign DNA. Decision-makers and consumers will find modified plants more palatable as a result of the next-generation CRISPR systems that enable precise gene expression fine-tuning, such as base editing, prime editing, and epigenome editing. A new era in crop genotype development that can withstand the catastrophic effects of climate change is made possible by the availability of various techniques for smart breeding and genome manipulation (Fig. 3).

9 Recommendations

1. Investment in advanced breeding technologies.
2. Implementation of speed breeding protocols.
3. Establish multidisciplinary breeding platforms.
4. Promotion of non-gm genome editing approaches.
5. Integration of microbiome applications.
6. Development of climate-resilient crop varieties.
7. Encouraging public and private sector collaboration.
8. Enhancing regulatory frameworks.
9. Capacity building and training.
10. Establishing pan-genome databases.
11. Implement robust monitoring and evaluation frameworks to assess the effectiveness of breeding programs.

References

1. Abdallah NA, Hamwieh A, Radwan K, Fouad N, Prakash P (2021) Genome editing techniques in plants: a comprehensive review and future prospects toward zero hunger. GM Crops Food 12(2):601–615. https://doi.org/10.1080/21645698.2021.2021724
2. Abdallah NA, Elsharawy H, Abulela HA, Thilmony R, Abdelhadi AA, Elarabi NI (2022b) Multiplex CRISPR/Cas9-mediated genome editing to address drought tolerance in wheat. GM Crops Food 1–17. https://doi.org/10.1080/21645698.2022.2120313
3. Alam MS, Kong J, Tao R, Ahmed T, Alamin M, Alotaibi SS, Abdelsalam NR, Xu J-H (2022) CRISPR/Cas9 mediated knockout of the OsbHLH024 transcription factor improves salt stress resistance in rice (Oryza sativa L.). Plants 11(9):1184. https://doi.org/10.3390/plants11091184
4. Amadou I, Gounga ME, Le GW (2013) Millets: nutritional composition, some health benefits and processing—a review. Emir J Food Agric 25:501–508. https://doi.org/10.9755/ejfa.v25i7.12045
5. Amiri AN, Bakhsh A (2019) An effective pest management approach in potato to combat insect pests and herbicide. 3 Biotech 9:16. https://doi.org/10.1007/s13205-018-1536-0
6. Arulganesh T, Kumam Y, Kumar K, Arul L, Kokiladevi E, Nakeeran S, Varanavasiappan S, Manonmani S, Sudhakar D (2021) Genome editing of elite rice cultivar CO51 for bacterial leaf blight resistance. Electron J Plant Breed 12:1060–1068
7. Bai Y, Guo Z, Wang X, Bai D, Zhang W (2009) Generation of double-virus-resistant marker-free transgenic potato plants. Prog Nat Sci 19(5):543–548
8. Bayer PE, Golicz AA, Tirnaz S, Chan CK, Edwards D, Batley J (2019) Variation in abundance of predicted resistance genes in the Brassica oleracea pangenome. Plant Biotechnol J 17(4):789–800
9. Ben-Asher J, Garcia y Garcia A, Hoogenboom G (2008) Effect of high temperature on photosynthesis and transpiration of sweet corn (Zea mays L. var. rugosa). Photosynthetica 46:595–603
10. Bhaskaran S, Savithramma DL (2011) Co-expression of *Pennisetum glaucum* vacuolar Na^+/H^+ antiporter and *Arabidopsis* H^+-pyrophosphatase enhances salt tolerance in transgenic tomato. J Exp Bot 62(15):5561–5570. https://doi.org/10.1093/jxb/err237
11. Brown TB, Cheng R, Sirault XRR, Rungrat T, Murray KD, Trtilek M, Furbank RT, Badger M, Pogson BJ, Borevitz JO (2014) Trait capture: genomic and environment modelling of plant phenomic data. Curr Opin Plant Biol 18:73–79
12. Butt H, Rao GS, Sedeek K, Aman R, Kamel R, Mahfouz M (2020) Engineering herbicide resistance via prime editing in rice. Plant Biotechnol J 18(12):2370
13. Casaretto JA, El-kereamy A, Zeng B, Stiegelmeyer SM, Chen X, Bi YM, Rothstein SJ (2016) Expression of OsMYB55 in maize activates stress-responsive genes and enhances heat and drought tolerance. BMC Genomics 17(1):1–15. https://doi.org/10.1186/s12864-016-2659-5
14. Concibido V, La Vallee B, Mclaird P, Pineda N, Meyer J, Hummel L, Yang J, Wu K, Delannay X (2003) Introgression of a quantitative trait locus for yield from Glycine soja into commercial soybean cultivars. Theor Appl Genet 106:575–582
15. Cook DE, Lee TG, Guo X, Melito S, Wang K, Bayless AM, Wang J, Hughes TJ, Willis DK, Clemente TE (2012) Copy number variation of multiple genes at Rhg1 mediates nematode resistance in soybean. Science 338(6111):1206–1209.
16. Danilevicz MF, Fernandez CGT, Marsh JI, Bayer PE, Edwards D (2020) Plant pangenomics: approaches, applications and advancements. Curr Opin Plant Biol 54:18–25
17. Davidson MM, Wratten RC, Wratten, DD, Conner AJ (2006) Field evaluation of potato plants transgenic for a cry1ac gene conferring resistance to potato tuber moth, *Phthorimaea operculella* (Zeller) (Lepidoptera: Gelechiidae). Crop Prot 25(3):216–224
18. Dolatabadian A, Bayer PE, Tirnaz S, Hurgobin B, Edwards D, Batley J (2020) Characterization of disease resistance genes in the Brassica napus pangenome reveals significant structural variation. Plant Biotechnol J 18(4):969–982

19. Dowd PF, Berhow MA, Johnson ET (2018) Enhanced pest resistance and increased phenolic production in maize callus transgenically expressing a maize chalcone isomerase-3 like gene. Plant Gene 13:50–55
20. Dunbar T, Tsakirpaloglou N, Septiningsih EM, Thomson MJ (2022) Carbon nanotube-mediated plasmid DNA delivery in rice leaves and seeds. Int J Mol Sci 23(8):4081
21. El-Esawi MA, Alayafi AA (2019) Overexpression of rice Rab7 gene improves drought and heat tolerance and increases grain yield in rice (Oryza sativa L.). Genes 10(1):56
22. Gao AG, Hakimi SM, Mittanck CA, Wu Y, Woerner BM, Stark DM, Shah DM, Liang J, Rommens CM (2000) Fungal pathogen protection in potato by expression of a plant defensin peptide. Nat Biotechnol 18(12):1307–1310. https://doi.org/10.1038/82436. PMID: 11101813
23. Ghosh S, Watson A, Gonzalez-Navarro OE, Ramirez-Gonzalez RH, Yanes L, Mendoza-Suárez M, Simmonds J, Wells R, Rayner T, Green P (2018) Speed breeding in growth chambers and glasshouses for crop breeding and model plant research. Nat Protoc 13(12):2944–2963
24. Gobu R, Shiv A, Kumar CA, Basavaraj PS, Harish D, Adhikari S, Vinita R, Umesh H, Sujatha M (2020) Accelerated crop breeding towards development of climate resilient varieties. Climate change and Indian Agriculture: Challenges and Adaptation Strategies (Not Available)
25. González FG, Capella M, Ribichich KF, Curín F, Giacomelli JI, Ayala F, Watson G, Otegui ME, Chan RL (2019) Field-grown transgenic wheat expressing the sunflower gene HaHB4 significantly outyields the wild type. J Exp Bot 70(5):1669–1681
26. Goswami A, Roy I, Sengupta S, Debnath N (2010) Novel applications of solid and liquid formulations of nanoparticles against insect pests and pathogens. Thin Solid Films 519(3):1252–1257
27. Gupta PK (2024) Drought-tolerant transgenic wheat HB4®: a hope for the future. Trends Biotechnol 42(7):807–809
28. Hao LI, Ruiying QIN, Xiaoshuang LIU, Shengxiang L, Rongfang XU, Jianbo Y, Pengcheng WEI (2019) CRISPR/Cas9-mediated adenine base editing in rice genome. Rice Sci 26(2):125–128
29. Harishchandra DL, Chethana KWT, Zhang W, Xing QK, Peng JB, Brooks S, Hyde KD, Li XH (2021) CRISPR/Cas9: contemporary designer nucleases for efficient genome editing in phytopathogenic fungi. Curr Res Environ Appl Mycol (J Fungal Biol) 11:341–363
30. He C, Yang A, Zhang W, Gao Q, Zhang J (2010) Improved salt tolerance of transgenic wheat by introducing betA gene for glycine betaine synthesis. Plant Cell Tissue Organ Cult 101(1):65–78
31. Hemming S, de Zwart F, Elings A, Righini I, Petropoulou A (2019) Remote control of greenhouse vegetable production with artificial intelligence—greenhouse climate, irrigation, and crop production. Sensors 19(8):1807
32. Henikoff S, Comai L (2003) Single-nucleotide mutations for plant functional genomics. Annu Rev Plant Biol 54(1):375–401
33. Houle D, Govindaraju DR, Omholt S (2010) Phenomics: the next challenge. Nat Rev Genet 11(12):855–866
34. Hu XJ, Chen D, Lynne MC, Fernanda Dreccer M, Zhang ZB, Drenth J, Kalaipandian S, Chang H, Xue GP (2018) Heat shock factor C2a serves as a proactive mechanism for heat protection in developing grains in wheat via an ABA-mediated regulatory pathway. Plant Cell Environ 41(1):79–98. https://doi.org/10.1111/pce.12957
35. Hua K, Jiang Y, Tao X, Zhu J (2020) Precision genome engineering in rice using prime editing system. Plant Biotechnol J 18(11):2167
36. Huang X, Su F, Huang S, Mei F, Niu X, Ma C, Zhang H, Zhu X, Zhu J, Zhang J (2021) Novel Wx alleles generated by base editing for improvement of rice grain quality. J Integr Plant Biol 63(9):1632–1638. doi: 10.1111/pce.12957
37. Huang XQ, Cöster H, Ganal MW, Röder MS (2003) Advanced backcross QTL analysis for the identification of quantitative trait loci alleles from wild relatives of wheat (*Triticum aestivum* L.). Theor Appl Genet 106(8):1379–1389

38. Hübner S, Bercovich N, Todesco M, Mandel JR, Odenheimer J, Ziegler E, Lee JS, Baute GJ, Owens GL, Grassa CJ (2019) Sunflower pan-genome analysis shows that hybridization altered gene content and disease resistance. Nature Plants 5(1):54–62
39. ISAAA Database (2021) GM approval database. Available online at: https://www.isaaa.org/gmapprovaldatabase/default.asp. Accessed 15 June 2023
40. Illouz-Eliaz N, Nissan I, Nir I, Ramon U, Shohat H, Weiss D (2020) Mutations in the tomato gibberellin receptors suppress xylem proliferation and reduce water loss under water-deficit conditions. J Exp Bot 71:3603–3612
41. Ishikawa HT, Aoki W, Hirano T, et al. (2022) Elemental abundances of nearby M dwarfs based on high-resolution near-infrared spectra obtained by the Subaru/IRD Survey: proof of concept. Astron J 163:72
42. Jeong JH, Resop JP, Mueller ND, Fleisher DH, Yun K, Butle EE, Timlin DJ, Shim KM, Gerber JS, Reddy VR (2016) Random forests for global and regional crop yield predictions. PLoS ONE 11(6):e0156571
43. Ji M, Wang K, Wang L, Chen S, Li H, Ma C, Wang Y (2019) Overexpression of a *S*-Adenosylmethionine Decarboxylase from sugar beet M14 increased *Araidopsis* salt tolerance. Int J Mol Sci 20(8):1990. https://doi.org/10.3390/ijms20081990
44. Ji Z, Sun H, Wei Y, Li M, Wang H, Xu J, Lei C, Wang C, Zhao K (2022) Ectopic expression of executor gene *Xa23* enhances resistance to both bacterial and fungal diseases in rice. Int J Mol Sci 23(12):6545. https://doi.org/10.3390/ijms23126545
45. Jiang D, Yang X, Clinton N, Wang N (2004) An artificial neural network model for estimating crop yields using remotely sensed information. Int J Remote Sens 25(9):1723–1732
46. Karthikeyan A, Pandian SK, Ramesh M (2011) Transgenic indica rice cv. ADT 43 expressing a Δ1-pyrroline-5-carboxylate synthetase (P5CS) gene from Vigna aconitifolia demonstrates salt tolerance. Plant Cell Tissue Organ Cult 107(3):383–395
47. Kim D, Alptekin B, Budak H (2018). CRISPR/Cas9 genome editing in wheat. Funct Integr Genomics 18(1):31–41. https://doi.org/10.1007/s10142-017-0572-x. Epub 2017 Sep 16. PMID: 28918562
48. Kumam Y, Rajadurai G, Kumar K, Varanavasiappan S, Reddy MK, Krishnaveni D, Mangrauthia SK, Raveendran M, Arul L, Kokiladevi E (2022) Genome editing of indica rice ASD16 for imparting resistance against rice tungro disease. J Plant Biochem Biotechnol 31:880–893
49. Kumari PH, Kumar SA, Sivan P, Katam R, Suravajhala P, Rao K, Varshney RK, Kishor PBK (2017) Overexpression of a plasma membrane bound Na+/H+ antiporter-like protein (SbNHXLP) confers salt tolerance and improves fruit yield in tomato by maintaining ion homeostasis. Front Plant Sci 7
50. Le DT, Chu HD, Sasaya T (2015) Creation of transgenic rice plants producing small interfering RNA of rice tungro spherical virus. GM Crops Food 6(1):47–53. https://doi.org/10.1080/21645698.2015.1025188
51. Li M, Chen R, Jiang Q, Sun X, Zhang H, Hu Z (2021) GmNAC06, a NAC domain transcription factor enhances salt stress tolerance in soybean. Plant Mol Biol 105:333–345
52. Li H, Yang Y, Hong W et al (2020) Applications of genome editing technology in the targeted therapy of human diseases: mechanisms, advances and prospects. Sig Transduct Target Ther 5:1. https://doi.org/10.1038/s41392-019-0089-y
53. Li Y, Meissle M, Romeis J (2008) Consumption of Bt maize pollen expressing Cry1Ab or Cry3Bb1 does not harm adult green Lacewings, Chrysoperla carnea (Neuroptera: Chrysopidae). PLoS One 3(8):e2909. https://doi.org/10.1371/journal.pone.0002909
54. Lin Q, Jin S, Zong Y, Yu H, Zhu Z, Liu G, Kou L, Wang Y, Qiu JL, Li J (2021) High-efficiency prime editing with optimized, paired pegRNAs in plants. Nat Biotechnol 39(8):923–927
55. Lin Q, Zong Y, Xue C, Wang S, Jin S, Zhu Z, Wang Y, Anzalone AV, Raguram A, Doman JL (2020) Prime genome editing in rice and wheat. Nat Biotechnol 38(5):582–585
56. Liu W, Feng J, Ma W, Zhou Y, Ma Z (2021) GhCLCg-1, a vacuolar chloride channel, contributes to salt tolerance by regulating ion accumulation in upland cotton. Front Plant Sci 12:765173. https://doi.org/10.3389/fpls.2021.765173

57. Liu L, Zhang J, Xu J, Li Y, Guo L, Wang Z, Zhang X, Zhao B, Guo YD, Zhang N (2020) CRISPR/Cas9 targeted mutagenesis of SlLBD40, a lateral organ boundaries domain transcription factor, enhances drought tolerance in tomato. Plant Sci 301:110683
58. Liu H, Zeng B, Zhao J, Yan S, Wan J, Cao Z (2023) Genetic research progress: heat tolerance in rice. Int J Mol Sci 24(8):7140. https://doi.org/10.3390/ijms24087140
59. Liu J, Yue J, Wang H, Xie L, Zhao Y, Zhao M, Zhou H (2023) Strategies for engineering virus resistance in potato. Plants 12:1736. https://doi.org/10.3390/plants12091736
60. Liu X, Ao K, Yao J, Zhang Y, Li Z (2022) Engineering plant disease resistance against biotrophic pathogens. Curr Opin Plant Biol 60:101987. https://doi.org/10.1016/j.pbi.2020.101987
61. Lobell DB, Hammer GL, McLean G, Messina C, Roberts MJ, Schlenker W (2013) The critical role of extreme heat for maize production in the United States. Nat Clim Chang 3(5):497–501
62. Ma X, Li Z (2020) Significantly improved recovery of recombinant Sonchus yellow net rhabdo-virus by expressing the negative-strand genomic RNA. Viruses 12:1459
63. Ma H, Liu C, Li Z, Ran Q, Xie G, Wang B, Fang S, Chu J, Zhang J (2018) ZmbZIP4 contributes to stress resistance in maize by regulating ABA synthesis and root development. Plant Physiol 178(2):753–770. https://doi.org/10.1104/pp.18.00436
64. Ma X, Xu Z (2020) Significantly improved recovery of recombinant sonchus yellow net rhabdovirus by expressing the negative-strand genomic RNA. Viruses 12(12):1459
65. Montenegro JD, Golicz AA, Bayer PE, Hurgobin B, Lee H, Chan CK, Visendi P, Lai K, Doležel J, Batley J (2017) The pangenome of hexaploid bread wheat. Plant J 90(5):1007–1013
66. Muthurajan R, Ramanathan V Bansilal Shillak A, Madhuri Pralhad S, Shankarrao CN, Rahman H, Kambale R, Nallathambi J, Tamilselvan S, Madasamy P (2021) Controlled over-expression of *AtDREB1A* enhances tolerance against drought and salinity in rice. Agronomy 11:159. https://doi.org/10.3390/agronomy11010159
67. Nguyen QH, Vu LTK, Nguyen LTN, Pham NTT, Nguyen YTH, Le S, Van Chu MH (2019) Overexpression of the GmDREB6 gene enhances proline accumulation and salt tolerance in genetically modified soybean plants. Sci Rep 9(1):19663. https://doi.org/10.1038/s41598-019-55895-0
68. Ogata T, Ishizaki T, Fujita M, Fujita Y (2020) CRISPR/Cas9-targeted mutagenesis of OsERA1 confers enhanced responses to abscisic acid and drought stress and increased primary root growth under nonstressed conditions in rice. PLoS ONE 15(12):e0243376
69. Pingali PL (2012) Green revolution: impacts, limits, and the path ahead. Proc Natl Acad Sci 109(31):12302–12308
70. Powell JP, Reinhard S (2016) Measuring the effects of extreme weather events on yields. Weather Clim Extremes 12:69–79
71. Qin L, Li J, Wang Q, Xu Z, Sun L, Alariqi M, Manghwar H, Wang G, Li B, Ding X (2020) High-efficient and precise base editing of C• G to T• A in the allotetraploid cotton (Gossypium hirsutum) genome using a modified CRISPR/Cas9 system. Plant Biotechnol J 18(1):45–56
72. Raliya R, Saharan V, Dimkpa C, Biswas P (2017) Nanofertilizer for precision and sustainable agriculture: current state and future perspectives. J Agric Food Chem 66(26):6487–6503
73. Ramírez Gonzales L, Shi L, Bergonzi SB, Oortwijn M, Franco-Zorrilla JM, Solano-Tavira R et al (2021) Potato CYCLING DOF FACTOR 1 and its lncRNA counterpart StFLORE link tuber development and drought response. Plant J 105:855–869. https://doi.org/10.1111/tpj.15093
74. Ravikumar G, Manimaran P, Voleti S, Subrahmanyam D, Sundaram R, Bansal K, Viraktamath BC, Balachandran SM (2014) Stress-inducible expression of AtDREB1A transcription factor greatly improves drought stress tolerance in transgenic indica rice. Trans Res 23(3):421–439
75. Razzaq A, Ajaz T, Li JC, Irfan M, Suksatan W (2021) Investigating the asymmetric linkages between infrastructure development, green innovation, and consumption-based material footprint: novel empirical estimations from highly resource-consuming economies. Resour Pol 74:102302. https://doi.org/10.1016/j.resourpol.2021.102302
76. Roy M, Wu R (2002) Overexpression of S-adenosylmethionine decarboxylase gene in rice increases polyamine level and enhances sodium chloride-stress tolerance. Plant Sci 163(5):987–992

77. Sanchis V (2011) From microbial sprays to insect-resistant transgenic plants: history of the biospesticide Bacillus thuringiensis A review. Agron Sustain Dev 31(1):217–231
78. Santillan Martinez MI, Bracuto V, Koseoglou E, Appiano M, Jacobsen E, Visser RGF, Wolters AA, Bai Y (2020) CRISPR/Cas9- targeted mutagenesis of the tomato susceptibility gene PMR4 for resistance against powdery mildew. BMC Plant Biol 20:284. https://doi.org/10.1186/s12870-020-02497-y
79. Schatz MC, Maron LG, Stein JC, Wences AH, Gurtowski J, Biggers E, Lee H, Kramer M, Antoniou E, Ghiban E (2014) Whole genome de novo assemblies of three divergent strains of rice, Oryza sativa, document novel gene space of aus and indica. Genome Biol 15:1–16
80. Schilling RK, Marschner P, Shavrukov Y, Berger B, Tester M, Roy SJ & Plett DC (2014) Expression of theArabidopsisvacuolar H+-pyrophosphatase gene (AVP1) improves the shoot biomass of transgenic barley and increases grain yield in a saline field Plant. Biotechnol J 12(3):378–386
81. Scott NR, Chen H, Cui H (2018) Nanotechnology applications and implications of agrochemicals toward sustainable agriculture and food systems. J Agr Food Chem 66(26):6451–6456. ACS Publications
82. Shah NH, Paulsen GM (2003) Interaction of drought and high temperature on photosynthesis and grain-filling of wheat. Plant Soil 257:219–226
83. Sharma S, Kumar G, Dasgupta I (2018). Simultaneous resistance against the two viruses causing rice tungro disease using RNA interference. Virus Res 15;255:157–164. https://doi.org/10.1016/j.virusres.2018.07.011. Epub 2018 Jul 18. PMID: 30031045.
84. Shen G, Wei J, Qiu X, Hu R, Kuppu S, Auld D, Blumwald E, Gaxiola R, Payton P, Zhang H (2015) Co-overexpression of AVP1 and AtNHX1 in cotton further improves drought and salt tolerance in transgenic cotton plants. Plant Mol Biol Rep 33(2):167–177. https://doi.org/10.1007/s11105-014-0739-8
85. Shi J, Gao H, Wang H, Lafitte HR, Archibald RL, Yang M, Hakimi SM, Mo H, Habben JE (2017) ARGOS 8 variants generated by CRISPR-Cas9 improve maize grain yield under field drought stress conditions. Plant Biotechnol J 15(2):207–216. https://doi.org/10.1111/pbi.12603
86. Shi H, Ishitani M, Kim C, Zhu JK (2000) The Arabidopsis thaliana salt tolerance gene SOS1 encodes a putative Na+/H+ antiporter. Proc Natl Acad Sci 97(12):6896–6901
87. Si X, Zhang H, Wang Y, Chen K, Gao C (2020) Manipulating gene translation in plants by CRISPR–Cas9-mediated genome editing of upstream open reading frames. Nat Protoc 15(2):338–363
88. Smith SM (2012) Food crisis in the horn of Africa: progress report, July 2011–July 2012. Oxfam International
89. Song JM, Guan Z, Hu J, Guo C, Yang Z, Wang S, Liu D, Wang B, Lu S, Zhou R (2020) Eight high-quality genomes reveal pan-genome architecture and ecotype differentiation of Brassica napus. Nat Plants 6(1):34–45
90. Su J, Wu R (2004) Stress-inducible synthesis of proline in transgenic rice confers faster growth under stress conditions than that with constitutive synthesis. Plant Sci 166:941–948. https://doi.org/10.1016/j.plantsci.2003.12.004
91. Syafrudin M, Kristanti RA, Yuniarto A, Hadibarata T, Rhee J, Al-Onazi WA, Algarni TS, Almarri AH, Al-Mohaimeed AM (2021) Pesticides in drinking water—a review. Int J Environ Res Public Health 18(2):468
92. Tang Y, Bao X, Zh Y, Wu Q, Guo Y, Yin X, Zeng L, Li J, Zhang J, He W (2019) Overexpression of a MYB family gene, OsMYB6, increases drought and salinity stress tolerance in transgenic rice. Front Plant Sci 10:168
93. Tashkandi M, Ali Z, Aljedaani F, Shami A, Mahfouz MM (2018) Engineering resistance against tomato yellow leaf curl virus via the CRISPR/Cas9 system in tomato. Plant Signal Behav 13(10):e1525996
94. Tettelin H, Masignani V, Cieslewicz MJ, Donati C, Medini D, Ward NL, Angiuoli SV, Crabtree JAL, Durkin AS (2005) Genome analysis of multiple pathogenic isolates of Streptococcus agalactiae: implications for the microbial pan-genome. Proc Natl Acad Sci 102(39):13950–13955

95. Thalapati S, Batchu AK, Neelamraju S, Ramanan R (2012) Os11Gsk gene from a wild rice, Oryza rufipogon improves yield in rice. Funct Integr Genomics 12:277–289
96. Thomazella DPT, Seong K, Mackelprang R, Dahlbeck D, Geng Y, Gill US, Qi T, Pham J, Giuseppe P, Lee CY, Ortega A, Cho MJ, Hutton SF, Staskawicz B (2021) Loss of function of a DMR6 ortholog in tomato confers broad-spectrum disease resistance. Proc Natl Acad Sci USA 118(27):e2026152118. https://doi.org/10.1073/pnas.2026152118
97. Tran MT, Doan DTH, Kim J, Song YJ, Sung YW, Das S, Kim EJ, Son GH, Kim SH, Van Vu T (2021) CRISPR/Cas9-based precise excision of SlHyPRP1 domain (s) to obtain salt stress-tolerant tomato. Plant Cell Rep 40:999–1011
98. Varshney RK, Roorkiwal M, Sun S, Bajaj P, Chitikineni A, Thudi M, Singh NP, Du X, Upadhyaya HD, Khan AW (2021) A chickpea genetic variation map based on the sequencing of 3,366 genomes. Nature 599(7886):622–627
99. Wang Y, Cheng X, Shan Q, Zhang Y, Liu J, Gao C, Qiu JL (2014) Simultaneous editing of three homoeoalleles in hexaploid bread wheat confers heritable resistance to powdery mildew. Nat Biotechnol 32(9):947–951
100. Wang H, Tang H, Yang C, Li Y (2019) Selective single molecule nanopore sensing of microRNA using PNA functionalized magnetic core–shell Fe3O4–Au nanoparticles. Anal Chem 91(12):7965–7970
101. Wang S, Zong Y, Lin Q, Zhang H, Chai Z, Zhang D, Chen K, Qiu JL, Gao C (2020) Precise, predictable multi-nucleotide deletions in rice and wheat using APOBEC–Cas9. Nat Biotechnol 38(12):1460–1465
102. Wang Y, Liang C, Meng Z, Li Y, Abid MA, Askari M, Wang P, Wang Y, Sun G, Cai Y (2019) Leveraging *Atriplex hortensis* choline monooxygenase to improve chilling tolerance in cotton. Environ Exp Bot 162:364–373. https://doi.org/10.1016/j.envexpbot.2019.03.012
103. Wang C, Zhang X, Fan Y, Gao Y, Zhu Q, Zheng C, Qin T, Li Y, Che J, Zhang M, Yang B, Liu Y, Zhao K (2015) XA23 is an executor R protein and confers broad-spectrum disease resistance in rice. Mol Plant 8(2):290–302. https://doi.org/10.1016/j.molp.2014.10.010. Epub 2014 Dec 15. PMID: 25616388
104. Wang T, Xun H, Wang W, Ding X, Tian H, Hussain S, Dong Q, Li Y, Cheng Y, Wang C (2021) Mutation of GmAITR genes by CRISPR/Cas9 genome editing results in enhanced salinity stress tolerance in soybean. Front Plant Sci 2752
105. Watson A, Ghosh S, Williams MJ, Cuddy WS, Simmonds J, Rey MD, Asyraf M, Hatta M, Hinchliffe A, Steed A, Reynolds D (2018) Speed breeding is a powerful tool to accelerate crop research and breeding. Nat Plants 4(1):23–29
106. Wei P, Che B, Shen L, Cui Y, Wu S, Cheng C, Liu F, Li MW, Yu B, Lam HM (2019) Identification and functional characterization of the chloride channel gene, GsCLC-c2 from wild soybean. BMC Plant Biol 19:1–15. https://doi.org/10.1186/s12870-019-1732-z
107. Xu R, Li J, Liu X, Shan T, Qin R, Wei P (2020) Development of plant prime-editing systems for precise genome editing. Plant Commun 1(3):100043
108. Yang L, Machin F, Wang S, Saplaoura E, Kragler F (2023) Heritable transgene-free genome editing in plants by grafting of wild-type shoots to transgenic donor rootstocks. Nat Biotechnol 1–10
109. Yang Y, Tang RJ, Mu B, Ferjani A, Shi J, Zhang H, Zhao F, Lan WZ, Luan S (2018) Vacuolar proton pyrophosphatase is required for high magnesium tolerance in *Arabidopsis*. Int J Mol Sci 19(11):3617. https://doi.org/10.3390/ijms19113617
110. Zhang Y, Bai Y, Wu G, Zou S, Chen Y, Gao C, Tang D (2017) Simultaneous modification of three homoeologs of Ta EDR 1 by genome editing enhances powdery mildew resistance in wheat. Plant J 91(4):714–724
111. Zhang H, Dong H, Li W, Sun Y, Chen S, Kong X (2009) Increased glycine betaine synthesis and salinity tolerance in AhCMO transgenic cotton lines. Mol Breeding 23(2):289–298
112. Zhang Y, Li J, Chen S et al (2020) An APETALA2/ethylene responsive factor, *OsEBP89* knockout enhances adaptation to direct-seeding on wet land and tolerance to drought stress in rice. Mol Genet Genomics 295:941–956. https://doi.org/10.1007/s00438-020-01669-7

113. Zhang A, Liu Y, Wang F, Li T, Chen Z, Kong D, Bi J, Zhang F, Luo X, Wang J (2019) Enhanced rice salinity tolerance via CRISPR/Cas9-targeted mutagenesis of the OsRR22 gene. Mol Breeding 39:1–10
114. Zhang YY, Li HX, Shu WB, Zhang CJ, Ye ZB (2011) RNA interference of a mitochondrial APX gene improves vitamin C accumulation in tomato fruit. Scientia Horticulturae 129(2):220–226. https://doi.org/10.1016/j.scienta.2011.03.025
115. Zhao Q, Feng Q, Lu H, Li Y, Wang A, Tian Q, Zhan Q, Lu Y, Zhang L, Huang T (2018) Pan-genome analysis highlights the extent of genomic variation in cultivated and wild rice. Nat Genet 50(2):278–284
116. Zhao C, Liu B, Piao S, Wang X, Lobell DB, Huang Y, Huang M, Yao Y, Bassu S, Ciais P (2017) Temperature increase reduces global yields of major crops in four independent estimates. Proc Natl Acad Sci 114(35):9326–9331
117. Zhong X, Hong W, Shu Y, Li J, Liu L, Chen X, Islam F, Zhou W, Tang G (2022) CRISPR/Cas9 mediated gene-editing of GmHdz4 transcription factor enhances drought tolerance in soybean (*Glycine max* [L.] Merr.). Front Plant Sci 13:988505
118. Zhou Y, Xu S, Jiang N, Zhao X, Bai Z, Liu J, Yao W, Tang Q, Xiao G, Lv C (2022) Engineering of rice varieties with enhanced resistances to both blast and bacterial blight diseases via CRISPR/Cas9. Plant Biotechnol J 20:876–885
119. Zong Y, Wang Y, Li C, Zhang R, Chen K, Ran Y, Qiu JL, Wang D, Gao C (2017) Precise base editing in rice, wheat and maize with a Cas9-cytidine deaminase fusion. Nat Biotechnol 35(5):438–440

Marine Protected Areas and Wetlands: Key Strategies for Climate Resilience and Carbon Sequestration

Are Marine Protected Areas Capable of Boosting Climate Change Resilience?

Wiame W. M. Emam and Kareem M. Soliman

Abstract Overfishing, pollution, habitat destruction, and climate change threaten marine ecosystems unprecedentedly. As these pressures continue to mount, marine ecosystems become more vulnerable to collapse, which could have disastrous effects on the millions of people who depend on them for their food, livelihoods, and cultural identity. In this context, marine protected areas (MPAs) have been established as a promising tool for conserving biodiversity, supporting sustainable fisheries, and building resilience to the impacts of climate change. In this chapter, we explore how MPAs can enhance resilience to climate change, review the research articles supporting this role, and provide examples from real-world case studies. It is worth mentioning that using MPAs as a strategy for coping with climate change has challenges and opportunities addressed in this chapter. Suggestions for future research and management initiatives were also provided. Ultimately, this book chapter aims to contribute to a better understanding of the crucial role that MPAs can play in constructing climate resilience and hitting the 30 $\times$ 30 target for biodiversity.

Keywords Mitigation · Adaptation · Mangroves · Saltmarshes · Seagrass · Coral reefs · Carbon sequestration · Biodiversity

Abbreviations and Definitions

MPAs	Marine protected areas
IPCC	Intergovernmental panel on climate change
CO_2-eq	Carbon dioxide equivalent
CBD	Convention on biological diversity
CPUE	Catch per unit effort

W. W. M. Emam (✉)
Department of Zoology, Faculty of Science, Ain Shams University, Abassia, Cairo, Egypt
e-mail: wiamewaheed@sci.asu.edu.eg

K. M. Soliman
Department of Zoology, Faculty of Science, Ain Shams University, Abassia, Cairo, Egypt
e-mail: dr_kariemsoliman@sci.asu.edu.eg

© The Author(s), under exclusive license to Springer Nature Switzerland AG 2025
M. T. Khalil et al. (eds.), *Climate Changes Impacts on Aquatic Environment*, Earth and Environmental Sciences Library, https://doi.org/10.1007/978-3-031-74897-4_9

1 Introduction

Marine ecosystems, which include a diverse array of habitats such as marshes, seagrass beds, coral reefs, mangrove forests, bird and fish rookeries, and more [10], are rich in biodiversity. However, these ecosystems are under escalating threats due to human activities. A significant portion, over 65% of the world's population, resides along coastlines, leading to increased marine and coastal biodiversity vulnerability to pressures such as overfishing, tourism, and deep-sea mining. These pressures result in pollution and ecological degradation [14]. A notable example is the decline of 71.1% in pelagic shark and ray populations between 1970 and 2018, which has been largely linked to increased fishing intensity [29, 37].

The Fifth Assessment Report of the "Intergovernmental Panel on Climate Change (IPCC)" highlighted the impacts of human activities on oceans, including rising sea temperatures, increased marine heatwaves, ocean acidification, and declining oxygen levels [16]. Such changes caused major disturbances in aquatic ecosystems—an increase in sea temperature, for instance, led to shifts in coral species diversity and abundance, contributing to the extinction of several coral species in the Indian Ocean [2, 19, 25]. Moreover, changes in marine zooplankton distribution due to rising sea temperatures profoundly impact marine food webs and ecosystem functioning [3, 31].

In response to these challenges, the concept of resilience has emerged as critical. Resilience denotes a marine ecosystem's capacity to withstand and rebound from the impacts of climate change while maintaining its structure, function, and ecosystem services.

Marine Protected Areas

Marine Protected Areas (MPAs), defined as "designated regions managed for the long-term conservation of marine resources, ecosystem services, or cultural heritage" [27], have received increasing attention as a potential strategy for bolstering resilience in marine ecosystems. Well-managed MPAs play a crucial role in safeguarding critical habitats, facilitating ecological connectivity, and providing a bulwark against the adverse effects of climate change by mitigating human pressures and safeguarding key areas and species.

The global initiative to conserve at least 30% of the world's land and oceans by 2030, known as the 30 $\times$ 30 target [5], has accelerated efforts to establish and manage MPAs effectively. Based on the allowance of certain activities (viz, mining, dredging, anchoring, infrastructure, aquaculture, fishing, and non-extractive activities) in marine areas and how these activities might affect ocean life (Table 1), the MPA Guide (https://mpa-guide.protectedplanet.net/) categorizes marine areas into four distinct levels of protection: fully protected, highly protected, lightly protected, and minimally protected. Fully protected areas (no-take zones) offer the highest level of conservation as all extractive activities like fishing are prohibited. In contrast, highly, lightly, and minimally protected areas allow progressively more activities.

Table 1 Impact of different activities on protection levels in marine areas, as per the MPA guide

Activity	Impact on protection level
Mining	Highly destructive, automatically disqualifies an area from MPA status
Dredging	The impact varies and may align with minimally or lightly protected areas
Anchoring	The impact varies; extensive anchoring lowers the protection level
Infrastructure	The impact varies according to the scale of the project: – Small-scale projects suitable for highly protected areas – Larger projects suitable only for minimally protected areas
Aquaculture	Varies in its environmental impact: – Ecosystem-restoring aquaculture, like oyster reef cultivation, helps restore habitats and enhance biodiversity. As a result, they are often compatible with marine areas designated as fully or highly protected under the MPA guide – Conversely, certain aquaculture practices, like salmon farming, can harm the environment by using chemicals, excessive feed, and releasing waste. Consequently, areas where such practices occur have their protection level downgraded
Fishing	In fully protected areas, fishing is completely prohibited In areas where fishing is permitted, the type of fishing gear used and its impact on the environment determine the level of protection assigned. For instance, certain types of gear may have less impact on marine life than others, influencing the level of protection needed Industrial fishing, characterized by large-scale operations with significant environmental impact, is particularly detrimental. Areas heavily impacted by industrial fishing are disqualified from being designated as MPAs due to the extensive harm inflicted on marine ecosystems

Effective management of MPAs can mitigate the impacts of overfishing, pollution, and habitat destruction, thereby enhancing ecological resilience [23].

In light of these considerations, this chapter will explore the mechanisms through which MPAs contribute to building climate resilience and advancing the 30 × 30 target, examine the factors influencing their effectiveness, and discuss the challenges and opportunities associated with establishing and effectively managing MPAs.

2 Mechanisms

MPAs play a crucial role in supporting marine ecosystems' resilience to climate change through various mechanisms. To identify the potential pathways through which MPAs could contribute to climate change impacts, Jacquemont et al. [17] screened more than 22,000 Web of Science research articles, out of which 378 articles were used for detailed evaluation, shedding light on 241 distinct MPAs. Most of the research articles were from Europe and Asia. Generally, MPAs contribute to resilience through climate mitigation and adaptation.

2.1 Climate Mitigation

Blue Carbon Sequestration

Blue carbon ecosystems, including mangrove forests, saltmarshes, and seagrass beds, are critical for climate mitigation due to their substantial potential for carbon sequestration and greenhouse gas offsets [22].

a. Mangrove Forests

Globally, mangrove forests occupy a spatial extent of 140,260 km^2 across 121 countries [4] in tropical and subtropical coastal areas. In Africa, mangroves cover a total area of 26,591.03 km^2, spanning 27 countries. Approximately 4% of the mangrove forests in Africa are found in Togo, Egypt, Mauritania, Sudan, Djibouti, the Republic of the Congo, Somalia, South Africa, Benin, Côte d'Ivoire, Eritrea, Liberia, Ghana, the Democratic Republic of the Congo, and Equatorial Guinea. Each of these countries encompasses a relatively small proportion, specifically less than one percent, of the total mangrove area within the continent. Conversely, more than 75% of Africa's mangrove forests are concentrated in the countries of West Africa.

Mangrove forests consist of trees and shrubs adapted to saline and brackish water conditions. These unique ecosystems are renowned for their extensive root systems that trap and stabilize sediments, effectively sequestering large amounts of carbon. Mangroves have been estimated to store up to four times more carbon per unit area than terrestrial forests [30]. This significant carbon storage capacity highlights their crucial role in mitigating climate change.

Due to their ecological importance, mangrove restoration initiatives have been ongoing since the 1970s, especially in Southeast Asia, East Asia, and South America. These efforts enhance blue carbon stocks [7]. Restoration projects, designed according to local policies and environmental conditions [18], typically use two main silvicultural strategies: reforestation and afforestation [32]. Reforestation focuses on immediately restoring mangroves in areas that have recently experienced degradation or deforestation due to human activities or natural causes [36], while afforestation involves establishing mangroves in areas that were previously devoid of mangrove plants [34].

Studies have extensively explored the efficacy of these restoration strategies in sequestering carbon. Song et al. [33] examined data from 370 restoration sites worldwide to compare the carbon sequestration potential of mangrove reforestation versus afforestation. The findings revealed that reforestation generally offers higher carbon storage potential per hectare than afforestation. Over 40 years, reforesting deforested mangrove regions globally could lead to a carbon uptake of 671.5–688.8 Tg CO_2-eq, which is 60% higher than afforesting the same area on tidal flats, which are considered more marginal sites. Several factors contribute to the greater carbon accumulation in reforestation sites, including favorable intertidal positioning, higher nitrogen availability, and lower salinity. These results highlight the importance of prioritizing mangrove reforestation to maximize carbon sequestration benefits and enhance the resilience of coastal ecosystems to climate change.

b. Saltmarshes

Saltmarshes occur in temperate and subtropical regions and are dominated by grasses and other herbaceous plants. They exhibit high carbon sequestration rates, with their vegetation and organic-rich soils trapping and storing carbon over time. Saltmarshes are particularly efficient at removing carbon dioxide from the atmosphere and transferring it to long-term storage.

Mason et al. [24] conducted a comprehensive analysis, including data from 431 research articles, to assess quantitatively the benefits of saltmarsh restoration in terms of carbon accumulation and greenhouse gas uptake. Their findings underscore the importance of prioritizing saltmarsh restoration initiatives. They found that saltmarshes globally store a substantial amount of carbon, estimated to be between 1.41 and 2.44 Petagrams (Pg). Moreover, restored marshes exhibit low greenhouse gas fluxes and rapid carbon accumulation. The mean net accumulation rate was calculated to be 64.70 metric tons of CO_2 equivalent per hectare per year. Based on the estimated accumulation and potential restoration rates, salt marsh regeneration could lead to significant carbon accumulation, ranging from 12.93 to 207.03 megatons (Mt) of CO_2 equivalent per year. This quantity of carbon sequestration might compensate for as much as half of the world's CO_2 emissions caused by energy production, which is a significant contribution considering that saltmarshes cover less than 1% of the Earth's surface.

c. Seagrass Beds

Seagrass beds are underwater meadows composed of seagrass species commonly found in coastal and estuarine environments. Like mangroves and saltmarshes, seagrass beds are critical in trapping sediment and storing organic carbon in their root systems, leading to significant long-term carbon storage. Despite their small oceanic footprint (less than 1%), seagrass meadows contribute approximately 10% of the annual carbon sequestration in the ocean [8].

According to Fourqurean et al. [13], coastal seagrass beds can store a substantial amount of carbon in the underlying sediment, estimated to be up to 83,000 metric tons per km^2. Seagrass meadows can offset approximately 0.42 tons of CO_2 equivalent per hectare per year [28].

Restoration projects, like that assessed by Oreska et al. [28], demonstrate the potential of seagrass meadows to offset CO_2 emissions. Though restoration efforts may inadvertently increase methane and nitrous oxide emissions, they still present environmentally and financially tangible benefits. Financially, the project yielded a benefit of $87,000, covering approximately 10% of the total restoration costs.

Overall, designating MPAs in regions with blue carbon ecosystems can significantly enhance their carbon sequestration potential. Moreover, supporting restoration activities, such as planting mangroves, restoring the hydrological connectivity of saltmarshes, and rehabilitating degraded seagrass beds within MPA boundaries, further contribute to climate change mitigation.

2.2 Climate Adaptation

MPAs play a crucial role in fostering ecological and social adaptation to the impacts of climate change.

2.2.1 Ecological Adaptation

Compared to unprotected sites, MPAs contribute to ecological adaptation by conserving critical habitats, increasing biodiversity, and enhancing reproductive output.

a. Protecting Critical and Coastal Habitats

MPAs play a crucial role in safeguarding critical habitats, such as mangroves, tidal marshes, coral reefs, and seagrass beds, which are essential for marine ecosystems' overall health and functioning.

Mangroves, in particular, dissipate wave energy and stabilize shorelines through soil accretion at a rate of 1.38 ± 0.88 cm/year more than in degraded areas [17]. Coral reefs and seagrass can also protect coastlines by reducing wave energy. While no studies have specifically measured if this effect is stronger in MPAs, wave attenuation is influenced by the habitat's vegetation density [12]. This implies that habitats protected from physical disturbance (like dredging and trawling) would offer better coastal protection than degraded habitats.

Accordingly, preserving these habitats contributes to the resilience of coastal communities and provides a buffer against coastal erosion, storm surges, and sea-level rise.

b. Enhancing Biodiversity Resilience

Jacquemont et al. [17] found that MPAs had higher species richness than unprotected areas. This can be attributed to MPAs serving as vital refuges for endangered and vulnerable marine species by minimizing direct human impacts such as overfishing, habitat destruction, and pollution. Protecting these species within MPA boundaries ensures their survival and stabilizes the ecosystem.

Cabo Pulmo National Park in the Gulf of California, Mexico, exemplifies the efficacy of MPAs. Established as a no-take marine reserve in 1995, it witnessed a remarkable 463% increase in fish biomass by 2009. Predator biomass experienced an 11-fold increase during this timeframe, while carnivore biomass quadrupled [1].

Similarly, in Australia, Turnbull et al. [35] highlighted that since its designation as a no-take zone in 2002, Cabbage Tree Bay has outperformed nearby no-take MPAs regarding fish richness and abundance, overall biomass, and targeted fish biomass. The biomass of all fish and large fish was four times higher, while the biomass of targeted fish was eleven times higher.

c. Reproductive Output

Reproductive capacity is critical to adaptation because it helps populations recover faster and allows larvae to disperse over greater distances [26]. This dispersal enhances connectivity between populations and improves the ability to colonize new habitats, vital for adapting to changing environmental conditions [15].

MPAs significantly boost the reproductive output of marine organisms, resulting in higher densities of larvae and more egg production compared to unprotected areas. This can be attributed to the presence of larger, older, and more individuals within MPAs, which are better at producing offspring. In contrast, recruitment rates showed no significant increase, due to higher predation rates on young recruits in MPAs [17].

2.2.2 Social Adaptation

a. Food Security and Livelihood Support

MPAs are crucial in enhancing food security and promoting sustainable livelihoods for coastal communities.

A key factor in this is the significant increase in catch per unit effort (CPUE) seen within highly protected MPAs, allowing fishermen to catch more fish with the same effort. This increase in CPUE is due to the recovery of fish populations within this protected area, which then spill over into adjacent fishing grounds, benefiting local fisheries [21]. Additionally, higher incomes for fishermen near these protected areas demonstrate that MPAs can offset the economic costs of restricting fishing activities [17]. Overall, MPAs offer sustainable livelihood opportunities for coastal communities, bolstering their ability to adapt to the impacts of climate change.

b. Community Engagement and Empowerment

Involving local communities in MPA management fosters a sense of ownership and stewardship. Participatory approaches empower communities to adapt to climate change by enabling them to make informed decisions about resource management and conservation.

c. Alternative Livelihoods

In areas of fully protected MPAs, communities are finding new ways to sustain themselves and be less dependent on exploiting marine resources, fostering economic diversification [17].

By promoting ecological resilience and supporting social adaptation, MPAs contribute to broader climate resilience efforts at both ecological and human levels. These dual benefits highlight the importance of integrating ecological and social considerations in MPA design and management to enhance overall effectiveness in climate change.

Case Study: "Pilar Municipal Marine Park" in the Philippines

In Pilar, a central Philippine town of 11,308 residents, the community manages the Pilar Municipal Marine Park (PMMP), established in 2005. Spanning 179 ha, the park includes a 29-ha no-take zone where all marine activities are banned, allowing fish populations to recover and spillover into the remaining 150 ha, where limited, non-destructive fishing is permitted. During Typhoon Haiyan in 2013, PMMP exemplified the potential of MPAs to enhance social adaptation, as its spillover fish were crucial for the community's survival when aid was inaccessible [6].

3 Factors Influencing the Climate Benefits of Marine Protected Areas

MPAs are critical tools for conserving marine biodiversity and mitigating the impacts of climate change. Their effectiveness, however, hinges on several key factors, including the level of protection, enforcement, age, size, and isolation. Edgar et al. [9] identified five criteria essential for MPA effectiveness:

1. Implementing no-take zones.
2. Regulations must be enforced properly.
3. MPA should be older than ten years.
4. It should cover an area larger than 100 km^2.
5. It should be physically separated from adjacent areas by natural barriers.

Case Study: "Papahānaumokuākea Marine National Monument"

One instance where MPAs have excelled is the 'Papahānaumokuākea Marine National Monument.' Established in 2006 around the Northwestern Hawaiian Islands, this site spans over 1.5 million km^2. Its no-take zones, which have been strictly protected since 1903, make it one of the most well-guarded areas for marine life on Earth. The extensive and strict protection measures implemented at this monument, coupled with its remote location, ensure minimal human disturbance, thus enhancing its effectiveness as a guard against disturbances to marine ecosystems.

Building on Edgar's work, Jacquemont et al. [17] investigated the relationship between MPA effectiveness and factors like protection level, age, and size in terms of providing climate-related benefits such as biodiversity conservation, CPUE, income generation or carbon sequestration.

a. Level of Protection

Undoubtedly, the level of protection is the most critical factor in determining the effectiveness of MPAs [17]. Fully or highly protected MPAs, in particular, provide the greatest benefits, especially in the context of climate change adaptation and mitigation. Fully protected areas show significant increases in species richness and fishers' income, while highly protected areas allow for low-impact fishing and boost CPUE and carbon sequestration.

Regrettably, the rush to meet international conservation targets has led to a decrease in the proportion of fully or highly protected MPAs. This trend is undermining their potential climate benefits, highlighting the urgent need to address this issue.

b. MPA Age

"MPA Age" refers to the duration an MPA has been established and operational. Jacquemont et al. [17] found that older MPAs demonstrate greater benefits in biodiversity, CPUE, income generation, and carbon sequestration. This positive correlation can be attributed to several factors. Firstly, over time, exploited fish populations within the MPA have the opportunity to recover and replenish their numbers. As fish stocks rebuild, they can spill into adjacent fishing grounds, benefiting nearby fisheries. Additionally, as MPAs mature, ecosystems such as mangroves and seagrass beds become more effective at carbon capture and storage due to habitat restoration and growth.

c. MPA Size

"MPA Size" refers to the physical area covered by an MPA. Larger MPAs generally exhibit higher CPUE values because they encompass a greater diversity of habitats and ecosystems, supporting a wider variety and larger populations of fish species. They also provide more refuge from fishing pressure outside the protected area, leading to higher fish densities within the MPA boundaries.

4 Exploring Challenges and Opportunities in Enhancing MPA Effectiveness

Despite MPAs' potential benefits, several challenges hinder their effectiveness in enhancing climate resilience. Addressing these challenges and leveraging opportunities is crucial for maximizing MPAs' contributions to climate change mitigation and adaptation.

Challenges

a. **Resource Limitations**

Limited financial and human resources pose significant challenges to effectively managing and enforcing MPAs. Many MPAs lack adequate funding for monitoring, enforcement, and community engagement activities, which can undermine their conservation goals [20].

b. **Governance and Policy**

Effective governance and policy frameworks are essential for the successful implementation of MPAs. Inconsistent policies, lack of political will, and weak enforcement mechanisms can hinder the establishment and management of MPAs. Moreover, some MPA management plans may consider climate change beyond their scope, further complicating efforts to address its impacts [20].

Opportunities

Amid these challenges, opportunities arise to enhance MPA management:

a. **Initiatives**

Initiatives like WildAid (https://wildaid.org/) provide a pathway to overcome resource limitations. By assisting developing nations in bolstering community engagement, enforcement measures, policy frameworks, training programs, and sustainable funding, WildAid has demonstrated tangible progress. Originating in the Galapagos Islands 25 years ago, WildAid's footprint now extends to 14 countries, showcasing its potential to address MPA management challenges on a global scale.

b. **Technological Advancements**

Advancements in technology, such as remote sensing, drones, and artificial intelligence, offer new opportunities for improving MPA monitoring and enforcement. These technologies can enhance the capacity of MPA managers to detect and respond to illegal activities and monitor ecological changes [11].

c. **Community-Based Management**

Community-based management approaches that involve local stakeholders in decision-making and enforcement can enhance the effectiveness of MPAs. These approaches can improve compliance and support for conservation efforts by fostering local ownership and stewardship.

5 Conclusion

In summary, MPAs have the potential to significantly enhance climate resilience through a combination of climate mitigation efforts (such as carbon sequestration) and adaptation strategies. These strategies yield ecological benefits, including coastal protection, biodiversity preservation, and enhanced reproductive capacity of marine organisms, as well as social mechanisms that improve the adaptive capacity of marine ecosystems and the livelihoods of millions of people who depend on them. It should be noted that these advantages are only realized when areas receive full or high levels of protection.

Recommendations

To enhance the climate resilience of MPAs, it is recommended to:

1. Ensure high protection levels,
2. Secure sufficient funds,
3. Support restoration activities, such as planting mangroves, rehabilitating saltmarshes with hydrological connectivity, and restoring degraded seagrass beds within MPA boundaries,
4. Establish effective governance involving local communities, and
5. Implement program evaluation and knowledge sharing.

References

1. Aburto-Oropeza O, Erisman B, Galland GR, Mascareñas-Osorio I, Sala E, Ezcurra E (2011) Large recovery of fish biomass in a no-take marine reserve. PLoS ONE 6(8):e23601. https://doi.org/10.1371/journal.pone.0023601
2. Ateweberhan M, McClanahan TR, Maina J, Sheppard C (2018) Thermal energy and stress properties as the main drivers of regional distribution of coral species richness in the Indian Ocean. J Biogeogr 45(6):1355–1366. https://doi.org/10.1111/jbi.13224
3. Brun P, Stamieszkin K, Visser AW, Licandro P, Payne MR, Kiørboe T (2019) Climate change has altered zooplankton-fuelled carbon export in the North Atlantic. Nat Ecol Evol 3:416–423. https://doi.org/10.1038/s41559-018-0780-3
4. Bunting P, Rosenqvist A, Hilarides L, Lucas RM, Thomas N (2022) Global mangrove watch: updated 2010 mangrove forest extent (v2.5). Remote Sens 14(4):1034. https://doi.org/10.3390/rs14041034
5. CBD (2022) Convention on biological diversity. COP15: nations adopt four goals, 23 targets for 2030 in landmark UN biodiversity agreement. Retrieved from https://shorturl.at/kqBU9
6. Chavez L (2021) With growing pressures, can the Philippines sustain its marine reserves? Mongabay series: Coral reefs, Oceans. https://news.mongabay.com/2021/06/with-growing-pressures-can-the-philippines-sustain-its-marine-reserves/
7. Duarte CM, Agusti S, Barbier E, Britten GL, Castilla JC, Gattuso J-P, Fulweiler RW, Hughes TP, Knowlton N, Lovelock CE, Lotze HK, Predragovic M, Poloczanska E, Roberts C, Worm B (2020) Rebuilding marine life. Nature 580:39–51. https://doi.org/10.1038/s41586-020-2146-7
8. EPA (2022) EPA scientists study the carbon-storing power of seagrass to fight climate change. https://www.epa.gov/sciencematters/epa-scientists-study-carbon-storing-power-seagrass-fight-climate-change
9. Edgar G, Stuart-Smith R, Willis T et al (2014) Global conservation outcomes depend on marine protected areas with five key features. Nature 506:216–220. https://doi.org/10.1038/nature13022
10. Emam WW, Khalil MT, Nassif MG, Soliman KM (2019) Applying geospatial technology in assessing the coastal vulnerability of Zaranik protectorate to sea-level rise. Egypt J Aquat Biol Fish 23(4):697–719
11. Emam WW, Soliman KM (2024) Integrating geospatial approach with citizen science to combat marine plastic pollution. In: Pal SC, Roy SS, Saha A, Abioui M (eds) Developments in environmental science: water resources monitoring management and sustainability-application of geostatistics and geospatial modeling (vol 16, Ch 13, pp 309–332). Elsevier. https://doi.org/10.1016/B978-0-443-23665-5.00013-2
12. Ferrario F, Beck MW, Storlazzi CD, Micheli F, Shepard CC, Airoldi L (2014) The effectiveness of coral reefs for coastal hazard risk reduction and adaptation. Nat Commun 5:3794. https://doi.org/10.1038/ncomms4794
13. Fourqurean JW, Duarte CM, Kennedy H, Marbà N, Holmer M, Mateo MA, Apostolaki ET, Kendrick GA, Krause-Jensen D, McGlathery KJ, Serrano O (2012) Seagrass ecosystems as a globally significant carbon stock. Nat Geosci 5:505–509. https://doi.org/10.1038/ngeo1477
14. Guzmán DH, Mier RL, Vergara A, Milanes CB (2023) Marine protected areas in Colombia: a historical review of legal marine protection since the late 1960s to 2023. Mar Policy 155:105726. https://doi.org/10.1016/j.marpol.2023.105726
15. Hixon MA, Johnson DW, Sogard SM (2014) BOFFFFs: on the importance of conserving old-growth age structure in fishery populations. ICES J Mar Sci 71(8):2171–2185. https://doi.org/10.1093/icesjms/fst200
16. IPCC (2021) Climate change is widespread, rapid, and intensifying—IPCC. Online. Available at https://www.ipcc.ch/2021/08/09/ar6-wg1-20210809-pr/
17. Jacquemont J, Blasiak R, Le Cam C, Le Gouellec M, Claudet J (2022) Ocean conservation boosts climate change mitigation and adaptation. One Earth 5(10):1015–1025. https://doi.org/10.1016/j.oneear.2022.09.002

18. Lee SY, Hamilton S, Barbier EB, Primavera J, Lewis III RR (2019) Better restoration policies are needed to conserve mangrove ecosystems. Nat Ecol Evol 3:870–872. https://doi.org/10.1038/s41559-019-0861-y
19. Linklater M, Jordan AR, Carroll AG, Neilson J, Gudge S, Brooke BP, Nichol SL, Hamylton SM, Woodroffe CD (2019) Mesophotic corals on the subtropical shelves of Lord Howe Island and Balls Pyramid, south-western Pacific Ocean. Mar Freshw Res 70(1):43–61. https://doi.org/10.1071/MF18151
20. Lopazanski C, Foshay B, Couture JL, Wagner D, Hannah L, Pidgeon E, Bradley D (2023) Principles for climate resilience are prevalent in marine protected area management plans. Conserv Lett 16(5):e12972. https://doi.org/10.1111/conl.12972
21. Di Lorenzo M, Guidetti P, Di Franco A, Calò A, Claudet J (2020) Assessing spillover from marine protected areas and its drivers: a meta-analytical approach. Fish Fish 21(5):906–915. https://doi.org/10.1111/faf.12469
22. Luisetti T (2021) Some countries donate blue carbon. Nat Clim Change 11:647–648. https://doi.org/10.1038/s41558-021-01103-9
23. Marzin C, Benzaken D, Otero MM, Quemmerais F, Bates A, Brown M, Hutto S, Brock R (2016) Marine protected areas and adaptation to climate change: how can MPAs increase climate resilience? In: Simard F, Laffoley D, Baxter JM (eds) 2016. Marine protected areas and climate change: adaptation and mitigation synergies, opportunities and challenges. IUCN, Gland, Switzerland, pp 29–39. https://portals.iucn.org/library/node/46398
24. Mason VG, Burden A, Epstein G, Jupe LL, Wood KA, Skov MW (2023) Blue carbon benefits from global saltmarsh restoration. Glob Change Biol 29(23):6517–6545. https://doi.org/10.1111/gcb.16943
25. McClanahan TR, Muthiga N (2021) Oceanic patterns of thermal stress and coral community degradation on the island of Mauritius. Coral Reefs 40:53–74. https://doi.org/10.1007/s00338-020-02015-4
26. Micheli F, Saenz-Arroyo A, Greenley A, Vazquez L, Espinoza Montes JA, Rossetto M, De Leo GA (2012) Evidence that marine reserves enhance resilience to climatic impacts. PLoS ONE 7:e40832. https://doi.org/10.1371/journal.pone.0040832
27. NOAA Ocean Exploration (2023) What is a marine protected area (MPA)? Online accessed on: June 2023, at https://oceanexplorer.noaa.gov/facts/mpas.html
28. Oreska MPJ, McGlathery KJ, Aoki LR, Berger AC, Berg P, Mullins L (2020) The greenhouse gas offset potential from seagrass restoration. Sci Rep 10:7325. https://doi.org/10.1038/s41598-020-64094-1
29. Pacoureau N, Rigby CL, Kyne PM, Sherley RB, Winker H, Carlson JK, Fordham SV, Barreto R, Fernando D, Francis MP, Jabado RW, Herman KB, Liu K-M, Marshall AD, Pollom RA, Romanov EV, Simpfendorfer CA, Yin JS, Kindsvater HK, Dulvy NK (2021) Half a century of global decline in oceanic sharks and rays. Nature 589:567–571. https://doi.org/10.1038/s41586-020-03173-9
30. Pham TD, Ha NT, Saintilan N, Skidmore A, Phan DC, Le NN, Viet HL, Takeuchi W, Friess DA (2023) Advances in earth observation and machine learning for quantifying blue carbon. Earth Sci Rev 243:104501. https://doi.org/10.1016/j.earscirev.2023.104501
31. Ratnarajah L, Abu-Alhaija R, Atkinson A, Batten S, Bax NJ, Bernard KS, Canonico G, Cornils A, Everett JD, Grigoratou M, Ishak NHA, Johns D, Lombard F, Muxagata E, Ostle C, Pitois S, Richardson AJ, Schmidt K, Stemmann L, Swadling KM, Yang G, Yebra L (2023) Monitoring and modelling marine zooplankton in a changing climate. Nat Commun 14:564. https://doi.org/10.1038/s41467-022-30511-9
32. Schlamadinger B, Boonpragob K, Janzen H, Kurz W, Lasco R, Smith P et al (2003) Supplementary methods and good practice guidance arising from the Kyoto Protocol. In: Penman J, Gytarsky M, Hiraishi T et al (eds) Good practice guidance for land use, land-use change and forestry (Chapter 4). Institute for Global Environmental Strategies for the IPCC. Retrieved from https://www.ipcc.ch/site/assets/uploads/2018/03/GPG_LULUCF_FULLEN.pdf
33. Song S, Ding Y, Li W, Meng Y, Zhou J, Gou R, Zhang C, Ye S, Saintilan N, Krauss KW, Crooks S, Lv S, Lin G (2023) Mangrove reforestation provides greater blue carbon benefit

than afforestation for mitigating global climate change. Nat Commun 14:756. https://doi.org/10.1038/s41467-023-36477-1
34. Soper FM, MacKenzie RA, Sharma S, Cole TG, Litton CM, Sparks JP (2019) Non-native mangroves support carbon storage, sediment carbon burial, and accretion of coastal ecosystems. Glob Change Biol 25(12):4315–4326. https://doi.org/10.1111/gcb.14813
35. Turnbull JW, Shah Esmaeili Y, Clark GF, Figueira WF, Johnston EL, Ferrari R (2018) Key drivers of effectiveness in small marine protected areas. Biodivers Conserv 27:2217–2242. https://doi.org/10.1007/s10531-018-1532-z
36. Vinh TV, Marchand C, Linh TVK, Vinh DD, Allenbach M (2019) Allometric models to estimate above-ground biomass and carbon stocks in Rhizophora apiculata tropical managed mangrove forests (Southern Viet Nam). For Ecol Manage 434:131–141. https://doi.org/10.1016/j.foreco.2018.12.017
37. WWF (2022) Living Planet Report 2022—Building a nature-positive society. In: Almond REA, Grooten M, Juffe Bignoli D, Petersen T (eds) WWF, Gland, Switzerland. Retrieved from https://wwfint.awsassets.panda.org/downloads/embargo_13_10_2022_lpr_2022_full_report_single_page_1.pdf

Carbon Sequestration Potential of Some Egyptian Wetlands for Mitigating Climate Change

Kamal H. Shaltout and Ebrahem M. Eid

Abstract Several studies on carbon sequestration potential (CSP) in some wetlands in Egypt were carried out by Shaltout, Eid, and other colleagues (2013–2021). This chapter aimed to evaluate the spatial diffusion of soil organic carbon (SOC) in vegetated and unvegetated areas in different wetlands of Egypt. The study focused on five northern Mediterranean lakes and Red Sea mangroves. The aim was to obtain a precise estimation of SOC stock and determine the potential for carbon sequestration in these wetlands, including estimates and monetary valuation of this potential. The average values for SOC stock and carbon sequestration rate (CSR) were significantly greater in mangroves (38.9 kg C/m^2 and 107.2 g C/m^2/yr) compared to the northern Mediterranean lakes (10.1 kg C/m^2 and 18.9 g C/m^2/yr). This implies that mangroves exhibit a higher efficiency in sequestering atmospheric carbon in their sedimentary environments. Regrettably, the mangrove areas in Egypt are relatively limited in size, encompassing a total of 28 sites with a combined area of 5.25 km^2. This is notably smaller compared to the smallest lake in North Egypt, namely Lake Mariut, which spans an area of 63 km^2. The monetary estimate of the carbon segregation service given by the five northern Mediterranean lakes in Egypt, concerning the stock of SOC measured in metric tons per total area, is evaluated to be approximately €1.96 billion. Among these lakes, Lake Manzalla exhibits the highest valuation, amounting to €0.89 billion, while Lake Mariut demonstrates the lowest, with €0.09 billion. Furthermore, the CSR in tons of carbon per total area per year is estimated to be approximately 2.27 million euros. Lake Manzalla recorded the highest CSR value of 1 million euros, while Lake Edku had the lowest CSR value of 0.56 million euros.

Keywords Carbon stock · Economic valuation · Mangroves · Mitigation · Northern lagoons · Services

K. H. Shaltout (✉)
Botany Department, Faculty of Science, Tanta University, Tanta, Egypt
e-mail: kamal.shaltout@science.tanta.edu.eg

E. M. Eid
Botany Department, Faculty of Science, Kafrelsheikh University, Kafr El-Sheikh, Egypt
e-mail: ebrahem.eid@sci.kfs.edu.eg

© The Author(s), under exclusive license to Springer Nature Switzerland AG 2025
M. T. Khalil et al. (eds.), *Climate Changes Impacts on Aquatic Environment*, Earth and Environmental Sciences Library, https://doi.org/10.1007/978-3-031-74897-4_10

1 Introduction

The rise in atmospheric carbon dioxide (CO_2) levels has prompted significant public and scientific interest in different ecosystems' carbon sequestration potential (CSP), particularly wetlands. Numerous scientific experts have proposed that sequestering carbon dioxide in soil organic carbon (SOC) holds substantial potential for aligning with the objectives of the Kyoto Protocol. This approach aims to stabilize the atmospheric CO_2 and other greenhouse gas levels, thereby mitigating the adverse effects of global warming [6]. The escalating levels of CO_2 on a global scale and the subsequent ramifications of climate change have prompted a greater focus on the critical role of ecosystems in addressing this issue. As a result, research efforts have intensified to underscore the significance of ecosystems in this endeavor.

There is a growing focus on preserving coastal ecosystems, particularly mangroves, due to their significant carbon storage capacity and the ongoing conversion of these areas for other purposes. The demand for precise information regarding SOC stock in Egypt has grown, considering the significance of SOC stock for the continual utilization of main resources and compliance with the Kyoto Protocol. Multiple research studies have been conducted on the CSP in Mediterranean lakes located in Egypt [2, 8, 9]. Additionally, the coastal Egyptian region of the Red Sea was deeply addressed [11, 13] as well as the Aqaba Gulf in South Sinai [12]. This chapter aimed to evaluate the spatial distribution of SOC in vegetated and unvegetated areas within various wetlands in Egypt, such as the northern Mediterranean lakes and Red Sea mangroves. The target was to obtain a precise estimation of SOC stock and determine its ecosystem service value by providing estimates and monetary valuation of its CSP.

2 Egyptian Wetlands

2.1 Classification and Description

The classification of Egyptian wetlands can be approached through two distinct patterns: a systematic pattern, which involves categorizing them based on their saltwater or freshwater characteristics, and a geographical pattern, which involves classifying them based on their location along the Red Sea and the Mediterranean coastlands in addition to their positioning as coastal or inland wetlands, and their association with the River Nile and its network of canals and drains. However, implementing effective environmental management and conservation practices challenges this taxonomy. A study conducted by Kassas [17] documented that there are 15 distinct wetland types in Egypt. These wetland types exhibit certain similarities, as illustrated in Fig. 1.

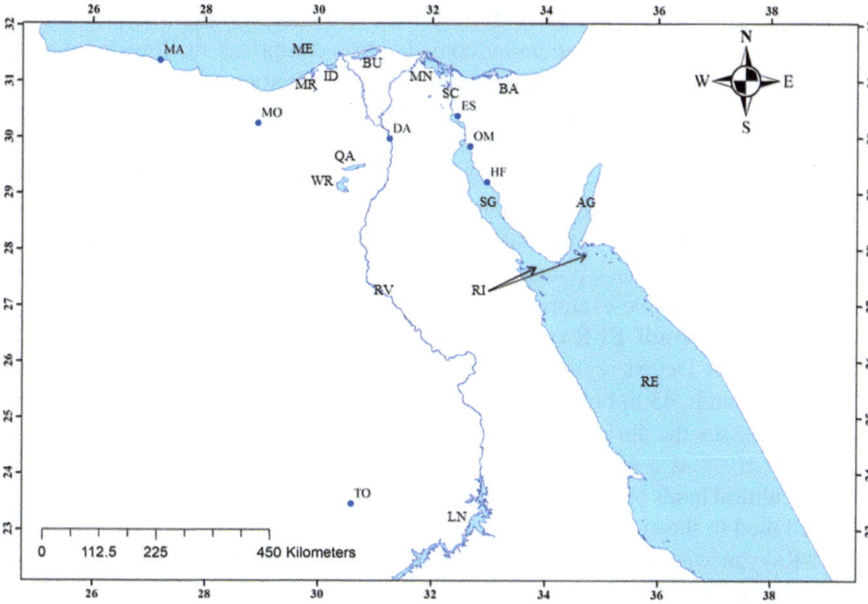

Fig. 1 Wetlands of Egypt; **BA**: Lake Bardawil, **MN**: Lake Manzalla, **BU**: Lake Burullus, **ID**: Lake Edku, **MR**: Lake Mariut, **MA**: Matrouh Lagoons, **MO**: Lake Moghra, **QA**: Lake Qarun, **WR**: Wadi El-Rayyan Lake, **DA**: Lake Dahshoor, **ES**: Ein Sokhna, **HF**: Hammam Faraon, **OM**: Oyon Mousa Springs, **RV**: River Nile, **LN**: Lake Nasser, **TO**: Toshka Depressions, **ME**: Mediterranean Sea, **RE**: Red Sea, **SG**: Suez Gulf, **AG**: Aqaba Gulf, **RI**: Red Sea Islands, and **SC**: Suez Canal System

a. The lakes located in northern Egypt include **Bardawil, Manzalla, Burullus, Edku,** and **Mariut**. These lakes exhibit varying origins and ecological characteristics [15]. All these locations possess natural or artificial connections to the Mediterranean, such as El-Boughaz. Additionally, they hold significant value as bird habitats, owing to their geographical positioning along migration routes. Besides, these fisheries hold significant importance in the Egyptian context. Khalil and Shaltout [19] elucidated that four entities are subjected to agricultural drainage and seawater, whereas Lake Bardawil does not receive any drainage water. The inclusion of Mallaha, located in Port Fouad, with its expansive salt mudflats, can be considered in this category.
b. **Matrouh Lagoons** are a prominent natural feature in the Matrouh Governorate of Egypt. These lagoons are a series of bodies of water geographically isolated from the Mediterranean Sea. These lagoons are supplied with water via a narrow barrier composed of limestone. A barrier near Marsa Matrouh was constructed to convert the existing lagoon into a functional port facility. The lagoons serve as valuable resources for fisheries, cage farming, and habitats for diverse and noteworthy biota.

c. **The Moghra and Wadi El-Natrun Lakes**. They are two prominent bodies of water in Egypt. The region under consideration comprises shallow depressions in the Western Desert's northern sector. The water is sourced from subterranean seepage. Moghra is situated in the eastern region of the Qattara Depression, whereas Wadi El-Natrun is situated in the western periphery of the Nile Delta. Moghra experiences seasonal habitation by pastoralists. Wadi El-Natrun serves as a location for a land reclamation project, although it has historically been recognized as the hub of the indigenous glass industry. In addition, it is possible to incorporate drainage ponds and pools within the diverse oases of the Western Desert, with notable examples found in Siwa Oasis.
d. **Qarun and Wadi El-Rayyan Lakes**. These two depressions are located in the Western Desert region. Lake Qarun is situated in the lowermost region, approximately 45 m below sea level, in the expansive depression that currently encompasses the agricultural territories of Fayoum Governorate. This body of water serves as a recipient of the excess drainage water originating from the agricultural lands of Fayoum. The hyper-saline nature of Lake Qarun is primarily attributed to the significant levels of evaporation occurring in its vicinity. Wadi El-Rayyan was an arid and uninhabited basin approximately 60 m below sea level. It contained a limited number of freshwater springs, giving rise to small reed swamps. During the 1970s, the Wadi El-Rayyan Depression became linked to the agricultural drainage system of the Fayoum Governorate. Two artificial brackish lakes were formed in this area [29].
e. **Abasa and Dahshoor Lakes**. Numerous small lakes are dispersed throughout the Delta region and its surrounding areas, primarily resulting from the accumulation of drainage water in depressions. Two lakes gained renown as locations for foul shooting, a popular winter sport. Located in the eastern region, Lake Abasa is a freshwater body that has retained its original purpose and is a hub for a research and training facility focused on fish farming. The western region of Dahshoor is characterized by its peripheral afforestation and the preservation of remnants of reed swamps.
f. **Ein Sokhna, Hammam Faraon, and Oyon Mousa Springs**. These locations are warm water springs along the Red Sea's littoral and coastal belts. Ein Sokhna lies on the western coast of the Gulf of Suez, Hammam Faraon on the eastern coast of the Suez Gulf, and Oyon Mousa lies in the southwestern part of Sinai. Water flows created small expanses of moist saline land covered with reed and rush growths.
g. **The River Nile** spans between the cities of Aswan and Cairo. The region encompasses many islands, characterized by their coastal and riverine areas offering diverse wetland habitats and vegetation, including floating reed formations. Within Aswan's vicinity is a collection of granitic islands known as the First Cataract Islands; they harbor remnants of riverine forests. The islands along the remaining stretch of the Nile River predominantly consist of alluvial deposits, with a limited number of them experiencing periodic inundation during certain seasons. The irrigation system comprises a network of over 47,000 km of canals

and drains interconnected with the main channel and its two Mediterranean branches, as documented in the study of **Khattab and El-Gharably** [20].

h. **Lake Nasser** is an artificial reservoir located in Egypt. It was created due to the construction of the High Dam's in Aswan. The water body is a substantial freshwater reservoir, ranking among the world's largest artificial lakes. It spans a length of 496 km, with 292 km located in Egypt and 204 km in Sudan. The total surface area of this reservoir is approximately 5000 square kilometers. The geographical location of the area under consideration, characterized by a high degree of aridity, presents a notable juxtaposition between desert and water, resulting in intriguing ecotone transitions [3]. Multiple shallow lobes characterize the western region, whereas the eastern region encompasses the mouths of various wadis, such as Wadi Allaqi.
i. **Toshka Depressions**. Several freshwater lakes were created in depressions in the Western Desert due to the overflow of Lake Nasser. Temporary freshwater bodies can be observed in highly arid desert environments. Wetland habitats prevail, including reed swamps. These depressions will eventually receive drainage of Toshka agricultural lands and become permanent.
j. **The Mediterranean Coast**. The west and east of the Nile Delta's Mediterranean coast provide little room for developed littoral salt marshes. The shoreline is in two distinct regions: the vicinity of the limestone cliffs to the west of Alameen (approximate longitude of 29° E) and the remaining coastal area characterized by coastal dunes. Beaches and near-shore strips support a wide range of diverse biota.
k. **The Suez Gulf**. The coastal region exhibits a significant presence of expansive salt marsh formations along its littoral zone. Typical zonation of coastal land vegetation is well recognized.
l. **The Red Sea** (including the Aqaba Gulf)**.** Its coastal lands have extensive patches of mangroves with a total area of 525 ha [25]. *Avicennia marina* prevails all over the coast, while *Rhizophora mucronata* is confined to the area south of Shalatin. The mangrove is an elaborating ecosystem with rich biota and provides refuge for fish spawning and various birds.
m. **The Red Sea coral reefs**. They exhibit elongated configurations that run near the coastline. The reefs under consideration encompass many coral species and their associated biota. These reefs are radical in the littoral and sublittoral zones' biological and physical ecological dynamics [16].
n. **The Red Sea Islands**. Two distinct types of habitats are present: namely, coral formations and volcanic islands. These islands' littoral and sub-littoral zones exhibit habitat characteristics like those found along the Red Sea coast, albeit with a lower degree of disturbance.
o. **The Suez Canal system** is a significant maritime transportation route connecting the Mediterranean Sea to the Red Sea. The region encompasses two prominent bodies of water: Lake Temsah, situated near Ismailia, and The Bitter Lake, located further south and boasts a larger expanse. The entire system facilitates the connection between the Mediterranean and the Red Seas, serving as a pathway for the migration of various organisms. Several Red Sea species have been

documented in the eastern Mediterranean, notably in Lake Bardawil in northern Sinai.

2.2 Threats upon the Egyptian Wetlands

a. The Egyptian wetlands, particularly the northern lakes, face various threats, notably, the conversion of these areas for alternative land uses such as land reclamation and urban development.
b. Despite experiencing significant loss in their respective areas, Lakes Manzalla and Burullus still maintain bodies of water that preserve their fundamental ecological characteristics. Lake Mariut has experienced a decline in its characteristics and has become fragmented into smaller basins significantly contaminated with pollutants. Lake Edku is subject to the impacts of both conversion and pollution. Additional threats to consider are the potential consequences stemming from land utilization practices in the surrounding areas of these lakes.
c. Land reclamation results in the discharge of excessive agricultural drainage into lakes, leading to a prevalence of brackish-fresh water conditions. Consequently, this phenomenon contributes to a reduction in habitat diversity. Introducing agricultural, domestic, and industrial effluents into lakes alters their chemical composition. This phenomenon is particularly significant due to the extensive catchment areas associated with each lake. The presence of these threats has a detrimental impact on the wetland functions and services they offer.
d. Wetlands are susceptible to the effects of natural sedimentation and silting processes in arid regions, specifically in the case of oases wetlands that experience sand encroachments.
e. Another concern impacting the lakes in the north Delta is the coastal erosion phenomenon that has become increasingly prominent since the twentieth century. This erosion has resulted in the formation of delicate sand barriers that now separate the lakes, particularly Lakes Manzalla and Burullus, from the adjacent sea. The ongoing process of erosion has the potential to transform the lakes into sea bays.
f. Climate change and the resulting increase in sea levels could lead to the submergence of lakes and their surrounding areas.
g. The primary factors contributing to the decline of mangroves include their conversion to aquaculture, particularly shrimp farming and agricultural and urban development. Additionally, extreme climatic events have emerged as a significant cause of mangrove loss [24].

2.3 The Services and Commodities Offered by the Wetlands in Egypt

a. **Water purification**. Wetland ecosystems fulfill a crucial function by effectively mitigating eutrophication and removing nitrogen and phosphorus compounds introduced via drainage processes. Aquatic vegetation, such as reeds and other submerged plants, can partially mitigate chemical pollutants, including heavy metals. Artificial wetlands have the potential to serve as an effective means for the purification of contaminated water sources.
b. **Mitigation strategies for sea surges**. The wetlands located in the northern Delta region serve as protective barriers, effectively buffering the sea from the adjacent low-lying farmlands. The absence of these lakes would expose agricultural areas to the risks associated with severe weather events and coastal inundation.
c. **Reservoirs of biodiversity**. Globally, wetlands harbor more than 40% of the total species found across the planet. Preserving coastal wetlands is crucial for the sustenance and survival of avian species that engage in migratory behaviors. Wetlands serve as sanctuaries for animal species during drought and other environmental challenges.
d. **Pristine balance** refers to the state of equilibrium or harmony in a system or entity. The coexistence of marine water in the northern sectors of Egypt and brackish water in the southern sectors contributes to diverse habitats, which in turn support a variety of biota, including various fish species.
e. **Products derived from wetlands**. Wetlands are recognized as highly productive ecosystems. The primary fishing grounds in Egypt consist of the northern lakes, viz., Lake Nasser, and the near-shore zones of coastal waters. Emergent wetland vegetation, such as reeds and rushes, offers valuable resources that support a diverse range of small-scale economic activities. Reeds serve many purposes in cultivating coastal sand formations, including but not limited to the establishment of shelterbelts and dune stabilization [26].
f. **Breeding and nursery habitats**. Wetlands are essential ecological components in various organisms' reproductive success and early life stages. These habitats serve as specialized environments where organisms engage in reproductive activities and provide optimal conditions for the mangrove swamps, tidal wetlands, and marine grasslands. These serve as crucial breeding and nursery habitats for numerous fish inhabiting these wetland ecosystems. The primary source of supplementary revenue for individuals engaged in fishing predominantly stems from the capture of waterfowl.
g. **Mangroves provide diverse ecosystem services**. Marine mammals, birds, and fish serve as crucial nursery habitats, effectively filtering nutrients. Additionally, they play a vital role in mitigating storm surges and supporting various rural economies [24].
h. **Carbon storage in sedimentary environments**. Addressing climate change necessitates a comprehensive approach encompassing emission reductions and removals. Mangrove forests possess the capacity to significantly contribute

to carbon removal, owing to their status as highly carbon-dense ecosystems. According to Sanderman et al. [24], the soils found in mangrove forests can serve as enduring carbon sinks when left undisturbed.

i. **The Storage of Carbon in Biomass**. Mangroves can store outstanding amounts of carbon in their biomass; however, most ecosystem carbon storage is detected in the soil. In a study conducted by Kauffman et al. [18], it was observed that soil carbon accounted for 78% of the overall carbon storage in tall mangroves. However, soil carbon contributed more than or equal to 96% of the total ecosystem carbon in low and medium-stature mangrove forests. Significantly, the researchers discovered that the transformation of these mangrove forests into shrimp ponds led to a substantial depletion of 90% of the carbon content within the uppermost 3 m of soil, amounting to a range of 612 to 1036 mega-grams of carbon per hectare.

j. Furthermore, the findings of Eid et al. [7] indicate that in mangroves, the stock of SOC is 147% greater than the stock recorded in shrimp farms, providing further evidence of the substantial contribution of anthropogenic factors to the value of SOC stock. In their study, Eid et al. [7] reported that the average cumulative potential CO_2 emission resulting from soil carbon stock depletion ascribed to mangroves' conversion into shrimp ponds was 34.9 kg CO_2/m^2. Furthermore, it is widely acknowledged that heavy metals play a significant role in inducing detrimental impacts on the biological characteristics of mangroves [4]. The impact of various forms of pollution on the productivity of mangroves has been identified in studies, resulting in reduced carbon sequestration and a less significant carbon sequestration rate (CSR) effect [1]. In their study along the southern Red Sea coast of Saudi Arabia, Arshad et al. [1] observed that the SOC stock of non-polluted mangrove locations is 116% higher than that of polluted mangrove locations.

k. **Minimizing the release of emissions**. Several studies, including Sanderman et al. [24], have observed that many mangrove soils are experiencing accretion because of rising sea levels. This process contributes to the ongoing carbon sequestration, with an estimated rate of 1.3–2.0 mega-grams per hectare per year.

l. **Climate benefit**. There exists a significant potential for climate mitigation by implementing measures to halt or reduce the rate of mangrove conversion. Preliminary estimates suggest that such actions could result in a CSR ranging from 25 to 122 tera-grams of carbon per year. The preservation and rehabilitation of extensive mangrove ecosystems in countries can significantly aid in achieving climate mitigation objectives.

m. **Recreation and ecotourism**. Wetlands offer diverse recreational opportunities, including angling, hunting, boating, and bird watching. The coastal regions of the Red Sea, along with its two adjacent gulfs, serve as significant locations for establishing and growing tourism infrastructure. The Egyptian coastal lands along the Red Sea and the Mediterranean Sea serve as locations for winter and summer resorts, respectively.

n. **Hydrological functions**. The potential utilization of wetlands for water storage has been explored, as evidenced by the consideration of using Lake Burullus as a reservoir during periods of high Nile flood. Moreover, wetlands can serve as a valuable source for replenishing underground aquifers in Egypt. Moreover, the lakes in the northern region serve as effective barriers, preventing subsurface seawater intrusion into the agricultural land in the southern areas.

o. **Climate change mitigation**. Certain wetland ecosystems can emit methane, which is recognized as a significant greenhouse gas. However, wetlands that exhibit high levels of biological productivity can function as carbon sinks. Consequently, preserving and rehabilitating these wetlands can enhance their ability to capture and store carbon. Coastal wetlands possess the potential to be incorporated into comprehensive strategies and schemes aiming at mitigating the projected increases in sea level.

p. **Education and research**. Wetlands serve as valuable locations for educational initiatives and public awareness campaigns. In addition, they offer platforms for conducting research studies on water-dependent ecosystem processes and addressing restoration requirements, maintenance strategies, and conservation methodologies.

3 Mediterranean Lakes

Eid and Shaltout [9] evaluated the spatial distribution of SOC in both vegetated and un-vegetated areas of Lake Burullus, a Mediterranean lake, to obtain a precise estimation of the SOC stock present in the lake, in alignment with the guidelines outlined in the Kyoto Protocol. Additionally, the study aimed to determine the values of Lake Burullus CSP. Compared to the un-vegetated locations, the study found that SOC content was notably greater in the vegetated localities, particularly in the uppermost soil layer. The stock of SOC exhibited a range of 9.3 kg C/m^2 in vegetated locations to 7.4 kg C/m^2 in un-vegetated localities, as indicated in Table 1. The vegetated sites exhibited a higher average CSR than the un-vegetated sites, with values of 14.9 and 8.6 g C/m^2/yr, respectively. The calculated CSP of Lake Burullus was determined to be 4.5 gigagrams of carbon per year, considering the geographical locality and factors of CSR.

In addition, Beshay [2] focused on evaluating Lake Mariut's contribution to the carbon sequestration process and its potential for mitigating atmospheric carbon levels. CSR exhibited significant variation across the three basins examined in the study. The average CSR of the basins under study can be ranked in the following order: SW basin > NW basin > FF basin. Moreover, the findings of the CSP revealed that the peak values were observed during the period spanning from 2008 to 2010, after which a gradual decline was observed in subsequent years. However, the southwestern basin exhibited a distinct pattern, with 1995–2008 displaying higher CSP values than 2008–2010. The SW basin exhibited the highest CSP with a recorded value of 117.2 Gg C/yr, succeeded by the NW basin with 30.3 Gg C/yr and the FF basin with 6.8 Gg C/yr.

Table 1 Total mean ± standard error of soil bulk density (SBD; g/cm^3), soil organic carbon (SOC) content (g C/kg), SOC density (kg C/m^3), SOC stock (kg C/m^2), carbon sequestration rate (CSR; g $C/m^2/yr$), and carbon sequestration potential (CSP; Gg C/yr) of the five Egyptian Mediterranean lakes.

Lake	Depth (cm)	SBD	SOC			CSR	CSP
			Content	Density	Stock		
Burullus—Veg*	40	1.67 ± 0.05	19.0 ± 2.8	24.4 ± 1.7	09.3 ± 1.0	14.9 ± 0.8	1.22 ± 0.07
Burullus—Uve*	40	1.80 ± 0.04	10.2 ± 0.5	18.2 ± 1.0	07.4 ± 0.8	08.6 ± 0.5	2.82 ± 0.16
Bardawil**	30	1.27 ± 0.04	25.2 ± 2.5	27.1 ± 2.2	08.1 ± 1.4	01.5 ± 0.1	0.95 ± 0.08
Manzala**	30	0.90 ± 0.03	32.9 ± 4.3	22.5 ± 1.9	06.7 ± 0.7	07.6 ± 0.7	7.79 ± 0.67
Burullus**	30	0.96 ± 0.03	28.5 ± 1.5	23.2 ± 1.8	06.9 ± 0.6	10.9 ± 0.9	4.47 ± 0.35
Edku**	30	1.08 ± 0.04	22.9 ± 0.9	22.4 ± 0.9	06.7 ± 0.4	07.9 ± 0.3	0.99 ± 0.04
Mariut**	30	1.06 ± 0.06	44.6 ± 1.7	42.5 ± 2.2	12.8 ± 1.1	80.8 ± 4.1	5.09 ± 0.26
Mean		**1.24 ± 0.04**	**26.2 ± 2.0**	**25.8 ± 1.7**	**10.1 ± 0.9**	**18.9 ± 1.1**	**3.33 ± 0.23**

Veg: vegetated sites; Uve: unvegetated sites; *: Eid and Shaltout [9], **: Eid et al. [8]

The potential for enhanced carbon storage in lake sediments may be contingent upon waterlogging, which can significantly impede the decomposition of organic matter and the burial of heightened primary production resulting from eutrophication.

Eid et al. [8] conducted a study on the five northern lakes in Egypt with the following objectives: (1) to evaluate the SOC content, the vertical distribution of soil, and the bulk density (SBD) in Bardawil, Manzalla, Burullus, Mariut, and Edku Lakes; (2) measure the CSP and the CSR of the aforementioned lakes and (3) assess a basic dataset on SOC stocks for further investigations considering the dynamics of SOC (Fig. 2). The hypothesis posited that the above mentioned parameters exhibited variation across the five lakes. The suspended particulate matter (SPM) concentration in Lake Bardawil exhibited the highest values, whereas Lake Manzalla displayed the lowest SPM concentration. The average SOC content in Lake Mariut exhibited the highest value, whereas Lake Edku demonstrated the lowest value. Upon examining the sediment profile spanning from 0 to 30 cm, it was observed that Lake Mariut exhibited the highest mean SOC density, whereas Lake Edku displayed the lowest. The study revealed notable disparities in SOC stocks across the five lakes under investigation. Lake Mariut exhibited the highest SOC value, while lakes Edku and Manzalla demonstrated the lowest SOC values. CSR of the five northern lakes in Egypt varied across the area, with Lake Bardawil exhibiting a CSR of 0.95 Gg C/yr, while Lake Manzalla recorded the highest CSR of 7.79 Gg C/yr, as shown in Table 1.

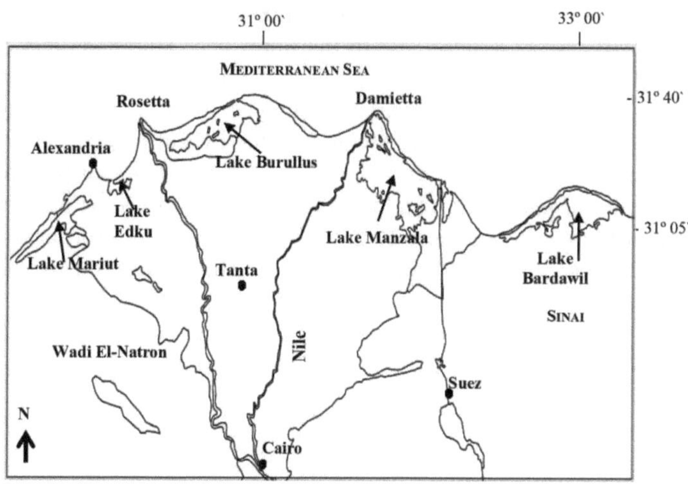

Fig. 2 Map of the five northern Mediterranean lakes in Egypt

4 Red Sea Coast

Several research studies addressed the mangrove ecosystem along the coast of the Red Sea. Eid and Shaltout [11] addressed the mangrove forests to assess the vertical allocation of SOC and SBD content in addition to SOC density, comparing them with a reference site along the Egyptian Red Sea coast. Moreover, the study aimed to estimate the CSR and CSP of mangrove forests in Egypt. Additionally, the study aimed to establish a baseline dataset on SOC stocks, which can be used for future investigations on the dynamics of SOC (Table 2). The average distribution of SBD exhibited a notable increase in mangrove and mudflat ecosystems as the depth increased. In the mangrove stands, SOC content notably decreased as the depth increased. Specifically, the SOC content decreased to 11.4 g C/kg at 20–30 cm deep from 20.0 g C/kg at 0–10 cm depth. In the mud flat, SOC content notably decreases as the depth increases. The SOC content decreases from 9.0 g C/kg at a depth of 0–10 cm to 1.9 g C/kg at a depth of 30–40 cm. The forest's type had a significant impact on the SOC stock. The mangrove forests' average SOC stock was higher (8.5 kg C/m^2) than the stands of the mud flat (2.6 kg C/m^2). The mean CSR of the mangrove ecosystems at 6.1 g C/m^2/yr exhibited a higher value than the mud flat ecosystems, which recorded a CSR of 2.0 g C/m^2/yr.

In their recent study, El-Hussieny et al. [13] estimated the carbon sequestration occurring in the mangrove sediments along the western coast of the Red Sea in Egypt. The study area spanned approximately 600 km^2, starting from Abu Minqar Island (27.216250° N, 33.876288° E) in the north near Hurghada and extending to Sharm El-Madfa'a (22.895165° N, 35.717757° E) near the Egyptian–Sudanese border. This study conducted a comparative analysis of the homogeneous population of *R. mucronata* and *A. marina*, along with the hybrid population comprising individuals of both species. SBD average values were 1.2 g/cm^3 for pure *A. marina*, 0.8 g/cm^3 for pure *R. mucronata*, and 0.7 g/cm^3 for mixed sites. Furthermore, the average values of SOC content were 10.2, 51.7, and 89.0 g C/kg for pure sites of *A. marina*, *R. mucronata*, and mixed sites, respectively. In contrast, the average values of SOC stock were respectively recorded as 60.5, 25.8, and 104.9 kg C/m^2 for pure *R. mucronata*, pure *A. marina*, and mixed locations of the two species. CSR of the three sites was measured to be 216, 77, and 338 g of carbon/square meter/year, respectively.

5 Aqaba Gulf

The research conducted by Omar [22] and El-Hussieny and Ismail [12] aimed to assess SOC stock in the sediments of fully developed mangrove (*Avicennia marina*) ecosystems. The study focused on three distinct zones: the intertidal, shoreline, and salt plains along the Aqaba Gulf. The investigation addressed two marine protected areas in South Sinai, Ras Mohammed and Naqb. A comparison was conducted to

Table 2 Total mean ± standard error of soil bulk density (SBD; g/cm^3), soil organic carbon (SOC) content (g C/kg), SOC density (kg C/m^3), SOC stock (kg C/m^2), carbon sequestration rate (CSR; g C/m^2/yr), and carbon sequestration potential (Mg C/yr) of mangrove forests distributed along the Egyptian Red Sea Coast (*Avicennia marina* and *Rhizophora mucronata*) and south Sinai (*A. marina*)

Mangrove	Depth (cm)	SBD	SOC			CSR	CSP
			Content	Density	Stock		
*North Red Sea**							
A. marina	40	1.40 ± 0.02	15.5 ± 0.6	21.2 ± 0.5	8.5 ± 0.1	6.1 ± 0.1	NA
Mud flat	40	1.72 ± 0.06	04.2 ± 0.7	06.4 ± 0.9	2.6 ± 0.2	2.0 ± 0.2	NA
*South Sinai***							
Intertidal mangrove	70	1.07	34.4	36.8	42.8	238.2	115.10
Shore line mangrove	70	1.27	07.2	09.1	28.4	054.5	0.85
Salt plain mangrove	70	1.12	14.5	16.2	65.6	104.1	0.76
Transplanted mangrove	70	1.41	05.7	08.0	18.9	048.0	0.18
Mud flat	40	1.37	03.6	04.9	09.8	013.7	NA
Hypersaline ecosystems	70	1.15	25.7	29.6	59.9	081.4	4.30
*South Red Sea****							
A. marina	60	1.20 ± 0.02	10.2 ± 1.1	11.7 ± 1.0	025.8 ± 1.8	077.0 ± 15.0	NA
R. mucronata	60	0.80 ± 0.06	51.7 ± 8.3	34.6 ± 4.3	060.5 ± 1.4	216.0 ± 47.0	NA
A. marina + *R. mucronata*	60	0.70 ± 0.04	89.0 ± 9.3	56.4 ± 4.6	104.9 ± 1.0	338.0 ± 14.0	NA
Mean		**1.20 ± 0.04**	**23.8 ± 4.0**	**21.4 ± 2.3**	**038.9 ± 0.9**	**107.2 ± 15.6**	**24.2**

*: Eid and Shaltout [11], **: El-Hussieny and Ismail [12], ***: El-Hussieny et al. [13], NA: not available

assess the similarities and differences considering the existence of SOC in sediments among samples collected from a hyper-saline ecosystem, mud flats, and a 10-year-old planted mangrove in the Salt Lake, the National Park of Ras Mohammed. Moreover, the research conducted an estimation of the capacity of these ecosystems to sequester atmospheric CO_2. In addition, sediment samples were subjected to analysis for SBD and the percentage of SOC content within a 10-cm depth interval up to the maximum depth attained. The results of these analyses are presented in Table 2.

A gradual increase was monitored in the SBD content of intertidal mangrove soil from the topsoil to the subsoil. However, a contrasting model was observed in the hyper-saline environment. SOC content for the six habitats under study exhibited a descending order as follows: intertidal mangrove (34.4 g C/kg), hyper-saline ecosystem (25.7 g C/kg), salt plain mangrove (14.5 g C/kg), shoreline mangrove (7.2 g C/kg), planted mangrove (5.7 g C/kg) and mud flats (3.6 g C/kg). The sediment of 10-year-old mangroves contained SOC content that was equivalent to 44.2% of the mature intertidal mangrove. Mangrove plantation is a highly effective measure for alleviating the influences of climatic variation.

Upon comparing the mean values of SOC stock, expressed in kilograms of carbon per square meter (kg C/m^2), and CSR, expressed in grams of carbon per square meter per year (g C/m^2/yr), between the northern lakes and mangroves (Tables 1 and 2), it becomes evident that both variables exhibit significantly higher values in mangroves (38.9 kg C/m^2 and 107.2 g C/m^2/yr), compared to the northern lakes (10.1 kg C/m^2 and 18.9 g C/m^2/yr). This implies that mangroves exhibit a higher efficiency in sequestering atmospheric carbon in their sedimentary environments. Regrettably, the mangrove areas in Egypt are relatively limited in size. According to Shaltout et al. [25], there are only 28 sites encompassing a total area of 525 hectares. This is notably smaller compared to the smallest lake in North Egypt, namely Lake Mariut, which spans an area of 63 square kilometers.

6 Valuation of Carbon Sequestration Service in the Five Lakes

The monetary evaluation of the carbon sequestration service offered by the five Mediterranean lakes in Egypt regarding the SOC stock in ton C per total area approximates € 1.96 billion, where Lake Manzalla had the maximum value of 0.89 € billion. However, Lake Mariut had a minimum of 0.09 € billion (Table 3). On the other hand, the CSR in ton C per total area per year approximates 2.27 € million, where Lake Manzalla had the maximum value of 1.00 € million, and Lake Edku had a minimum of 0.56 € million.

Table 3 Monetary valuation of the carbon sequestration in the five Mediterranean lakes in Egypt

Lake	Area		SOC stock				CSR			
	km^2	ha	kg C/m^2	ton C/ha	Ton C/area	Value (€)	g C/m^2/yr	ton C/ha/yr	ton C/area/yr	Value (€)
Mariut	63	6300	12.8	128	806,400	88,704,000	80.8	0.808	5090	555,944
Edku	126	12,600	6.7	67	844,200	92,862,000	7.9	0.079	995	109,494
Burullus	410	41,000	6.9	69	2,829,000	311,190,000	10.9	0.109	4469	491,590
Manzala	1200	120,000	6.7	67	8,040,000	884,400,000	7.6	0.076	9120	1,003,200
Bardawil	650	65,000	8.1	81	5,265,000	579,150,000	1.5	0.015	975	107,250
Total	2449	244,900	–	–	17,784,600	1,956,306,000	–	–	11,529	2,267,478

SOC: soil organic carbon; **CSR**: carbon sequestration rate

7 Estimation of Carbon Sequestration Service in the Five Lakes

The primary flows within the biogeochemical carbon cycle of Lake Burullus can be succinctly outlined as documented in the studies conducted by Shaltout and Khalil [26] and Plan Bleu [23].

a. The carbon in the lake ecosystem is derived from three primary sources: the dissolution of atmospheric CO_2 in the water, the absorption of atmospheric CO_2 by green plants, predominantly common reeds, and the influx of carbon through waste-water inflow from nine agricultural drains that discharge into the lake.
b. The internal dynamics of the lake ecosystem involve the transformation into dissolved organic carbon (DOC) from dissolved inorganic carbon (DIC) through photosynthesis by aquatic plants. Additionally, organic matter derived from the decomposed marine organisms undergo sedimentation in the lake.
c. The carbon in the lake ecosystem is released through various processes, including plant respiration, the utilization of reed beds, the capture of fish, and the extraction of water for offshore aquaculture operations.

Temporal variations are observed in most carbon fluxes occurring in the lake ecosystem. The fluxes associated with common reeds are contingent upon the plant's life cycle. For the period from December to April, the stems, panicles, and leaves undergo senescence and decompose as litter. The plant assumes a rhizome form during this period, exhibiting reduced activity. The peak of primary production occurs during the spring growing season, characterized by the greatest level of CO_2 absorption. A carbon portion that the reeds absorbed throughout the dormant time will subsequently contribute to the sedimentary reservoir [10].

The process of phytoplankton photosynthesis, which converts DIC into DOC, is influenced by various aspects, including water temperature, nutrient availability, salinity, and turbidity. The hydrological regime of Lake Burullus is influenced by various factors, primarily through the contribution of nine drains that supply the lake with approximately 3.9 million cubic meters of water per year [14]. The opening of drain mouths has a significant impact on the biophysical characteristics of the lake. This action facilitates the entry of nutrient-rich water containing organic matter, particularly during low seawater inflow from the El-Boughaz channel, which serves as an outlet between the lake and the sea.

The investigation of the effects of human management on carbon sequestration in lakes has received limited attention due to the intricate nature of these interactions. The introduction of drainage water tends to result in eutrophication. This process can stimulate the growth of phytoplankton and green algae such as *Scenedesmus*, consequently causing an increase in turbidity. Under equal circumstances, the increase in phytoplankton abundance is expected to enhance the process of photosynthesis and subsequently promote carbon sequestration. However, the rise in green algae populations has a contrasting impact, as it restricts photosynthesis by reducing light availability. Furthermore, introducing saline seawater into the lake results in an elevation of the salinity gradient of the water and a subsequent decrease in temperature, particularly in the eastern region. These two phenomena can potentially restrict the process of phytoplankton photosynthesis, consequently impeding carbon sequestration in the El-Boughaz channel region.

7.1 Carbon Stock Quantification

Estimating the current carbon stock in the lake was conducted by considering the two primary compartments of carbon sequestration on the location, including the biomass of marine plants and sediment, with a particular focus on the common reeds. The assessment of SOC was conducted by incorporating the findings of Eid and Shaltout [9], specifically examining the impacts of alterations in vegetated regions. The analysis findings indicated a notable correlation between the plant cover in a certain area and the estimated amount of carbon stored in its sediment. The phenomenon of root excretion is characterized by elevated levels of carbon transfer in sediment areas that are vegetated compared to bare ones.

7.2 Calculations that Allow Reaching a SOC Stock of 3375 Gg C

The investigation conducted by Plan Bleu [23] involved the identification of plant-covered and non-plant-covered regions, which have been present since 2011. This determination was made by analyzing maps derived from satellite image processing techniques employed by the Tour du Valat. The densities of plants were determined by calculating the average values of the Normalized Difference Vegetation Index (NDVI) spectral index during the winter and summer periods for each year within the analyzed timeframe of 2011–2015. According to the findings of Plan Bleu [23], the estimated carbon stock in sediment in 2015 was 3375 Gg C. In contrast, Eid and Shaltout [9] reported a carbon stock of 3181 Gg C. This discrepancy in the recorded values may be attributed to variations in the extent of plant coverage in the respective study areas. Plan Bleu [23] focused on an area of 17,929 ha predominantly covered by *Phragmites australis*, whereas Eid and Shaltout [9] utilized surface data from 2005, where plant cover accounted for 8200 ha. Based on the estimates provided in Table 4, it was observed that the SOC per unit area exhibited a higher value in plant-covered regions (9.3 kg C/m^2) compared to non-plant-covered regions (7.4 kg C/m^2).

Table 4 Estimate of organic carbon stored in the sediment (SOC) of vegetated and non-vegetated areas of Lake Burullus in 2015 (after [23])

Component	Vegetated zone	Non-vegetated zone	Total
SOC per unit area (kg C/m^2)	9.3	7.4	
Estimated surface area (ha)	17,929	23,071	41,000
Percentage of surface area	44	56	100
SOC stock (Gg C)	1667	1707	3375

7.3 *Carbon Stock in Biomass of Common Reed*

In the analysis conducted by Plan Bleu [23] on carbon stored in plant biomass, the researchers deemed helophyte coverage comparable to reed coverage (*P. australis*). This decision was made because *P. australis* is the predominant angiosperm species found in the lake, as highlighted by Eid et al. [10]. Furthermore, *P. australis* tends to establish dense monospecific stands rapidaly under favorable environmental conditions. Comprehensive data regarding the precise distribution of other helophytes, such as species belonging to the *Typha* genus, must be available. It is important to acknowledge that *P. australis* reeds are utilized by the local community as a fuel source [26], causing the direct release of carbon stored in the plant into the atmosphere. However, this aspect has yet to be considered in the scope of this work.

P. australis carbon content was determined by multiplying the dry matter mass per square meter by the carbon percentage in the above-ground (including leaf, stem, and panicle) and underground parts (including rhizome and root) of the plant in the same spatial extent Eid et al. [10]. The carbon mass per square meter was subsequently divided based on the three density levels, as indicated in Table 5. In their study, Eid et al. [10] ascribed the quantities of dry matter per square meter to areas with a high-density cover of *P. australis*. Subsequently, the quantities for areas with a low and medium-density cover were comparably extrapolated. In conclusion, the carbon mass per square meter was multiplied by the surface area corresponding to each density category, thereby facilitating the estimation of the overall carbon mass. The carbon stock in the sediment and reed biomass can be approximately 3706 Gg C (equivalent to 3.7 million tons) in 2015, as indicated in Tables 4 and 5. Therefore, sediment constituted 91% of the carbon stock.

7.4 *Measuring Carbon Exchanges*

Estimating the net ecosystem exchange (NEE) should ideally consider the CO_2 and CH_4 fluxes originating from various carbon cycle compartments, such as sediment, plants, phytoplankton, macroalgae, and the water column. Nevertheless, in practical terms, the unavailability of data regarding gas exchanges in the lake and the inherent difficulties associated with conducting new in situ measurements pose significant

Table 5 Carbon stock in *Phragmites australis* (after [23])

Component	Mass (kg DM/m^2)	C content (%)	C mass (kg C/m^2)	Total C mass (Gg C)
Low plant density				
Above-ground parts (leaf, stem and panicle)	0.83	0.43	0.36	10.89
Underground parts (rhizome and root)	0.25	0.44	0.11	3.30
Subtotal- low density	1.08		0.47	14.19
Medium plant density				
Above-ground parts (leaf, stem and panicle)	2.08	0.43	0.89	64.04
Underground parts (rhizome sand root)	0.62	0.44	0.27	19.42
Subtotal-medium density	2.70		1.16	83.47
High plant density				
Above-ground parts (leaf, stem and panicle)	5.40	0.43	2.32	179.02
Underground parts (rhizome and root)	1.60	0.44	0.70	54.28
Subtotal- high density	7.00		3.02	233.30
Grand total				330.96

challenges in accurately and comprehensively estimating carbon fluxes. However, it is anticipated (according to expert analysis) that substantial methane emissions are likely to occur in such a setting, potentially leading to a decrease in the sedimentary carbon reservoir.

Without empirical field measurements, the most dependable information regarding this species' carbon balance and dynamics in Lake Burullus can be obtained from the model of Eid et al. [10]. It is worth mentioning that the original model of Soetaert et al. [27] was modified using field information of a specific location. Carbon assimilation into the interior cycle of the plant primarily occurs through rhizome mobilization and photosynthesis. The emission of outgoing exchanges was primarily attributed to respiration and the deposition of deceased plant components, including the panicle, leaf, rhizome, and root.

7.5 Monetary Worth of Carbon Sequestration Service

A range of methodologies have been employed in scholarly discourse to determine the commercial importance of carbon. Among these approaches, the Social Cost of Carbon Method (SCC) emerges as the most suitable framework for evaluating the carbon value of Lake Burullus. Another approach, the Clean Development Mechanism (CDM), is available to countries listed in Annex I of the Kyoto Protocol. This mechanism serves as a means for developing nations to secure funding for establishing infrastructure to prevent or reduce greenhouse gas emissions in their territories. Another method known as Joint Implementation (JI) resembles the CDM, where shareholders purchase carbon credits to enhance their status concerning emissions and fund clean framework projects.

The SCC method is founded on a theoretical cost that quantifies the reduction in utility resulting from the emanation of an additional metric ton of carbon under optimal contamination levels. This cost is determined by optimizing a growth trajectory, considering factors such as interest and population growth rates, among other relevant variables. The concept in question has been extensively employed in the field of literature to assess the economic worth of ecosystem services [28].

7.6 Evaluating the Societal Costs of Carbon

The concept of social cost of carbon (SCC) pertains to the economic repercussions experienced by a community because of emitting an additional metric ton of carbon into the air. This cost is measured by comparing it to a predetermined emissions trajectory, such as a scenario that reflects the continuation of present demographic and economic patterns, commonly known as the business-as-usual scenario. In more accurate terminology, SCC refers to the alteration in the reduced utility value of consumption for each surplus metric ton of carbon dioxide comparable, expressed, and emitted concerning present consumption levels. SCC estimation is primarily derived from computational simulations conducted using three prominent models: FUND, PAGE, and DICE, as stated in the study of Nordhaus [21]. The models under consideration are called Integrated Assessment Models (IAMs). Each of these models comprises a geophysical component responsible for estimating climate sensitivity—that is, the correlation between climatic alterations and the emission of greenhouse gases. Additionally, IAMs incorporate a monetary component that quantifies the impact of global warming in terms of economic damage.

7.7 *The Commercial Significance of the Carbon Sequestration Service*

a. Based on a price of €30 for carbon per ton of CO_2 (equals €110/ ton of carbon), the valuation of the carbon storage service offered by Lake Burullus can be calculated as follows: €110 multiplied by 3,706,000, resulting in a total value of €407,660,000.
b. The annual monetary value of carbon sequestration by *P. australis* can be estimated as €45,243,000, calculated by multiplying 110 tons of atmospheric carbon sequestered by *P. australis* by a conversion factor of 411,300 euros per ton.
c. The annual sedimentation process quantifies the presence of organic carbon, which can be evaluated at a value of €512,600 per year, calculated as 110 multiplied by 4660.

As a component of the Med-ESCWET Project, an economic assessment was conducted to evaluate three regulating ecosystem services linked to the adaptation to climatic variation. The study focused on Lake Burullus in Egypt, as documented in the study of Dubreuil and Dutreix [5]. The services under consideration encompassed carbon sequestration services, food control, and coastal storm protection. Four locations in the Mediterranean region were selected to assess the value of these services (Fig. 3). These sites include the Lonjsko polje floodplain in Croatia, the Vic coastal lagoon in France (Hérault), Lake Burullus in Egypt and the Yeniçağa peatlands in Turkey. It is important to note that the intention here is not to assign a monetary value to services that do not have a market price. Rather, the aim is to establish a shared terminology that enables policymakers to recognize the environment as a form of natural capital essential for the functioning of various business sectors [5].

The evaluation of Egyptian and Turkish sites is conducted using distinct methodologies. These factors result in varying prices per metric ton of CO_2. The methodologies employed in this study yield comparable results for the Yeniçağa peatland, which is subject to strict exploitation restrictions and the overexploited Lake Burullus (Table 6). The perceived economic value assigned to the protection service of the coasts for the Étang de Vic is relatively low due to the limited level of human activity in this area. As a result, the estimation of the negative effects of coastal degradation on local communities has decreased. However, it is noteworthy that the conservative economic estimate of coastal protection underscores the efficacy of this buffer zone in offering storm protection. Additionally, the flood protection service offered by the Lonjsko Polje floodplain in Croatia is highly valued. Managing the retention potential in natural areas necessitates human intervention [5].

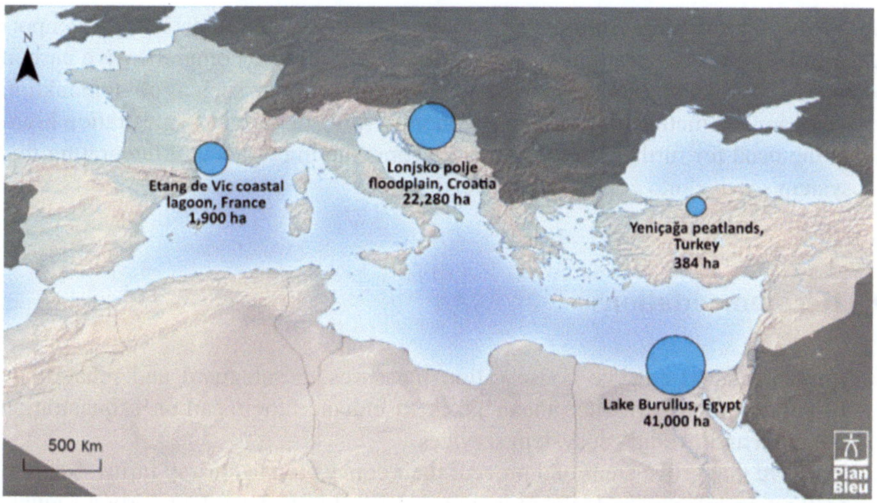

Fig. 3 The geographical distribution and magnitude of the pilot sites, as outlined in the **Plan Bleu report of 2016**

Table 6 Comparison of the monetary values of carbon sequestration in Lake Burullus in Egypt and other Asian and European Mediterranean lakes (after [5])

Wetland	Country	Area (ha)	Total value (€)	Unit value (€/ha)
Carbon sequestration				
Lake Burullus	Egypt	41,000	45,755,600/yr	1,116/yr
Yençağa peatlnds	Turkey	383	664,967/yr	1,734/yr
Coastal protection				
Étange de Vic	France	1,900	2.273,680	1,197
Flood control				
L. P. floodplain	Croatia	22,280	1,516,272,085	68,055

8 Conclusion

The carbon cycle in Egypt's five northern Mediterranean lakes, including Lake Burullus, is complex, involving multiple compartments such as plants, sediments, and phytoplankton, along with interactions with the atmosphere and surrounding environment. In Lake Burullus, human impacts have significantly altered the hydrological regime, potentially leading to eutrophication. The carbon sequestration service in Lake Burullus has been assessed primarily through the carbon stock in sediments and reed beds, with an estimated total of approximately 3706 Gg of carbon. While precise estimates of net ecosystem exchange (NEE) are limited by data constraints, the reedbed's net annual carbon absorption is estimated at 411.3 Gg C/yr. The significant size of Lake Burullus and its dominant reed bed underscore its importance in carbon sequestration. However, to achieve a more comprehensive carbon balance, additional research is needed on other components, such as phytoplankton, macroalgae, and methane fluxes. The economic value of carbon sequestration highlights the need for further study and underscores the importance of integrating this ecosystem service into conservation decisions.

9 Recommendations

1. Implement and enforce conservation measures to safeguard and rehabilitate Egypt's northern Mediterranean lakes to enhance their carbon sequestration potential and overall ecosystem services.
2. Preserve mangrove areas and prevent their conversion to shrimp farms. Support restoration efforts for depleted mangrove sites to improve their carbon sequestration efficiency.
3. Conduct further research to develop a comprehensive carbon budget for Egyptian ecosystems, including coastal areas, inland lakes, the River Nile, and canal systems. Focus on understanding the impacts of water temperature, salinity, and methane emissions of carbon dynamics.
4. Include additional components like phytoplankton and macroalgae in carbon cycle assessments. Invest in technology to accurately measure methane emissions and other relevant factors.
5. Use research findings to inform and enhance local conservation and management strategies, ensuring effective regulation of hydrological regimes and management of plant populations.

Acknowledgements Authors wish to thank Ms. Heba Bedair, Assistant Lecturer in Botany Department, Faculty of Science, Tanta University, for the drawing of the map of Egyptian wetlands (Fig. 1).

References

1. Arshad M, Alrumman SA, Eid EM (2018) Evaluation of carbon sequestration in the sediment of polluted and non-polluted locations of mangroves. Fundam Appl Limnol 192(1):53–64. https://doi.org/10.1127/fal/2018/1127
2. Beshay NS (2013) Impact of the different pollution sources on the carbon storage potentialities of Lake Mariut. M.Sc. Thesis, Faculty of Science, Alexandria University, Alexandria
3. Bishai HM, Abdel-Malek SA, Khalil MT (2000) Lake Nasser. Publication of National Biodiversity Unit No. 11, Egyptian Environmental Affairs Agency (EEAA), Cairo
4. Defew LH, Mair JM, Guzman HM (2005) An assessment of metal contamination in mangrove sediments and leaves from Punta Mala Bay, Pacific Panama. Mar Pollut Bull 50(5):547–552. https://doi.org/10.1016/j.marpolbul.2004.11.047

5. Dubreuil C, Dutreix N (2017) Mediterranean wetlands: an economic valuation of their services to climate change adaptation and regulation. Building the Mediterranean future together: ware resources and natural environment. Plan Bleu Notes #33, Plan Bleu, Valbonne. https://planbleu.org/wp-content/uploads/2017/04/note_33_en_web_avril2017.pdf
6. Eid EM, Arshad M, Alrumman SA, Al-Bakre DA, Ahmed MT, Almahasheer H, Keshta AE (2022) Evaluation of soil organic carbon stock in coastal sabkhas under different vegetation covers. J Mar Sci Eng 10(9):1234. https://doi.org/10.3390/jmse10091234
7. Eid EM, Arshad M, Shaltout KH, El-Sheikh MA, Alfarhan AH, Picó Y, Barcelo D (2019) Effect of the conversion of mangroves into shrimp farms on carbon stock in the sediment along the southern Red Sea coast, Saudi Arabia. Environ Res 176:108536. https://doi.org/10.1016/j.envres.2019.108536
8. Eid EM, Keshta AE, Shaltout KH, Baldwin AH, Sharaf El-Din AA (2017) Carbon sequestration potential of the five Mediterranean lakes of Egypt. Fundam Appl Limnol 190(2):87–96. https://doi.org/10.1127/fal/2017/0993
9. Eid EM, Shaltout KH (2013) Evaluation of carbon sequestration potentiality of Lake Burullus, Egypt, to mitigate climate change. Egypt J Aquat Res 39(1):31–38. https://doi.org/10.1016/j.ejar.2013.04.002
10. Eid EM, Shaltout KH, Al-Sodany YM, Soetaert K, Jensen K (2010) Modeling growth, carbon allocation and nutrient budgets of *Phragmites australis* in Lake Burullus, Egypt. Wetlands 30:240–251. https://doi.org/10.1007/s13157-010-0023-0
11. Eid EM, Shaltout KH (2016) Distribution of soil organic carbon in the mangrove *Avicennia marina* (Forssk.) Vierh. along the Egyptian Red Sea Coast. Reg Stud Mar Sci 3:76–82. https://doi.org/10.1016/j.rsma.2015.05.006
12. El-Hussieny SA, Ismail IM (2017) Role of *Avicennia marina* (Forssk.) Vierh. of South Sinai, Egypt in atmospheric CO_2 sequestration. Int J Sci Res 6(2):1935–1946. https://www.ijsr.net/archive/v6i2/ART20171097.pdf
13. El-Hussieny SA, Shaltout KH, Alatar AA (2021) Carbon sequestration potential of *Avicennia marina* (Forssk.) Vierh. and *Rhizophora mucronata* Lam. along the Western Red Sea Coast of Egypt. Rendiconti Lincei Scienze Fisiche e Naturali 32:599–607. https://doi.org/10.1007/s12210-021-01005-0
14. El-Shinnawy I (2002) Al-Burullus Wetland's hydrological study. MedWet Coast, Egyptian Environmental Affairs Agency (EEAA), Cairo
15. Galal TM, Shaltout KH, Hassan LM (2012) The Egyptian Northern lakes: habitat diversity, vegetation and economic importance. LAP Lambert Academic Publishing, Saarbrücken
16. Habib M (2004) Corals of Egypt. Academy for Educational Development (AED) and Egyptian Environmental Affairs Agency (EEAA), Cairo
17. Kassas M (2004) National wetlands. Strategy and plan of action for Egypt. MedWet Coast, EEAA, Cairo
18. Kauffman J, Heider C, Norfolk J, Payton F (2014) Carbon stocks of intact mangroves and carbon emissions arising from their conversion in the Dominican Republic. Ecol Appl 24(3):518–527. https://doi.org/10.1890/13-0640.1
19. Khalil MT, Shaltout KH (2006) Lake Bardawil: Zaranik protected area. Publication of National Biodiversity Unit No. 15, Egyptian Environmental Affairs Agency (EEAA), Cairo
20. Khattab A, El-Gharably Z (1984) The problem of aquatic weeds in Egypt and methods of management. In: Proceedings of EWRS 3rd symposium on weed problems in Mediterranean area, Lisbon, pp 104–113
21. Nordhaus W (2014) Estimates of the social cost of carbon: concepts and results from the DICE-2013R model and alternative approaches. J Assoc Environ Resour Econ 1:273–312. https://doi.org/10.1086/676035
22. Omar SA (2017) Evaluation of atmospheric carbon dioxide sequestration in Mangrove ecosystem in South Sinai, Egypt. Ph.D. Thesis, Faculty of Science, Mansoura University, Mansoura
23. Plan Bleu (2016) Economic assessment of ecosystem services provided by Mediterranean wetlands in terms of climate regulation. Plan Bleu, Valbonne

24. Sanderman J, Hengl T, Fiske G, Solvik K, Adame MF, Benson L, Bukoski JJ, Carnell P, Cifuentes-Jara M, Donato D, Duncan C, Eid EM, zu Ermgassen P, Ewers Lewis CJ, Macreadie PI, Glass L, Gress S, Jardine SL, Jones TG, Nsombo EN, Rahman MM, Sanders CJ, Spalding M, Landis E (2018) A global map of mangrove forest soil carbon at 30 m spatial resolution. Environ Res Lett 13(5):055002. https://doi.org/10.1088/1748-9326/aabe1c
25. Shaltout KH, El-Bana MI, Eid EM (2018) Ecology of the Mangrove forests along the Egyptian Red Sea Coast. LAP Lambert Academic Publishing, Saarbrücken
26. Shaltout KH, Khalil MT (2005). Lake Burullus: burullus protected area. Publication of National Biodiversity Unit No. 13, Egyptian Environmental Affairs Agency (EEAA), Cairo
27. Soetaert K, Hoffmann M, Meire P, Starink M, Oevelen D, Regenmortel S, Cox T (2004) Modeling growth and carbon allocation in two reed beds (*Phragmites australis*) in the Scheldt estuary. Aquat Bot 79(3):211–234. https://doi.org/10.1016/j.aquabot.2004.02.001
28. Stern N (2006) Stern review: the economics of climate change. Government of the United Kingdom, London
29. WRPA (2002) Wadi el Rayan: gateway to the Western desert. Wadi el Rayan Protected Area (WRPA), Egyptian Environmental Affairs Agency (EEAA), Cairo

Towards Resilient Aquatic Ecosystems: Climate Change and Sustainable Development

Climate Change and Sustainable Development

Abdelfattah Badr and Hanaa H. El-Shazly

Abstract Climate change is a long-term shift in temperatures and climatic conditions, resulting mainly from the release of Green House Gases (GHGs) from activities such as burning fossil fuels, creating coal and petrol, industry output, travelling, development, and agriculture. These GHGs are major influences on global warming, accelerating the increase in the Earth's average temperature. The recognition of climatic variation as an existent menace to those inhabiting the Earth began at the 1979 Climate Conference, where the importance of international collaboration was articulated. In reaction, the Intergovernmental Panel on Climate Change (IPCC) was formed in 1988, containing three working groups dealing with scientific knowledge, socioeconomic impact, and countermeasures. Moreover, the United Nations put in place the UN Framework on Climate Change **(UNFCC)** in 1994, which culminated in the 2015 Paris Pact. The intent of this arrangement is to keep the temperature increase for the twenty-first century well below the threshold of 2 °C and ensure it does not surpass 1.5 °C above pre-industrial measurements. Climate alternation presents a perilous menace to fundamental necessities such as water, nutrition, and energy. It is also integral to the 2030 Sustainable Development Goals (SDGs) prescribed by the UN, which strive to abolish poverty, avert starvation, and guarantee a better quality of life for everyone. In 2015, the United Nations adopted the Sustainable Development Goals, which emphasize the interconnectedness of social, economic, and environmental sustainability. Nonetheless, climate change could impede progress toward the achievement of these objectives, particularly SDGs 1 (No Poverty), 2 (Zero Hunger), and 3 (Great Health and Well-being). Furthermore, the negative effects of climatic alteration reach to other SDGs including, SDG 6 "Clean Water and Sanitation", SDG 7 "Affordable and Clean Energy", SDG 12 of "Responsible Consumption and Production", SDG 14 (Life Below Water) and SDG 15 (Life on Land). This study delved into various facets of climate change, such as outlines, markers, origins, and

A. Badr (✉)
Faculty of Science, Helwan University, Cairo, Egypt
e-mail: abadr@science.helwan.edu.eg

H. H. El-Shazly
Faculty of Education, Ain Shams University, Cairo, Egypt
e-mail: hanaahegazy@edu.asu.edu.eg

© The Author(s), under exclusive license to Springer Nature Switzerland AG 2025
M. T. Khalil et al. (eds.), *Climate Changes Impacts on Aquatic Environment*, Earth and Environmental Sciences Library, https://doi.org/10.1007/978-3-031-74897-4_11

repercussions, while calling attention to the potential implications of climate change on UN SDGs.

Keywords Climate change · Greenhouse gases · High temperature · Sustainable development · Biodiversity · and genetic resources

1 Introduction

1.1 What is Climate Change?

Long-term changes in temperature and weather patterns brought on by the release of Greenhouse gases (GHGs) from burning fossil fuels are known as climate change. Changes in this pattern could be attributed to variations in the solar cycle. But since the nineteenth century, human activity has increased significantly as a contributor to greenhouse gas emissions, and as a result, it is believed that human activity is to blame for climate change (https://www.un.org/en/climatechange/what-is-climate-change). Since the Earth's formation 4.5 billion years ago, the Sun's intensity, the positions of the continents and oceans, Earth's orbits, and volcanic eruptions have all contributed to changes in the climate. Nonetheless, the recent climate shifts in the Earth have been acknowledged by international organizations, who have expressed concern over their resolve to continue studying climate change through the creation of the Intergovernmental Panel on Climate Change (IPCC). Over the past three decades, the IPCC has increased its efforts to evaluate the body of scientific data on climate change, identify its effects on the environment and society, and develop mitigation plans.

1.2 Greenhouse Gases and Global Warming

The second decade of the twenty-first century (2011–2020) was the warmest decade on record, with an average temperature of 1.1°C above pre-industrial levels in 2019, according to the 5th IPCC synthesis report published in 2021. Presently, the rate of increase in global warming caused by human activity is 0.2°C every ten years. Rising sea levels, melting glaciers, altering wind and precipitation patterns, decreasing snowfall, shifting animal migration and life cycles, shifting plant life cycles, and damage to coral reefs are the most significant and well-known indicators. The Earth's temperature rose above its natural rates due to an increase in the rate of absorption of infrared radiation, which resulted in a change in the world's climate. These gases are listed below. An increase in the rate of emissions of so-called greenhouse gases and an increase in their concentrations in the atmosphere caused global warming. Although estimates of these gases' relative proportions vary [22], CO_2 is the main greenhouse gas (GHG) at roughly 76%, followed by methane (16%), nitrous acid (6%), and fluorocarbon gases (2%). Additionally, equipment that uses these gases emits fluorinated gases. According to Hager et al. [14], these emissions can have a warming effect that is up to 23,000 times stronger than CO_2.

According to Ritchie et al. [27], the distribution of global greenhouse gas emissions by sector in 2020 shows that electricity and heat production were the largest contributors, accounting for 15.18 billion tonnes of CO_2e, followed by the transport sector with 7.29 billion tonnes (Fig. 1). Other significant contributors included manufacturing and construction (6.22 billion tonnes), agriculture (5.87 billion tonnes), and fugitive emissions (3.22 billion tonnes). These figures highlight the critical sectors where emission reduction efforts should be concentrated to address global climate change effectively.

Global warming refers to an increase in the Earth's average temperature, both in the atmosphere and oceans. Rising temperatures are a significant concern due to the associated risks, particularly the potential rise in sea levels that threatens coastal cities worldwide. Figure 2 illustrates the long-term synchronization between CO_2 concentrations, global average temperatures, and sea levels over the past 400,000 years. This issue is crucial because CO_2 is a primary greenhouse gas driving climate change. Historically, CO_2 concentrations fluctuated between 180 and 280 ppm, closely aligning with temperature changes. However, due to fossil fuel combustion and deforestation, CO_2 levels have surged to over 425 ppm as of 2024—a dramatic increase of more than 50%. Englander [8] notes that during the last 55 million years, CO_2 levels reached close to 1000 ppm, leading to significantly higher global temperatures and polar ice melt, which raised sea levels by about 250 feet (75 m) compared to today.

Climate has fluctuated for hundreds of thousands of years, but the irregularity of precipitation changes makes it challenging to directly link long-term precipitation patterns to specific external forces [14]. However, weather station data suggest that the observed pattern of precipitation response to warming is consistent with climate models predicting these changes under various scenarios. Long-term warming has also caused significant shifts in daily weather variability, according to European weather station data. Historical records of extreme events provide vital insights into the mechanisms and potential future occurrences of such events [14, 22]. Extreme climate events, such as heat waves, droughts, floods, cyclones, and water scarcity, lead to crop losses and declining pasturelands, negatively impacting agricultural productivity and contributing to food insecurity worldwide. These events disproportionately affect smallholder farmers, who make up 10–15% of the global population but supply 50% of the world's food needs [15]. In developing nations in Africa and Asia, smallholder farmers focus on ensuring food security through their farming practices [18].

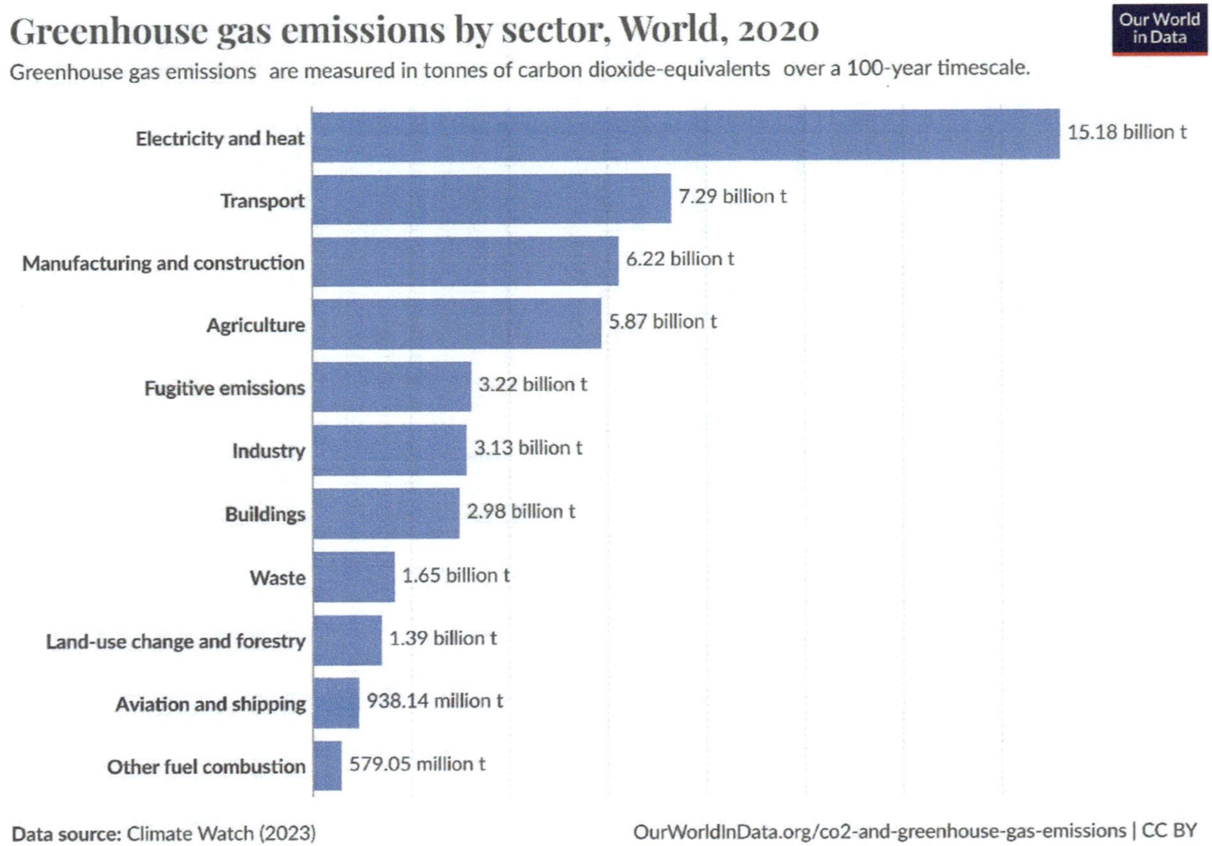

Fig. 1 Global greenhouse gas emissions by sector in 2020, measured in billion tonnes of carbon dioxide-equivalents (CO_2e). *Data source* Climate Watch, 2023 [27]

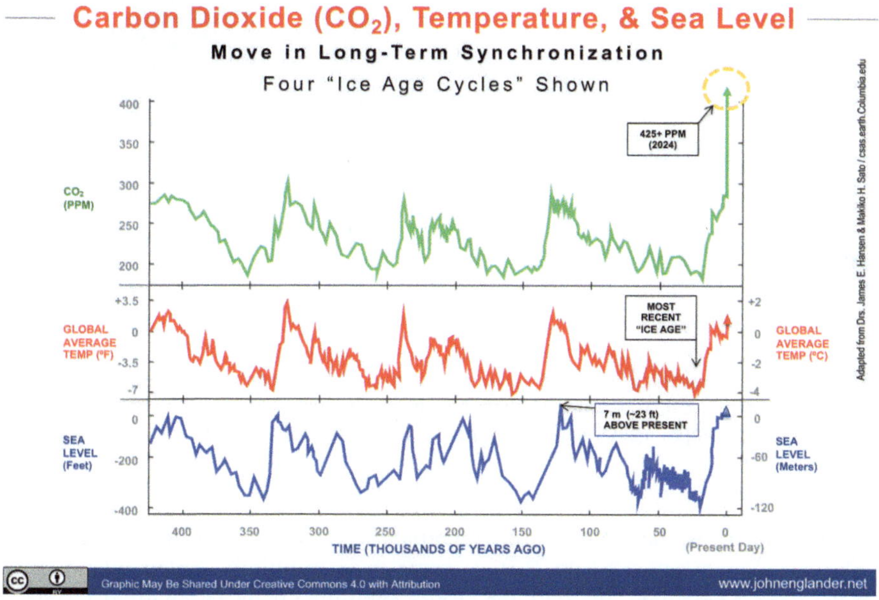

Fig. 2 A graph illustrating the association of the global temperature increases (red line curve) and sea level rise (blue line curve), with the increase in the atmospheric CO_2 concentration (green line curve). *Source* Englander [8]

1.3 Multilateral Cooperation to Curb Climate Change

Enacted in 2015, the Paris Agreement is an international treaty that was approved by 196 countries and came into force in November 2016. The United Nations Framework on Climate Change (UNFCC) was founded in 1994 and is nearly universally represented among the UN's member states. With a target of only 1.5 °C above pre-industrial levels, this global agreement seeks to keep the rise in global temperature this century well below 2°C. In 2018, the IPCC published one of its most significant reports, which considered a 1.5 °C temperature rise as a committed temperature goal. It also recommended action to reach net-zero GHG emissions by 2050 and called for climate action to keep global warming at this level. A Special Report on Climate Change and Land, published by the IPCC in 2019, also examined the links between climate change, food security, and sustainable land management. The report also discussed how climate change is affecting natural ecosystems that support human communities by providing them with essential resources for daily living, such as coastal regions, oceans, polar ecosystems, and mountain ecosystems [16].

For the first time, all countries came together to share experiences in battling climate change and adjusting to its impacts through the international climate change

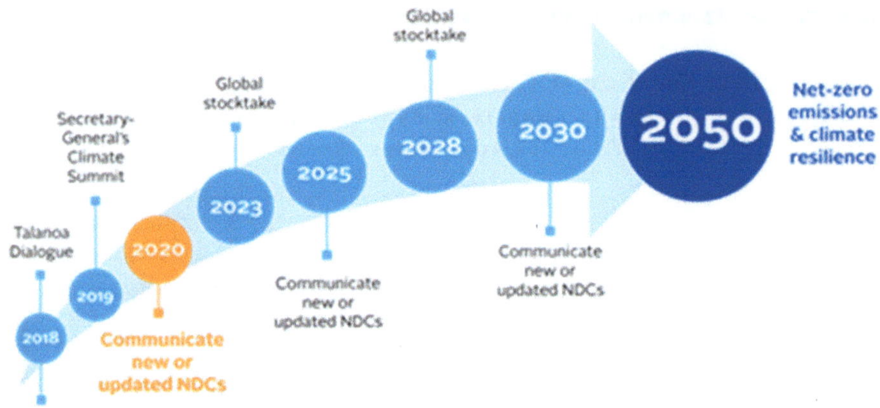

Fig. 3 Diagram illustrating the Paris Agreement's time plan for countries to review and revise their NDCs until 2050, reporting on their efforts and progress to the international community. https://www.unpri.org/news-and-press/paris-agreement-cop24-update-everything-you-need-to-know/3853.article

process known as the IPCC Paris Agreement. A five-year cycle of ever-more-ambitious climate action by the Parties serves as an ambitious implementation plan for the Paris Agreement. In 2020, the parties submitted their nationally determined contributions (NDCs) and reaffirmed their commitment to this ambitious agenda. The COP27 in Egypt decided to ask all Parties to reevaluate and reinforce the 2030 targets in their NDCs in order to bring them into line with the Paris Agreement temperature goal by the end of 2023. The decision acknowledged that the global warming limit is 1.5 °C. Figure 3 shows how nations will evaluate and update their NDCs in accordance with the Paris Agreement until 2050.

The Paris Rulebook, which was adopted during the 2019 UN Secretary-General's Climate Summit, and ongoing communication and/or updating of the NDCs by the Parties are the foundations for climate change management, which is frequently accomplished through adaptation and mitigation [26]. Climate change is caused by both natural and man-made factors, but the effects of the latter are more noticeable in certain places. For instance, East Africa is experiencing an increase in the frequency and severity of extreme events like floods and droughts. Additionally, the region is experiencing high levels of environmental stress brought on by human activity, such as deforestation and extensive land use [20]. These activities exacerbate environmental changes brought on by climate change and rural households' incapacity to adapt to its effects. On the other hand, according to Doty et al. [6], every nation in North Africa faces a high risk of drought and rising temperatures.

Climate change and rapid population growth are likely to worsen the already dire water shortage conditions in many countries, and this is seen as a major threat in Africa [29]. Africa's vulnerability to climate change is exacerbated by a number of non-climatic factors, such as widespread poverty, hunger, a high incidence of disease, protracted conflicts, low levels of development, and a low capacity for adaptation, as stated in the [34] on the Millennium Development Goals. According to reports by Niang et al. [24] and Welborn [35], Sub-Saharan Africa is predicted to bear the greatest burden of the expected reduction in agricultural productivity and increase in water insecurity, as well as the increased frequency of exposure to extreme weather events, flooding along the coast, and health risks. In the Sahel region of Africa, temperature increases are expected to be 50% higher than the global average, according to a 2017 USAID report. Six million people in the region experience severe food insecurity, and 1.6 children are at risk of suffering from severe acute malnutrition [35].

2 Sustainable Development

Development that meets current needs without jeopardizing those of future generations is referred to as sustainable development. In order to spur action over a 15-year period in areas of critical importance for humanity and the planet, the United Nations adopted the term "sustainable development" and made it public following the historic 2015 summit of world leaders. This resulted in the 2030 United Nations Strategic Goals for Sustainable Development (UNSDGs). These objectives represent the global community's commitment to eradicating poverty and hunger in all of its manifestations and to guaranteeing that everyone on the planet can meet their potential needs in an atmosphere of equality and stability while also maintaining dignity. In order for the Earth to support the needs of both the present and future generations, the UN parties to the UNSDGs agreement declared their resolve to prevent environmental degradation, ensure sustainable resource consumption, achieve food security, manage natural resources sustainably, and take action against climate change.

The UNSDGs represent the commitment of all UN members to ensuring that all peoples can live prosperous lives and advance socially, economically, and technologically while maintaining the integrity of the environment. The adoption of the UNSDGs is another way that all countries' aspirations to promote inclusive, equitable, and peaceful societies free of violence and fear are made clear. Through a revitalized Global Partnership focused on the needs of the poorest and most vulnerable and with the participation of all countries, all stakeholders, and all people to realize all human ambitions across the full extent of the UNSDGs, the Partnership for Sustainable Development, grounded in a spirit of strengthened global solidarity, mobilized the means required to implement the UNSDGs. In Fig. 4, the 17 UNSDGs for 2030 are listed.

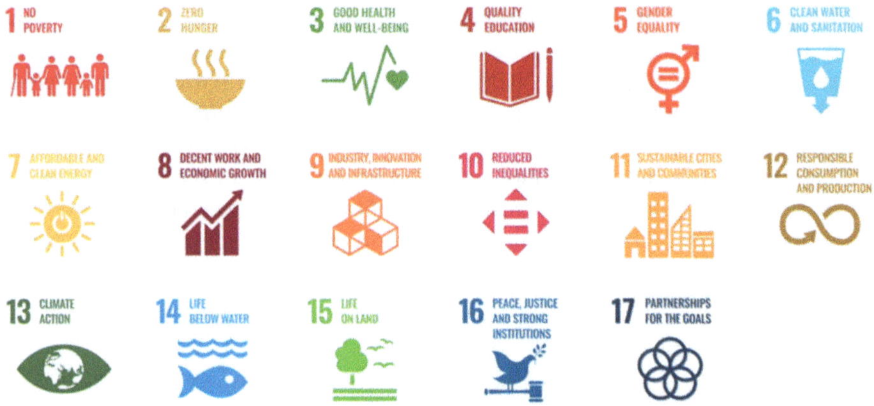
1 NO POVERTY
2 ZERO HUNGER
3 GOOD HEALTH AND WELL-BEING
4 QUALITY EDUCATION
5 GENDER EQUALITY
6 CLEAN WATER AND SANITATION
7 AFFORDABLE AND CLEAN ENERGY
8 DECENT WORK AND ECONOMIC GROWTH
9 INDUSTRY, INNOVATION AND INFRASTRUCTURE
10 REDUCED INEQUALITIES
11 SUSTAINABLE CITIES AND COMMUNITIES
12 RESPONSIBLE CONSUMPTION AND PRODUCTION
13 CLIMATE ACTION
14 LIFE BELOW WATER
15 LIFE ON LAND
16 PEACE, JUSTICE AND STRONG INSTITUTIONS
17 PARTNERSHIPS FOR THE GOALS

Fig. 4 Diagrams illustrating the United Nations 2030's 17 Sustainable Development Goals (SDGs), which are an approved call for action by all UN countries in a global partnership for ending poverty and hunger and improve health and education, reduce inequality and achieve economic growth while acting on combating climate change and working to preserve oceans and forests

2.1 Achieving Sustainable Development Goals

To attain sustainable development, three fundamental components—economic expansion, social integration, and environmental preservation—must be balanced. These tasks need to be completed with sound governance. Social inclusion and economic growth are interdependent and essential to the welfare of individuals and society as a whole. However, the health of ecosystems is closely linked to environmental protection. These aspects of sustainability are closely related to agriculture and water as essential life resources and human ability to maintain development resources. The relationship between these resources and the entire ecosystem is sensitive to changes in the amount and frequency of extreme events, as well as changes in the climate, according to a report published in 2013 by the African Climate Policy Center [1]. The Addis Ababa Action Agenda was created during the 3rd International Conference on Financing for Development, which took place in Ethiopia in 2015, with the goal of financing global efforts to achieve the UNSDGs. The 21st Conference of the Parties (COP) action plan, which aims to prioritize the UNSDGs in national development plans for all nations globally, is supported by the Addis Ababa finance agenda.

The United Nations approved extensive environmental and social reform programs to move toward stable sustainable development within 15 years (2015–2030), with the adoption of the 2030 sustainable development agenda. Sustainable development is built on four pillars to achieve societal and economic development, environmental protection, and good governance, despite the United Nations 2030 agenda having 17 goals (Fig. 4).

(1) The SDGs 1 through 6 are covered by social development, which is attained through investments in human capital and the realization of every individual's human rights. These objectives provide for the various needs of the populace, including food, health, and education, as well as preserving human capital's knowledge and skills, which are primarily the duty of the educational system and businesses that offer vital training opportunities.
(2) Economic growth is the result of balanced investments in business capital, human capital, and infrastructure, which leads to economic development. By increasing people's knowledge and skill levels, human capital influences economic growth and helps to create a thriving economy. The Organization for Economic Co-operation and Development (OECD) Parties concur that business investment and consumer spending drive economic growth, which in turn determines the quantity of skilled labor required to improve employment conditions in economies across the globe for a higher standard of living [25].
(3) By ensuring that environmental sustainability is necessary, an ecological balance between resource conservation and consumption can be achieved. In light of this, it is possible to achieve environmental protection in line with the UNSDGs, with a focus on striking a balance between mitigating climate change and ecological conservation [2]. This goal could be interpreted as fulfilling two distinct tasks, such as consuming and demanding energy, which are two essential components of economic growth. Nevertheless, as greater environmental damage is seen as a result of climate change activities, worries about the environment have grown. Controlling greenhouse gas emissions was crucial in achieving a consensus at the 21st Conference of Parties in Paris (2015) to prioritize the UN Sustainable Development Goals (SDGs) in national development plans [6].
(4) Good governance in sustainable development (GGSD) was approved to help societies establish a democratic system in implementing the 2030 agenda for sustainable development and addressing important climate and environmental issues through global partnership. This will help societies create effective development plans. Flexible planning for sustainable development is made possible by governance, and effective governance ensures that the current use of resources causes the least amount of harm to those resources. To effectively execute the 2030 sustainable development goals, governance issues require increased dialogue and action at all levels and by all institutions.

2.2 Vulnerability of Sustainable Development Goals to Climate Change

The six Sustainable Development Goals (SDGs) of the 2030 agenda of the United Nations member states are directly impacted negatively by climate change. These goals are closely related to the growing global population as well as the difficulties and pressures placed on global food security. Individuals are worried regarding people's health, well-being, and the demand for food.

- SDG 1 “No Poverty”
- SDG 2 “Zero Hunger”
- SDG 3 “Good Health and Well-Being”
- SDG 6 “Clean Water and Sanitation” SDG 7 "Affordable and Clean Energy", SDG 12 of “Responsible Consumption and Production”
- SDS 13 “Climate Action” SDG 14 "Life Below Water" SDG 15 "Life on Land"
- SDG 15 “Life on Land”.

The UNSDs cannot be achieved by 2030 owing to the insecurity of the world’s food supply. This year’s World Food Program annual report [38] shows an unexpected rise in the number of individuals experiencing food insecurity. The Global Network Against Food Crises (GNAFC) and the Food Security Information Network (FSIN) have released alarming reports that show that in 2022, there will be approximately 258 million people experiencing acute food insecurity across 58 countries and territories, up from 193 million in 2021 across 53 countries and territories. In the seven years that the WFP reports have been released, this has been the highest number. According to the WFP 2023 report, over 40% of people in seven countries are either at risk of severe acute hunger or starvation and destitution. Of those, extreme conditions occurred in Afghanistan, Yemen, South Sudan, Burkina Faso, parts of Nigeria, and Haiti (for the first time in the country’s history), but more than half (57%) were in Somalia. According to a report in the British newspaper “The Guardian” in May 2023, 10% of the world’s population suffers from hunger, and this could result in more people experiencing acute food insecurity due to rising costs of food production from plants and animals to meet an increase in food production by 70% by 2050, compared to 2009 food demand. The COVID-19 pandemic in 2020–2021 and the effects of the Russian–Ukrainian War on the food supply since February 2022 further exacerbated the situation.

The increasing global population’s demands for food, fuel, and fiber present further worrying challenges to reaching the UNSDs by 2030. Croplands in agriculture have been extended into the forests to meet these demands. Due to forest encroachment, vital global public goods found in forest ecosystems—such as carbon sequestration and biodiversity—are lost [17]. The United Nations Environment Program (UNEP) has supported a recent push for a sustainable development goal of zero deforestation by 2030 in order to lessen the impact of croplands encroaching on forests. The primary impacts on food security and agricultural productivity are anticipated to be a rise in production variability and a contraction in some regions. According to projections, crop net returns could decline by 80% by 2100, with yield reductions of up to 50% anticipated in some countries [24]. Small-scale farmers would be the most negatively impacted. Food security would suffer as a result in many African nations.

Climate change is probably going to affect the ecology of some disease vectors, which will affect the temporal-spatial spread of infectious diseases like dengue fever, cholera, and meningitis, among others. Human health has already acknowledged that this has a negative impact on malaria in the highlands of East Africa and southern Africa [7, 35]. According to predictions, rising sea level may cause flooding along the coasts of seas and oceans, which would harm mangroves and coral reefs near coastal settlements and have negative effects on fishing and tourism [1, 37]. According to the 2013 World Bank report, Morocco, Tunisia, and Egypt are the three African nations with the largest populations that are most vulnerable to sea level rise. These nations' arid environments make agricultural productivity insufficient to feed their rapidly expanding populations. Due to their current circumstances, these nations are incredibly vulnerable to failing to meet the Sustainable Development Goals (SDGs). This emphasizes the necessity of improving the food and agriculture sectors in order to achieve Zero Hunger and eradicate extreme poverty, as these issues are key to ending both hunger and poverty.

Intense climate threats and more erratic rainfall patterns may become more common as the climate warms and the sea level rises. Human security will be compromised, and society will be more vulnerable to the negative effects of climate change. It is anticipated that the most adverse effects of climate change will affect African nations. Welborn [35] suggested that the best way to stop more needless deaths from droughts, floods, and other natural and man-made disasters would be to improve disaster risk governance, which would provide Africa with an adaptive capability. Around 70% of smallholder farmers in Sub-Saharan Africa primarily rely on agriculture as their primary source of income, according to the World Food Program [38]. Other environmental concerns such as pest and disease outbreaks, desertification, degradation, soil fertility loss, and the potential rise in livestock and crop diseases are already endangering African crop production systems. Small-scale livestock production has also been impacted by the loss of grazing areas brought on by overuse of land and drought [32]. Due to their reliance on rain-fed agriculture, low yields, and frequent crop failure, African smallholder farmers may be the most vulnerable to the effects of climate change [12].

3 Management of Climate Change by Adaptation and Mitigation

Responses to climate change can be broadly defined as adaptation, which is the process by which vulnerable communities adjust to conditions that are naturally changing, including opportunities, risks, and hazards presented by a variety of natural stimuli [30]. By creating adaptation and mitigation plans, climate response actions can be implemented either before or after the effects of the climate become evident. When it comes to responding to the negative consequences of climate change, society can take a variety of short- and long-term measures, which together represent adaptation. According to Agrawal [3], adaptation can take on various forms and dimensions, including being proactive or reactive, individual or group-oriented, and planned or unplanned. Conversely, Epule et al. [9] pointed out that both climatic and non-climatic drivers have the ability to initiate the response actions.

Multiple authors have put forth diverse approaches to address the effects of climate change. According to Rodima-Taylor et al. [28], there are two main categories of response systems used by African countries to deal with environmental change: (i) informal responses, primarily from local actors, and (ii) formal responses from the government and other external actors. Local communities apply their own values and perspectives through informal responses, which are bottom-up adaptations. These are primarily driven by local actors making use of their knowledge of the local ecosystem, which is derived from social actors' experiences with its resources and cultural traditions and their ability to support livelihoods. Conversely, formal responses happen to be top-down actions taken in anticipation of climate change by entities like government agencies, non-governmental organizations, and civic groups, frequently to support independent planned adaptation [4]. The integration of climate change adaptation responses into national development planning has been encouraged by the Network of African Science Academies in a number of African countries [23].

Steffen et al. [31] provided concepts for estimating the various impact sectors of climate change at the global level as well as critical limits for safe operating spaces. However, in order to synthesize the body of scientific knowledge across disciplines and offer a better understanding of the combined risks, Cramer et al. [5] addressed combined changes in land use by pollution increase and biodiversity decline for five interconnected impact domains (water, ecosystems, food, health, and security) in the Mediterranean region. Habib-Ur-Rahman et al. [13] provided an overview of the opportunities, including mitigation and adaptation strategies, for sustainable agriculture production systems in Asia. To guarantee food security, the suggested plan incorporates crop-specific adaptation, technological approaches, and impact assessments. Opportunities include carbon sequestration, breeding climate-resilient livestock and crop varieties, and promoting agroforestry and mixed livestock and cropping systems.

In the agriculture industry, adaptation strategies can be transformative or incremental. According to Zinyemba et al. [39], incremental adaptation refers to the gradual actions taken in response to the effects of climate change that are planned based on different scenarios based on hazards and guided by climate predictions. On the other hand, transformative adaptation refers to adjustments that fundamentally modify the ecological, social, and/or cultural characteristics and functions of the system. This kind of vulnerability to climate change is determined by evaluating current climate risks in order to estimate future climate change. By transforming them into more equitable, sustainable, or resilient states, it seeks to lessen the core causes of climate change vulnerabilities, such as social, cultural, economic, environmental, and power relations [11]. Accordingly, through multi-stakeholder engagement, climate policies are recognized as the mainstream approaches to adapting to climate change at the national and sectoral levels [11]. Building resilience to the changing climate is made possible by putting adaptation interventions into practice and keeping an eye on their development.

The biological ability of plants and animals to adapt more quickly to harsher and more extreme weather conditions is enhanced by biodiversity. In the meantime, genetic biodiversity serves as a significant gene pool for the genes that govern how well plant and animal species are able to adapt to changing environmental conditions and endure hard and receptive environments. However, the following three important steps must be taken into account in order to fully utilize the potential of biodiversity in enhancing genetic resources and agricultural crops.

(1) Steer clear of activities that could wipe out biodiversity or damage agricultural ecosystems, like using pesticides that could kill pollinators.
(2) Enhancing understanding and practices regarding the preservation and utilization of crop wild relatives in order to increase biodiversity.
(3) Increase the effort put into utilizing biodiversity as a source of genes and traits for enhancing genetic resources and creating novel cultivars. To prevent pointless action, policies that support this kind of approach are vital.

The majority of forests have higher levels of biodiversity than other ecosystems, making them vital parts of the planet's biodiversity. Figure 5 depicts the global distribution of forests, highlighting the nations with the greatest forest area in 2020 (million hectares) and percentage of the world's total forest cover. Tropical forests account for half of all forests on Earth, with a share of 45%, followed by boreal forests at 27%, and temperate and subtropical forests at 16% and 11%, respectively.

Earth is rapidly running out of natural forest vegetation owing to the fact that when a new land is needed for agriculture, forest trees are cut down and replaced by food crops to produce food for consumption by the ever-increasing human population. Deforestation and biodiversity loss are all accelerated by climate change. According to McAlpine et al. [19], increased food consumption is a factor in deforestation and the decline of biodiversity. Major global forests are at risk as a result of these activities. For instance, the Tri-national Paraná Atlantic Forest in South America, which spans Brazil, Argentina, and Paraguay, is one of the world's most diverse ecosystems and is home to 5% of vertebrate species, which includes fish, amphibians, birds, and reptiles, and approximately 7% of plant species [36]. Nevertheless, according to

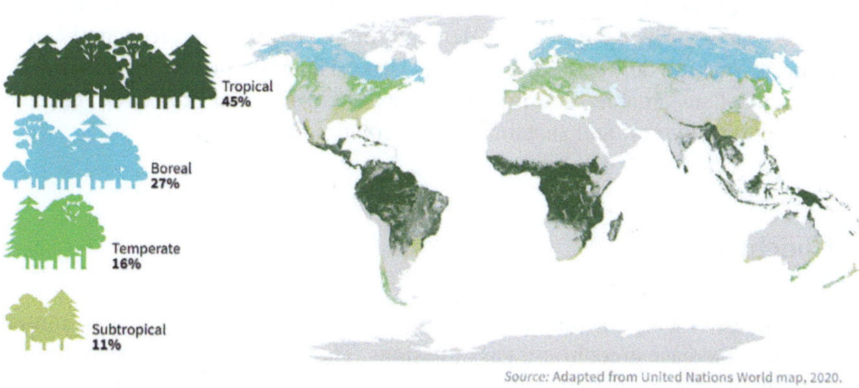

Fig. 5 World map showing the proportion and distribution of global forest cover by climatic domain in 2020 (FAO [10], pp. 1)

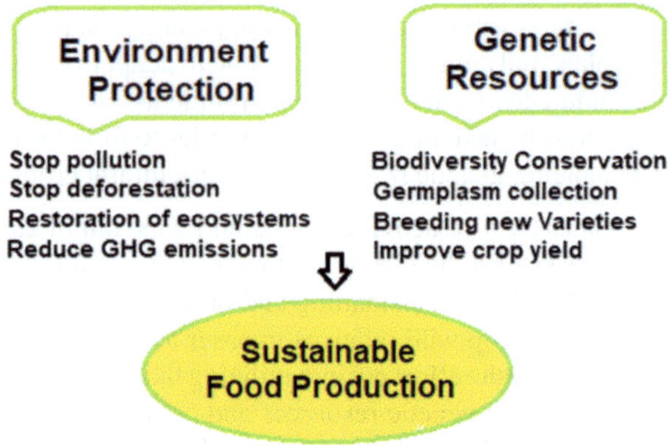

Fig. 6 Diagram illustrating recommended actions for sustainable food production by improving genetic resources and environment protection

Mohebalian et al. [21], this forest is also among the world's most susceptible to deforestation.

The conversion of natural ecosystems into farmland needs to stop, or at least be rationalized, in order to meet the environmental goals of the UNSDGs. Restoring degraded forest land to its original ecological integrity and productivity is one way to accomplish this. Restoring forest trees and other natural vegetation to a landscape while integrating production systems is an alternative approach to forest land restoration, which does not necessarily entail returning the forest vegetation to its pre-agricultural state. Long-term sustainability and productivity frequently rank higher in systems that are integrated with trees and other plants. According to a 2023 article in the Guardian newspaper, Davis highlighted that 18 nations in the Caribbean and South America, including Brazil and Argentina, have made a commitment to restore 50 million hectares of land by 2030. Agroforestry techniques are being introduced to cocoa and coffee farms in Colombia and Nicaragua through a few projects included in the initiative. The goal is to encourage farmers to plant more trees on their land in addition to growing crops. Due to its involvement in 90% of global deforestation and nearly a third of carbon emissions, food production is also a significant contributor to the climate crisis. Growing agriculture demands more land, which is frequently taken from forests, making deforestation a serious issue. The main factors influencing the achievement of sustainable food production are environmental protection, efficient use of genetic resources, and sustainable conservation (Fig. 6).

4 Conclusion

Climate change is a significant and urgent global issue primarily driven by human activities that increase greenhouse gas emissions. The impacts of climate change are widespread, affecting weather patterns, sea levels, biodiversity, and human health.

The scientific community, through organizations like the IPCC, has made substantial efforts to understand and mitigate these impacts. The Paris Agreement represents a global commitment to limit temperature increases and reduce greenhouse gas emissions, emphasizing the need for collective action.

Sustainable development aims to balance economic growth, social inclusion, and environmental protection, ensuring that future generations can meet their needs. The United Nations' 2030 Agenda for Sustainable Development outlines 17 goals to address critical global challenges, including poverty, hunger, health, and climate action. However, climate change poses a significant threat to achieving these goals, particularly in vulnerable regions like Africa, where the impacts on food security, health, and livelihoods are most severe.

5 Recommendations

1. Strengthen climate policies and international cooperation.
2. Invest in renewable energy and energy efficiency.
3. Enhance climate resilience and adaptation.
4. Promote sustainable agricultural practices.
5. Strengthen governance and institutional capacity.
6. Raise public awareness and education.
7. Support research and innovation.
8. Ensure social equity and justice.

References

1. ACPC (African Climate Policy Centre) (2013) Vulnerability to climate change in Africa: challenges and recommendations for Africa, ClimDev-Africa policy brief No. 2. Copyright © 2013, African Climate Policy Centre (ACPC). All rights reserved. ClimDev-Africa website at http://www.climdev-africa.org
2. Agboola PO, Bekun FV, Agozie DQ et al (2022) Environmental sustainability and ecological balance dilemma: accounting for the role of institutional quality. Environ Sci Pollut Res 29:74554–74568. https://doi.org/10.1007/s11356-022-21103-2
3. Agrawal A (2008) The role of local institutions in adaptation to climate change. World Bank. https://doi.org/10.1596/28274
4. Armatas CA, Venn TJ, McBride BB, Watson AE, Carver SJ (2016) Opportunities to utilize traditional phenological knowledge to support adaptive management of social-ecological systems vulnerable to changes in climate and fire regimes. Ecol Soc 21(1)
5. Cramer W, Guiot J, Fader M, Garrabou J, Gattuso JP, Iglesias A, Lange MA, Lionello P, Llasat MC, Paz S, Peñuelas J (2018) Climate change and interconnected risks to sustainable development in the Mediterranean. Nat Clim Change 8:972–980
6. Doğan B, Saboori B, Can M (2020) Does economic complexity matter for environmental degradation? An empirical analysis for different stages of development. Environ Sci Pollut Res 26(31):31900–31912. https://doi.org/10.1007/s11356-019-06333-1

7. Doty D, Grajeda E, Phillips P, Shrestha A (2011). Climate change and African political Stability (CCAPS). Busby J, White K, Smith T (eds) Vulnerability to climate change. An assessment of East and Central Africa. Student working paper no. 2. Robert S. Strauss Center for International Security and Law. All rights reserved
8. Englander J (2021) Moving to higher ground: rising sea level and the path forward. The Science Bookshelf
9. Epule TE, Ford JD, Lwasa S, Lepage L (2017) Climate change adaptation in the Sahel. Environ Sci Policy 75:121–137
10. FAO (2020) Income security for smallholder farmers in Zimbabwe. http://www.fao.org/in-action/income-security-farmers-zimbabwe/en/
11. Fedele G, Donatti CI, Harvey CA, Hannah L, Hole DG (2019) Transformative adaptation to climate change for sustainable social-ecological systems. Environ Sci Policy 101:116–125
12. Grey MS, Manyani A (2020) Integrating local indigenous knowledge to enhance risk reduction and adaptation strategies to drought and climate variability: the plight of smallholder farmers in Chirumhanzu district, Zimbabwe. J Disaster Risk Stud (Jàmbá) 12(1)
13. Habib-Ur-Rahman M, Ahmad A, Raza A, Hasnain MU, Alharby HF, Alzahrani YM, Bamagoos AA, Hakeem KR, Ahmad S, Nasim W, Ali S, Mansour F, El Sabagh A (2022) Impact of climate change on agricultural production; issues, challenges, and opportunities in Asia. Front Plant Sci 10(13):925548. https://doi.org/10.3389/fpls.2022.925548
14. Hager GC, Brönnimann S, Cowan T, Friedman AR, Hawkins Ed, Iles C, Müller W, Schurer A, Undorf S (2019) Causes of climate change over the historical record. Environ Res Lett 14:123006. https://doi.org/10.1088/1748-9326/ab4557
15. IFAD (2020) Why rural people? https://www.ifad.org/en/investing-in-rural-people
16. IPCC (2019) Climate Change and Land: an IPCC special report on climate change, desertification, land degradation, sustainable land management, food security, and greenhouse gas fluxes in terrestrial ecosystems. [PR Shukla, J Skea, E Calvo Buendia, V Masson-Delmotte, H-O Pörtner, DC Roberts, P Zhai, R Slade, S Connors, R van Diemen, M Ferrat, E Haughey, S Luz, S Neogi, M Pathak, J Petzold, J Portugal Pereira, P Vyas, E Huntley, K Kissick, M Belkacemi, J Malley (eds)]. file:///C:/Users/Usuario/Downloads/2021-1_
17. Laurance WF, Sayer J, Cassman KG (2014) Agricultural expansion and its impacts on tropical nature. Trends Ecol Evol 29(2):107–116
18. Mbow C, Halle M, El Fadel R, Thiaw I (2020) Land resources opportunities for a growing prosperity in the Sahel. Curr Opin Environ Sustain 48:85–92
19. McAlpine CA, Etter A, Fearnside PM, Seabrook L, Laurance WF (2009) Increasing world consumption of beef as a driver of regional and global change: a call for policy action based on evidence from Queensland (Australia), Colombia and Brazil. Glob Environ Change 19(1):21–33. https://doi.org/10.1016/j.gloenvcha.2008.10.008
20. Mkonda MY (2019) A novel assessment of the impacts, vulnerability, and adaptation of climate change in Eastern Africa. Licensee Intech Open. http://creativecommons.org/licenses/by/3.0
21. Mohebalian PM, Lopez LN, Tischner AB, Aguilar FX (2022) Deforestation in South America's tri-national Paraná Atlantic Forest: trends and associational factors. For Policy Econ 137:102697
22. Morice CP, Kennedy JJ, Rayner NA, Jones PD (2012) Quantifying uncertainties in global and regional temperature change using an ensemble of observational estimates: the HadCRUT4 data set. Geophys Res Atmos (First published: 17 April 2012). https://doi.org/10.1029/2011JD017187
23. NASAC (2015) Climate change adaptation and resilience in Africa. Recommendations to policymakers. Netw Afr Sci
24. Niang E, Ruppel OC, Abdrabo MA, Essel A, Lennard C, Padgham J, Urquhart P (2014) Africa. In: Barros VR, Field CB, Dokken DJ, Mastrandrea MD, Mach KJ, Bilir TE, Chatterjee M, Ebi KL, Estrada YO, Genova RC, Girma B, Kissel ES, Levy AN, MacCracken S, Mastrandrea PR, White LL (eds) Climate change 2014: impacts, adaptation, and vulnerability. Part B: regional aspects. Contribution of working group II to the fifth assessment report of the intergovernmental panel on climate change. Cambridge University Press, Cambridge, United Kingdom and New York, NY, USA, pp 1199–1265

25. OECD (2020) Education at a glance 2020: OECD indicators. OECD Publishing, Paris. https://doi.org/10.1787/69096873-en
26. Privitera R, La Rosa D, Pappalardo V, Martinico F (2021) Climate change management through adaptation and mitigation. ISBN: 978-88-916-4307-0
27. Ritchie H, Rosado P, Roser M (2020) Breakdown of carbon dioxide, methane and nitrous oxide emissions by sector. Our world in data. https://ourworldindata.org/emissions-by-sector
28. Rodima-Taylor D, Olwig MF, Chhetri N (2012) Adaptation as innovation, innovation as adaptation: an institutional approach to climate change. Appl Geogr 33:107–111
29. Schilling J, Hertig E, Tramblay Y, Scheffran J (2020) Climate change vulnerability, water resources and social implications in North Africa. Reg Environ Change 20:15. https://doi.org/10.1007/s10113-020-01597-7
30. Smit B, Pilifosova O (2003) Adaptation to climate change in the context of sustainable development and equity. Sustain Dev 8(9):9
31. Steffen W et al (2015) Planetary boundaries: guiding human development on a changing planet. Science 347:6223
32. Tarchiani V, Rossi F, Camacho J, Stefanski R, Mian KA, Pokperlaar DS, Coulibaly, H, Adamou AS (2017) Smallholder farmers facing climate change in West Africa: decision-making between innovation and tradition. J Innov Econ Manage (3):151–176
33. The Guardian newspaper (2023) https://www.theguardian.com/global-development/2023/may/03
34. United Nations Report (2015) The millennium development goals. New York, USA
35. Welborn L (2018) Africa and climate change: projecting vulnerability and adaptive capacity. Africa Report 14 | November 2018, Institute For Security Studies
36. Willis KJ (2017) State of the world's plants 2017. Report. Royal Botanic Gardens, Kew, Richmond, Surrey, England
37. World Bank (2013) Turn down the heat: climate extremes, regional impacts, and the case for resilience. http://www-wds.worldbank.org/external/default/WDSContentServer/WDSP/IB/2013/06/1
38. World Food Program (2023) https://www.wfp.org/news/global-report-food-crises
39. Zinyemba C, Archer E, Rother HA (2021) Climate change, pesticides, and health: considering the risks and opportunities of adaptation for Zimbabwean smallholder cotton growers. Int J Environ Res Public Health 18(1):121

Climate-Resilient Aquatic Ecosystems: A Roadmap for Sustainable Development

Waheed M. Emam, Kareem M. Soliman, and Wiame W. M. Emam

Abstract Biodiversity, peoples' livelihoods, and climate regulation are the core reasons for the significance of Egypt's aquatic ecosystems. Climate change, habitat destruction, pollution, and overfishing threaten them, though. This chapter therefore seeks to develop a practical roadmap towards their resilience to climate change by focusing on aquaculture, fisheries, blue food supply chains, consumer behavior, and marine protected areas (MPAs). The roadmap has specific objectives, desired outcomes, strategic targets, and priority actions focusing on resilience building, sustainability promotion, and long-term health of Egyptian blue food systems. Recommendations included improving policy frameworks; investing in research; capacity-building enhancement; promoting sustainable practices; and enhancing monitoring and evaluation. These strategies will help Egypt achieve its 2030 Sustainable Development Vision while aligning with global climate change and biodiversity targets, thus providing a planned method of addressing current challenges for a safe future for its aquatic ecosystems.

Keywords Aquaculture · Fisheries · Blue food supply chain · Consumer behaviour · Marine protected areas · Policy and governance · Egypt

W. M. Emam
Professor, Department of Zoology, Faculty of Science, Ain Shams University, Abassia, Cairo, Egypt
e-mail: waheedemam@sci.asu.edu.eg

K. M. Soliman · W. W. M. Emam (✉)
Department of Zoology, Faculty of Science, Ain Shams University, Abassia, Cairo, Egypt
e-mail: wiamewaheed@sci.asu.edu.eg

K. M. Soliman
e-mail: dr_kariemsoliman@sci.asu.edu.eg

© The Author(s), under exclusive license to Springer Nature Switzerland AG 2025
M. T. Khalil et al. (eds.), *Climate Changes Impacts on Aquatic Environment*, Earth and Environmental Sciences Library, https://doi.org/10.1007/978-3-031-74897-4_12

1 Introduction

Aquatic ecosystems, including seas, rivers, lakes, and wetlands, are fundamental to biodiversity, supporting livelihoods, and climate regulation. Coastal wetlands, including mangroves, seagrass meadows, and tidal marshes, are vital for climate change mitigation and adaptation as they can sequester and store significant amounts of atmospheric CO_2 in their biomass and soils for thousands of years, thus reducing greenhouse gas emissions [6]. Additionally, they protect coastlines from flooding and erosion caused by storm surges [2, 7, 10]. However, these ecosystems face threats from climate change, overexploitation, habitat loss, pollution, and invasive species [1]. To address these challenges, immediate action is required to build resilience and promote sustainable management.

2 Main Impacts of Climate Change on Aquatic Environments

The first step in developing a roadmap for sustainable development is to gain a thorough understanding of how climate change is affecting aquatic ecosystems.

2.1 *Ocean Warming and Acidification*

Over the last fifty years, the ocean has absorbed over 90% of Earth's heat, raising global sea surface temperature by 0.11 °C (0.19 °F) from 1950 to 2020 [11]. This warming affects marine species' distribution, breeding patterns, and survival rates. Coral reefs, which are particularly sensitive to temperature changes, face widespread bleaching events that threaten their existence. Furthermore, increased CO_2 levels lead to ocean acidification, harming calcifying organisms like corals and molluscs. Projections suggest ocean warming will increase by 0.6–2.0 °C by century's end [11].

2.2 *Sea Level Rise*

Global sea level rise due to ice melting and seawater thermal expansion is threatening coastal ecosystems and causing saltwater intrusion into freshwater systems. This impacts coastal habitats (like mangroves and salt marshes, essential for coastal protection and marine nurseries) and degrades freshwater habitats by displacing species and reducing water quality and availability.

2.3 *Changes in Hydrological Cycles*

Climate change alters the water cycle, impacting water availability, quality, and distribution globally [8]. It disrupts traditional precipitation patterns, leading to more frequent and severe floods or droughts, negatively impacting freshwater ecosystems. Floods can cause runoff that carries pollutants into water bodies, while droughts reduce water availability, concentrating pollutants and putting stress on aquatic life. Additionally, changes in snowmelt and rainfall patterns alter river flow regimes, affecting species that depend on specific flow conditions for spawning and migration. Disrupted flow patterns also influence sediment transport which is crucial for maintaining habitat structures in rivers and deltas.

2.4 *Extreme Weather Events*

Climate change is likely to increase the frequency and severity of extreme weather events like typhoons and hurricanes [5], which poses a threat to food security [3]. To address these risks, it is crucial to implement immediate and thorough measures to enhance prevention, adaptation, and resilience [9], thereby strengthening agri-food systems and improving their ability to cope with changing climate conditions.

3 Roadmap to Sustainable Aquatic Ecosystems Resilient to Climate Change. Case Study: Egypt

Understanding the main impacts of climate change on aquatic environments is crucial for devising effective strategies to mitigate these effects. Egypt, one of the top 10 global aquaculture producers in 2022 [4], faces significant threats from these climate-induced changes. The Nile Delta, in particular, is highly vulnerable to rising sea levels and saltwater intrusion. A potential sea level rise of 50 cm could severely impact the low-lying lands of the Delta and densely populated cities such as Alexandria and Port Said. This could lead to substantial migration from affected areas, increasing strain on services and escalating the financial burden of development.

At the same time, rising sea temperatures and bleaching events threaten the Red Sea's coral reefs. Pollution, overfishing, and habitat degradation compound these issues.

In response, this chapter proposes a practical roadmap for building climate-resilient aquatic ecosystems in Egypt. It outlines specific objectives, desired outcomes, strategic targets, and priority actions. By emphasizing sustainable practices, conservation efforts, and strong governance, Egypt can safeguard the long-term health and productivity of its blue food systems, paving the way for a positive and hopeful future.

The proposed roadmap aims to support Egypt's 2030 Sustainable Development Vision, the 2050 National Climate Change Strategy, and the updated National Action Plan for Biodiversity Conservation. It also aligns with the UN Sustainable Development Goals (SDGs) 2030, particularly Goals 1, 2, 5, 12, 13, 14, and 15, by promoting efficient, resilient, and sustainable blue food systems.

The roadmap relies on science-based management and robust regulatory frameworks to effectively tackle challenges such as overfishing, habitat destruction, and pollution while reducing the carbon footprint of aquatic food production. It draws inspiration from the FAO Strategy for the Blue Transformation—Roadmap 2022–2031 and the 2021 Declaration for Sustainable Fisheries and Aquaculture. The roadmap is designed to advance sustainable practices across five key sectors: aquaculture, fisheries, the blue food supply chain, consumer behavior, and marine protected areas.

Sector 1: Aquaculture Roadmap

Objective

To achieve sustainable aquaculture production that satisfies 35% of Egypt's demand by 2030, in line with FAO recommendations (FAO 2020).

Outcomes by 2030

- Attain a 35% increase in sustainable aquaculture production from Egyptian freshwater and marine sources.
- Increase green jobs in blue food and improve livelihoods through high-skilled employment opportunities for women and men.

Strategic Targets (T) and Priority Actions (PA)

T1: Enhancing sustainable aquaculture production

PA1.1 Develop and disseminate guidance and tools for implementing good aquaculture practices.
PA1.2 Strengthen national governance processes to support sustainable aquaculture development.
PA1.3 Improve seed quality to boost production efficiency.
PA1.4 Update policies related to small-scale aquaculture and integrate them into the national development agenda.
PA1.5 Promote responsible governance of land and water resources to ensure equitable access and sustainability.

T2: Advancing innovative technology

PA2.1 Foster the development of cutting-edge, climate-smart technologies for aquaculture operations.
PA2.2 Support the adoption of technologies that enhance the genetic resources of seeds.
PA2.3 Use modern technology to collect and manage data efficiently.

PA2.4 Encourage public–private partnerships to stimulate innovation and cooperation.

T3: Securing livelihoods in aquaculture

PA3.1 Provide small- and medium-sized fish farmers with the skills, financing, and information they need.
PA3.2 Create more job opportunities in aquaculture for women and youth.

T4: Minimizing environmental impacts

PA4.1 Adopt sustainable practices to protect biodiversity and ecosystems.
PA4.2 Improve the efficiency of resource use, including water and feed.
PA4.3 Invest in infrastructure development to support sustainable practices.
PA4.4 Enhance biosecurity measures, disease control, and aquatic health management.
PA4.5 Monitor and manage pollution and disease outbreaks in farmed fish populations.

T5: Regular monitoring and reporting

PA5.1 Support the development of early warning systems for climate impacts on aquaculture.
PA5.2 Utilize smart technology for comprehensive monitoring and reporting of aquaculture's ecological, social, and economic impacts.
PA5.3 Develop and refine indicators to measure the sustainability of aquaculture practices.

Additional considerations

a. Employ "Aquaculture Governance Indicators" (AGIs) to evaluate and enhance governance practices and ensure they support sustainable aquaculture.
b. Effective management of water quality, coastal habitats, and wild species health requires the engagement of all stakeholders, including farmers, NGOs, researchers, and government bodies. By working together, we can achieve comprehensive management and ensure the health and sustainability of Egypt's aquatic ecosystems.
c. Locate aquaculture facilities away from sensitive habitats and use carrying capacity information to manage industry size and arrangement. Government policies typically regulate the farm's location, so ecosystem-based policies and strong enforcement are key to sustainable aquaculture.
d. Source feed ingredients responsibly and reduce reliance on wild-caught fish. Governments should set sustainability standards for feed production and support ongoing research for alternative nutrient sources.
e. Reduce nutrient waste, drug and chemical use, and prevent species escapes to protect local ecosystems.
f. Implement policies and strategies that support sustainable feeding practices, farm infrastructure, and wastewater treatment.

g. Prioritize farming low-carbon footprint species such as seaweeds, bivalves (e.g., oysters, mussels, and clams), and small pelagic fish (e.g., herring, sardines, and anchovies) over higher-footprint fed species like salmon, shrimp, trout, and sea bass. Fed species have higher carbon footprints because their fish feed can contribute up to 80% of their total emissions. Therefore, selecting species not relying on fish feed can significantly reduce environmental impacts.
h. Utilize seaweeds to absorb excess nutrients and provide habitats for marine life.

Sector 2: Fisheries Roadmap

Introduction

Sustainable fisheries are essential to maintaining healthy fish stocks, protecting biodiversity, and supporting the livelihoods of fishing communities. Achieving this requires ecosystem-based fisheries management that addresses the complex interactions within marine environments. This approach avoids over-exploitation, protects threatened species, and ensures continued productivity and stability of fish populations. It reduces bycatch and harmful environmental changes, such as trophic cascades, while protecting the diversity and genetic integrity of wild stocks. It supports the participation of small-scale producers and blue food businesses in decision-making, resource management, and value chain development. It also promotes responsible fishing practices by equipping fishers and fish workers with the necessary knowledge and data.

Objective

Ensure effective fishery management to sustain Egypt's blue food supply with healthy, non-overexploited stocks while securing equitable livelihoods.

Outcomes

- By 2027, adopt good fishing practices that benefit fish populations and their habitats in alignment with the National Biodiversity Strategy and Action Plan (NBSAP) 2030.
- Phase out all illegal fishery activities by 2030.
- Ensure gender equality in fisheries by 2030.

Strategic Targets and Priority Actions

T1: Effective governance and policies

PA1.1 Ensure that the latest and most efficient fishing technologies and policies are used and that coordination is maintained at regional levels.
PA1.2 Manage fishing rights and access to resources fairly and sustainably, ensuring everyone has a fair chance to benefit from fisheries.
PA1.3 Provide training and support to small-scale fishers to improve their technical and business capabilities.

PA1.4 Ensure fisheries policies are considered in broader national development plans, including food systems and risk management.

T2: Enhance the livelihoods of fishers and fish workers

PA2.1 Improve the welfare and working conditions of people working in the fisheries sector.
PA2.2 Encourage more women to participate in decision-making roles and provide them with the necessary tools and information.
PA2.3 Help fishers and fish workers obtain financial support to improve their livelihoods.

T3: Effective fisheries management systems that support ecological and economic benefits

PA3.1 Develop innovative data systems for policy and management.
PA3.2 Regular monitoring and reporting on fisheries.
PA3.3 Develop comprehensive management plans that balance environmental, social, and economic goals.
PA3.4 Implement measures to protect biodiversity, support ecosystem restoration, and enhance resilience.

T4: Efficient and safe fishing vessels

PA4.1 Gather data on vessel performance and profitability.
PA4.2 Support and enhance safety standards for fishing vessels.
PA4.3 Maintain and rehabilitate fishing infrastructure due to natural disasters or crises.
PA4.4 Introduce technical innovations in fishing operations to improve economic viability and reduce ecosystem loss.

Key strategies to effectively combat overfishing include: (1) conducting regular stock assessments to monitor fish populations and ensure their sustainability closely; (2) enforcing catch limits to maintain healthy population levels and support the recovery of overfished stocks; (3) restricting certain types of fishing gear to reduce bycatch significantly; and (4) implementing seasonal closures, spatial restrictions, and regulations on the entry of new fishermen and vessels. By integrating ecosystem-based management practices, promoting good governance, enhancing the welfare of fishers, and ensuring the safety and efficiency of fishing operations, Egypt can secure a sustainable and equitable future for its blue food supply.

Sector 3: Blue Food Supply Chain

Objective

Developing a sustainable blue food supply chain while strengthening its ability to adapt to and withstand the impacts of climate change.

Outcomes by 2030

- Adoption of environmentally friendly and sustainable practices throughout the supply chain.
- Increased capacity of the blue food sector to adapt to climate change and other environmental stresses.

Strategic Targets and Priority Actions

T1: Sustainable practices

T1a: Achieve 80% of blue food sourced from certified sustainable fisheries and aquaculture operations within 18 months

PA1.1 Partner with certified sustainable fisheries and aquaculture farms.

T1b: Reduce waste in the blue food supply chain by 20% within 24 months

PA1.2 Develop and implement waste reduction strategies and recycling programs.
PA1.3 Regularly assess and mitigate the environmental impacts of supply chain activities.

T2: Climate resilience

T2a: Integrate climate-adaptive practices and technologies into supply chain operations

PA2.1 Sourcing raw materials from suppliers who use climate-resilient practices.
PA2.2 Diversifying sourcing and supply chains to reduce dependency on single sources that may be vulnerable to climate impacts.
PA2.3 Investing in energy-efficient technologies and renewable energy sources to reduce the carbon footprint of supply chain operations.

T2b: Develop and enforce climate-resilience policies for 90% of blue food operations within 18 months

PA2.4 Create and enforce policies to support climate resilience in the blue food sector
PA2.5 Collaborate with stakeholders to identify climate risks and develop adaptation strategies

Sector 4: Consumer Behaviour

Objective

Promote consumer participation in achieving sustainable blue food and enhance resilience in the face of climate change.

Outcomes by 2030

1. Increased consumer awareness of the sustainability challenges in the seafood industry.

2. Enhanced consumer ability to make informed decisions regarding sustainable blue food.
3. Reduced carbon footprint associated with blue food consumption.
4. Improved support for local economies through the consumption of locally sourced blue food.
5. Increased consumption of a diverse range of blue food to promote biodiversity and food security.

Strategic Targets and Priority Actions

T1: Increase consumer awareness

PA1.1 Develop educational campaigns to inform consumers about the environmental and social impacts of their seafood choices, emphasizing the low carbon footprint of wild-caught fish (1–5 kg CO_2 per kilogram) and farmed fish (4–6 kg CO_2 per kilogram) compared to beef (around 60 kg CO_2 per kilogram).

PA1.2 Partner with certification bodies to highlight the importance and meaning of sustainability certifications and seafood rating systems, which help consumers recognize sustainable seafood in the market.

T2: Enable informed decision-making

PA2.1 Provide clear labeling on seafood products, indicating their sustainability status, carbon footprint, and certifications from organizations like the "Aquaculture Stewardship Council" (ASC), "Best Aquaculture Practices" (BAP), and "Marine Stewardship Council" (MSC).

PA2.2 Promote the use of mobile apps and online resources that help consumers identify sustainable seafood options and understand the limitations of current certification processes, such as the exclusion of small-scale producers and the complexity and expense of certification.

T3: Reduce environmental impact of consumption

PA3.1 Encourage the consumption of species with lower environmental impacts and the utilization of the whole fish to reduce waste. Highlight culinary traditions, such as those in Japan, where various fish parts (heads, bones, gills, fins, and internal organs) are consumed.

PA3.2 Educate consumers on the benefits of buying local, sustainably managed fish to reduce the carbon footprint associated with exports along major trade routes. Emphasize the importance of verifying the sustainability of locally sourced products.

T4: Promote local and sustainable options

PA4.1 Support local fisheries and aquaculture operations by promoting their products as sustainable and eco-friendly choices. Encourage consumers to ask where the products come from and how they are caught to ensure sustainable practices.

PA4.2 Raise public awareness about the limitations of seafood rating systems. These systems often fail to account for differences between individual producers and do not typically include indicators to assess a product's carbon footprint.

T5: Enhance blue food diversity and food security

PA5.1 Encourage the inclusion of a diverse range of blue food species in diets to maintain ecological balance, reduce pressures on overexploited species, and promote food security, especially for communities relying on blue food threatened by ecological shifts and global warming.

PA5.2 Highlight the nutritional benefits of consuming a variety of blue food species and promote culinary traditions that utilize different parts of the fish, reducing waste and maximizing nutritional benefits.

Efforts to reduce emissions from blue food must be accelerated in the next few years as the human population increases and the demand for protein grows. More must be done to raise public awareness, send clear policy signals, and increase investment in the enabling environment.

Sector 5: Marine Protected Areas (MPAs)

When they receive full or high levels of protection, marine protected areas (MPAs) have the potential to significantly enhance climate resilience through a combination of climate mitigation efforts (such as carbon sequestration) and adaptation strategies.

Egypt has a network of six MPAs mainly located in the Gulf of Aqaba and the Red Sea, covering a combined area of approximately 11,716 km^2 (~5% of Egypt's marine area)[1]. This relatively limited percentage reflects the country's challenges and opportunities in marine conservation. To meet Aichi Target 11, Egypt would need to expand its MPA network and enhance the effectiveness of existing MPAs to reach the 10% protection goal for coastal and marine areas.

Objective

By 2030, increase Egypt's Marine Protected Areas (MPAs) coverage to at least 10% of the marine area, improve the effectiveness of existing MPAs by achieving international management standards, and integrate climate change adaptation strategies into 100% of MPAs to enhance their resilience to climate impacts.

Outcomes by 2030

1. MPAs cover at least 10% of Egypt's marine areas by 2030.
2. Enhanced biodiversity conservation and ecosystem health within MPAs, with improved habitat quality and species abundance.
3. Through adaptive management practices, MPAs are resilient to climate change impacts, such as rising sea temperatures and ocean acidification.

Strategic Targets and Priority Actions

T1: Expand MPA coverage to 10% of Egypt's marine areas by 2030

[1] https://www.protectedplanet.net/en/thematic-areas/marine-protected-areas

PA1.1 Conduct assessments to identify and prioritize additional marine areas for protection based on biodiversity value, ecological importance, and threats. Designating MPAs in regions with blue carbon ecosystems can significantly enhance their carbon sequestration potential.

PA1.2 Collaborate with local communities, scientists, and policymakers to gain support and ensure the inclusion of diverse interests in the MPA expansion process.

PA1.3 Incorporate the new MPAs into marine spatial planning to optimize their conservation impact.

PA1.4 Officially designate new MPAs, ensuring legal and institutional frameworks are in place for effective management.

T2: Achieve effective management and international standards for All MPAs by 2026

PA2.1 Create and update comprehensive management plans for each MPA, including objectives, zoning, and enforcement strategies.

PA2.2 Implement and maintain high protection levels within at least half of the existing MPAs to enhance their conservation effectiveness.

PA2.3 Offer training and resources to improve the skills and capabilities of MPA staff and stakeholders.

PA2.4 Establish monitoring programs to assess marine ecosystems' health and management actions' effectiveness.

T3: Implement climate adaptation measures in 100% of MPAs by 2027

PA3.1 Conduct assessments to identify climate change risks and vulnerabilities for each MPA.

PA3.2 Initiate and support marine restoration projects to replenish coral reefs, fish stocks, and other species. Additionally, restoration activities, such as planting mangroves, restoring the hydrological connectivity of saltmarshes, and rehabilitating degraded seagrass beds within MPA boundaries, further contribute to climate change mitigation.

PA3.3 Support research on climate impacts and resilience strategies and incorporate findings into MPA management practices.

4 Conclusion

The roadmap outlined in this chapter highlights a strategic approach to enhancing the climate resilience of Egypt's aquatic ecosystems. These ecosystems are crucial for biodiversity, livelihoods, and climate regulation but face significant threats from climate change, habitat degradation, pollution, and overfishing. The proposed strategies aim to address these challenges by promoting sustainable practices, strengthening governance frameworks, and encouraging innovation across key sectors, including aquaculture, fisheries, the blue food supply chain, consumer behavior, and marine protected areas.

For the long-term health and productivity of Egypt's blue food systems, climate adaptation measures, sustainable management practices, and effective governance and monitoring systems must be integrated. In terms of the country's 2030 Sustainable Development Vision and global climate and biodiversity targets, the roadmap becomes Egypt's cross-cutting framework to guide it by aligning with national and international goals.

Recommendations

1. Strengthen Policy and Governance
2. Invest in Research and Innovation
3. Enhance Capacity Building
4. Promote Sustainable Practices
5. Expand and Improve MPAs
6. Implement Monitoring and Evaluation Systems
7. Foster Community Engagement

By embracing these recommendations, Egypt can build climate-resilient and sustainable aquatic ecosystems.

References

1. Bellard C, Marino C, Courchamp F (2022) Ranking threats to biodiversity and why it doesn't matter. Nat Commun 13:2616. https://doi.org/10.1038/s41467-022-30339-y
2. de Paula D, Costa M, Macreadie PI (2022) The evolution of blue carbon science. Wetlands 42:109. https://doi.org/10.1007/s13157-022-01628-5
3. FAO (Food and Agriculture Organization) (2015) Climate change and food security: risks and responses. Rome, FAO. https://www.fao.org/3/a-i5188e.pdf
4. FAO (Food and Agriculture Organization) (2022) Strategy on climate change 2022–31. Rome, pp 39. https://www.fao.org/3/cc2274en/cc2274en.pdf
5. Ferreira S (**2024**) Extreme weather events and climate change: economic impacts and adaptation policies. Annu Rev Resour Econ 16. https://doi.org/10.1146/annurev-resource-101623-095314
6. IPCC (2019) IPCC special report on the ocean and cryosphere in a changing climate. Cambridge University Press, Cambridge
7. Moore JW, Schindler DE (2022) Getting ahead of climate change for ecological adaptation and resilience. Science 376(6600):1421–1426. https://doi.org/10.1126/science.abo3608
8. Tabari H (2020) Climate change impact on flood and extreme precipitation increases with water availability. Sci Rep 10:13768. https://doi.org/10.1038/s41598-020-70816-2
9. United Nations (2020) Executive summary: United Nations common guidance on helping build resilient societies, New York (UN). https://unsdg.un.org/download/4522/71673
10. Van Dolah ER, Miller Hesed CD, Paolisso MJ (2020) Marsh migration, climate change, and coastal resilience: human dimensions considerations for a fair path forward. Wetlands 40:1751–1764. https://doi.org/10.1007/s13157-020-01388-0
11. Venegas RM, Acevedo J, Treml EA (2023) Three decades of ocean warming impacts on marine ecosystems: a review and perspective. Deep Sea Res Part II 212:105318. https://doi.org/10.1016/j.dsr2.2023.105318